Formulation, Characterization, and Stability of Protein Drugs

Case Histories

Pharmaceutical Biotechnology

Series Editor: Ronald T. Borchardt

The University of Kansas
Lawrence, Kansas

Recent volumes in this series:

Volume 2   STABILITY OF PROTEIN PHARMACEUTICALS,
Part A: Chemical and Physical Pathways of Protein
Degradation
Edited by Tim J. Ahern and Mark C. Manning

Volume 3   STABILITY OF PROTEIN PHARMACEUTICALS,
Part B: *In Vivo* Pathways of Degradation and Strategies
for Protein Stabilization
Edited by Tim J. Ahern and Mark C. Manning

Volume 4   BIOLOGICAL BARRIERS TO PROTEIN DELIVERY
Edited by Kenneth L. Audus and Thomas J. Raub

Volume 5   STABILITY AND CHARACTERIZATION OF
PROTEIN AND PEPTIDE DRUGS: Case Histories
Edited by Y. John Wang and Rodney Pearlman

Volume 6   VACCINE DESIGN: The Subunit and Adjuvant
Approach
Edited by Michael F. Powell and Mark J. Newman

Volume 7   PHYSICAL METHODS TO CHARACTERIZE
PHARMACEUTICAL PROTEINS
Edited by James N. Herron, Wim Jiskoot,
and Daan J. A. Crommelin

Volume 8   MODELS FOR ASSESSING DRUG ABSORPTION
AND METABOLISM
Edited by Ronald T. Borchardt, Philip L. Smith,
and Glynn Wilson

Volume 9   FORMULATION, CHARACTERIZATION, AND
STABILITY OF PROTEIN DRUGS: Case Histories
Edited by Rodney Pearlman and Y. John Wang

Formulation, Characterization, and Stability of Protein Drugs

Case Histories

Edited by

Rodney Pearlman

Megabios Corporation
Burlingame, California

and

Y. John Wang

Scios Nova, Inc.
Mountain View, California

Plenum Press • New York and London

Library of Congress Cataloging-in-Publication Data

On file

ISBN 0-306-45332-0

© 1996 Plenum Press, New York
A Division of Plenum Publishing Corporation
233 Spring Street, New York, N. Y. 10013

10 9 8 7 6 5 4 3 2 1

Printed in the United States of America

To Jessica and Lynn

Contributors

Irina Beylin • Development, Alza Corporation, Palo Alto, California 94303

Thomas C. Boone • Process Science, Amgen, Inc., Thousand Oaks, California 91320

Lisa S. Bouchard • Pharmaceutical Research Institute, Bristol-Myers Squibb, Seattle, Washington 98101

John M. Brown • Pharmaceutical Development, Centocor Inc., Malvern, Pennsylvania 19355

Mark Busch • Pharmaceutical Research and Development and Quality Control, Scios Inc., Mountain View, California 94043

Gert Eberlein • Research and Development, Matrix Pharmaceutical Inc., Menlo Park, California 94025

John Geigert • Quality, IDEC Pharmaceuticals Corporation, San Diego, California 92121

Barbara F. D. Ghrist • Quality Control, Genentech, Inc., South San Francisco, California 94080

Wayne R. Gombotz • Department of Drug Delivery and Formulation, Immunex Corporation, Seattle, Washington 98101

Alan C. Herman • Analytical Research and Development, Amgen Inc., Thousand Oaks, California 91320

Maninder S. Hora • Department of Formulation Development, Chiron Corporation, Emeryville, California 94608

Madhav S. Kamat • Centocor Inc., Malvern, Pennsylvania 19355; *present address*: World Wide Pharmaceutical Technology, Bristol-Myers Squibb and Company, New Brunswick, New Jersey 08903

Michael G. Kunitani • Department of Analytical Development, Chiron Corporation, Emeryville, California 94608

Leo S. Lin • Department of Analytical Development, Chiron Corporation, Emeryville, California 94608

Hsieng S. Lu • Protein Structure, Amgen Inc., Thousand Oaks, California 91320

Alan P. MacKenzie • Mercer Island, Washington 98040

Dorothy Marquis-Omer • Department of Vaccine Pharmaceutical Research, Merck Research Laboratories, West Point, Pennsylvania 19486

C. Russell Middaugh • Department of Vaccine Pharmaceutical Research, Merck Research Laboratories, West Point, Pennsylvania 19486

Tue H. Nguyen • Department of Pharmaceutical Research and Development, Genentech, Inc., South San Francisco, California 94080

Susan C. Pankey • Pharmaceutical Research Institute, Bristol-Myers Squibb, Seattle, Washington 98101

Duke H. Phan • Pharmaceutical Research Institute, Bristol-Myers Squibb, Seattle, Washington 98101

Michael F. Powell • Department of Pharmaceutical Research and Development, Genentech, Inc., South San Francisco, California 94080

Gautam Sanyal • Department of Vaccine Pharmaceutical Research, Merck Research Laboratories, West Point, Pennsylvania 19486

Zahra Shahrokh • Department of Pharmaceutical Research and Development, Genentech, Inc., South San Francisco, California 94080

Steven J. Shire • Department of Pharmaceutical Research and Development, Genentech, Inc., South San Francisco, California 94080

Glen L. Tolman • Pharmaceutical Development, Centocor Inc., Malvern, Pennsylvania 19355

Sriram Vemuri • Pharmaceutical Research and Development and Quality Control, Scios Inc., Mountain View, California 94043

David B. Volkin • Department of Vaccine Pharmaceutical Research, Merck Research Laboratories, West Point, Pennsylvania 19486

Y. John Wang • Pharmaceutical Research and Development and Quality Control, Scios Inc., Mountain View, California 94043

Preface to the Series

A major challenge confronting pharmaceutical scientists in the future will be to design successful dosage forms for the next generation of drugs. Many of these drugs will be complex polymers of amino acids (e.g., peptides, proteins), nucleosides (e.g, antisense molecules), carbohydrates (e.g., polysaccharides), or complex lipids.

Through rational drug design, synthetic medicinal chemists are preparing very potent and very specific peptides and antisense drug candidates. These molecules are being developed with molecular characteristics that permit optimal interaction with the specific macromolecules (e.g., receptors, enzymes, RNA, DNA) that mediate their therapeutic effects. Rational drug design does not necessarily mean rational drug delivery, however, which strives to incorporate into a molecule the molecular properties necessary for optimal transfer between the point of administration and the pharmacological target site in the body.

Like rational drug design, molecular biology is having a significant impact on the pharmaceutical industry. For the first time, it is possible to produce large quantities of highly pure proteins, polysaccharides, and lipids for possible pharmaceutical applications. Like peptides and antisense molecules, the design of successful dosage forms for these complex biotechnology products represents a major challenge to pharmaceutical scientists.

Development of an acceptable drug dosage form is a complex process requiring strong interactions between scientists from many different divisions in a pharmaceutical company, including discovery, development, and manufacturing. The series editor, the editors of the individual volumes, and the publisher hope that this new series will be particularly helpful to scientists in the development areas of a pharmaceutical company (e.g., drug metabolism, toxicology, pharmacokinetics and pharmacodynamics, drug delivery, preformulation, formulation, and physical and analytical chemistry). In addition, we hope this series will help to build bridges between the development scientists and scientists in discovery (e.g., medicinal chemistry, pharmacology, immunology, cell biology, molecular biology) and in manufacturing (e.g., process chemistry, engineering). The design of successful dosage forms for the next generation of drugs will require not only a high level of expertise by individual scientists, but also a high degree of interaction between scientists in these different divisions of a pharmaceutical company.

Finally, everyone involved with this series hopes that these volumes will also be useful to the educators who are training the next generation of pharmaceutical scientists. In addition to having a high level of expertise in their respective disciplines, these young scientists will need to have the scientific skills necessary to communicate with their peers in other scientific disciplines.

RONALD T. BORCHARDT
Series Editor

Preface

This volume represents the second compilation of case histories of formulation, stabilization, and characterization of protein drugs. The first volume, *Stability and Characterization of Protein and Peptide Drugs: Case Histories*, was published in 1993. For both of these volumes, it has been the intent of the editors to offer practical approaches and examples for the design of formulations for therapeutic proteins. Also, we have chosen proteins that are already available on the market or in various stages of clinical testing. Many excellent texts and papers exist that detail the theoretical aspects of protein stability, and the reader is encouraged to refer to these sources, which are referenced in earlier volumes of this series, as well as the bibliography sections in each chapter.

With the large amount of interest in biotechnology-derived products, we believe it is important to keep current with information on formulation design and development of protein drugs. We have asked the contributing authors to apply relevant examples from their laboratories, so that recent data of a useful nature will be accessible to formulation scientists. What has been exciting about putting this second volume together has been the response from our authors in providing information on how they developed their particular formulations. They have provided excellent illustrations of the recent advances made in the area of protein analytical methods, characterization, and formulation. Also, there is a rich variety both in the nature of the proteins presented in this volume as well as in the type of formulations that have been developed. In addition to sterile parenteral formulations, a number of proteins have been formulated as gels for topical application, in microspheres for prolonged release, in collagen matrices for wound healing, or even as aerosols for inhalation.

The first chapter is an unusual one in that it is a compilation of information on degradation of over 70 proteins from the work of many laboratories. Contributors have generously shared previously unpublished data on the sites of degradation of a wide variety of proteins. The degradation reactions described are the principal reactions that proteins may undergo in aqueous solution at pH ranges from 4.5 to 7.5. The reactions studied include deamidation, cyclic imide formation, iso-asp formation, and oxidation. Although proteins experience other reactions in solution (aggregation, racemization, hydrolysis, and disulfide exchange, etc.), these are often found to occur at extremes of pH, or are the result of specific interactions, and are not included in this chapter.

For each protein listed, sequence information, predicted "hot spots" for degradation, and a hydroflex plot are supplied, as well as experimental findings of degradation. From these results, a picture emerges of which sites to look for as being reactive in any protein sequence. While there is no certain way to predict degradation *a priori* by such an approach, the trends presented by this informative chapter will help guide the formulator to identify the most likely pathway of degradation. Thus, having a conception of the most likely sites of degradation should be of value to the formulator when first inspecting the sequence of a new protein.

The remaining chapters are devoted to the stability and formulation of individual proteins. The second chapter deals with the stabilization of basic fibroblast growth factor (bFGF), which represents one of several growth factors being developed as therapeutic agents. Various growth factors are being tested for a wide variety of indications, including wound healing, bone regeneration, and protection of the gastrointestinal tract during chemotherapy, thus necessitating a range of very different delivery systems. A discussion of the analytical techniques used to study bFGF and its degradation route is presented. The power of HPLC as an analytical tool is shown where a minor modification in protein structure (a cyclic imide formed at an iso-asparagine residue) can readily be detected in a protein.

Although heparin or heparinlike substances stabilize bFGF against heat-induced denaturation, these stabilizers failed to prolong the shelf life of bFGF in solution. Such observations of the role of thermodynamic versus kinetic factors in predicting stability are common in the development of small-molecule drugs, and they are also seen in protein development. The authors describe the stability of bFGF in solution and in lyophilized form, along with the identity of the principal degradation products. Several formulations are described, including a powder form, a microsphere preparation, and a gel formulation.

The chapter on acidic FGF (aFGF) describes a series of biophysical studies that define the reactivity and behavior of the protein under temperature- and denaturant-induced stress conditions. Such studies are useful in the preformulation phases of development in order to obtain a sense of the relative reactivity of the protein. Again, stabilization is effected by employing heparinlike molecules to bind to aFGF. The authors compare agents and the nature of the interaction.

An interesting point is raised in these and several other chapters, one that anyone designing protein formulations will readily appreciate. When developing a formulation, one needs to maintain a delicate balance between often-divergent factors. For example, conditions that give rise to the highest degree of conformational stability may be deleterious toward chemical or physical stability. Furthermore, in designing formulations that will be administered to a patient, concern over the safety and biocompatability of excipients and the formulation as a whole must also be considered.

Transforming growth factor-β_1 (TGF-β_1) has markedly different properties than the FGFs. It exists as a 24-kDa homodimer, and thus has unique requirements for analysis, stability, and formulation. TGF-β_1 is stable in solution at low pH values, and because of its cysteine-rich structure care must be taken in formulation to avoid disulfide bond rearrangement. This agent is being evaluated for different indications, and, consequently, it is presented in a variety of formulations. Some of these formulations rely on using a stable solution or lyophilized form of the protein as a basis for mixing with a gel or semisolid matrix for further flexibility in dosage form design. Examples of loss of protein to adsorption in solution and the development of a freeze-dried product are described in this chapter.

Relaxin is an important hormone in reproductive biology. One of its actions is to help induce ripening of the cervix during childbirth. Relaxin shares some structural features similar to insulin, possessing an A and B chain linked by two disulfide bonds, as well as an internal disulfide bond on the A chain. The primary degradation products result from oxidation of methionine residues, and analysis of degraded samples led to the identification sites of oxidation. The authors describe the stability profile of relaxin in solution over the pH range 3–9, followed both by bioassay and by HPLC. They also show that the Arrhenius approach can be used over a limited temperature range for this protein, and that the two degradation pathways are indicated by the plot. A description of a stabilized gel formulation of relaxin indicates care must be used in selecting excipients since heavy metals may catalyze oxidative degradation pathways.

The chapter on interferon-β-1b describes the formulation approach for this cytokine as a model for similar hydrophobic proteins. This protein is a mutant, in that a cysteine at position 17 has been replaced by a serine. This substitution is made because of the possibility of disulfide exchange occurring with a free cysteine residue, leading to aggregation. Because of its hydrophobic nature, the authors screened a number of surfactants for use as formulation adjuvants in enhancing the apparent solubility of the protein. A lyophilized formulation of interferon-β-1b (sold as Betaseron®) is described, along with formulation and structural strategies used to prolong the half-life of the compound upon administration.

Granulocyte-colony stimulating factor (GCSF, sold as Neupogen®) is being used to combat the neutropenia often associated with aggressive chemotherapy. GCSF has two intramolecular disulfide bonds as well as a free cysteine, and thus the potential for disulfide bond exchange is a possibility. Formulation at low pH values is used to prevent oxidation of the free-cysteine residue. The authors describe a number of important analytical techniques employed in the characterization and stability monitoring of GCSF. Such a panel of assays is used to probe different aspects of the stability profile of the protein, and this chapter clearly provides a pragmatic example of this orthogonal analytical approach.

Another interesting aspect of the GCSF formulation design has to do with ensuring that the protein is not exposed to freezing conditions, which may cause aggregation. To ensure that the final dosage form has not been subjected to freezing during shipping and storage, Neupogen® is packaged in a unique outer packing carton and the package contains an indicator to tell if the container has been exposed to freezing conditions.

Granulocyte–macrophage colony-stimulating factor (GM-CSF, sold as LEU-KINE®) is also used to stimulate white blood cell production. GM-CSF is a glycoprotein produced by yeast. The analytical methods for following stability are described, and they involve a spectrum of assays to define the product's degradation profile. GM-CSF is supplied as a stable solution or as a lyophilized formulation.

The next chapter describes the formulation and stability of a monoclonal antibody used as a radioimaging diagnostic. The product is rather unusual as compared to a therapeutic protein in that it contains a stabilized fragment of the antibody which is complexed with a radio-immunoscintigraphic agent—technetium 99m—prior to administration. Typically, the final product has a utilization time of 2 hr from reaction to administration, so this entails a unique challenge for formulation and preparation. Thus, stability and formulation of the antibody fragment have to be studied, as well as the conditions for the preparation of the final product. The authors describe the need to prevent oxidation of the protein in solution prior to lyophilization by degassing procedures, to maximize the reactivity of the antibody fragment with the technetium.

Chimeric proteins are ones in which two proteins are joined (usually by recombinant DNA techniques) to offer bifunctional properties of the resulting hybrid protein. A fusion between transforming growth factor-α and *Pseudomonas* exotoxin results in a protein with anticancer properties that targets cancer cells rich in the growth factor receptor. Since such a protein is not found in nature, there is always a possibility of unusual reactions occurring or difficulties in its production. Again the authors report on the use of a mutant protein to overcome problems with disulfide scrambling. They also describe a thorough biophysical analysis of structural changes encountered in the protein in response to certain stress conditions, using techniques such as quasi-elastic light scattering, circular dichroism, fluorescence spectroscopy, and others. Such studies can prove to be invaluable in the preformulation investigation of protein denaturation and aggregation, and this work contains a good description of the typical studies that should be considered. The final formulation is made as an irrigation solution for instillation into the bladder.

The final chapter describes the stabilization and formulation of deoxyribonuclease (DNase). This protein is aerosolized by an air jet nebulizer for local administration to the lungs of cystic fibrosis patients. Unusual requirements were needed for this formulation because many patients with this disease have hyperreactive airways, and thus formulation components had to be kept to a minimum. Bivalent metal ions, such as calcium and magnesium, were found to be necessary for the activity of DNase, and they also were found to have a stabilizing effect on the molecule. Because DNase is a glycoprotein, it possesses charge heterogeneity, which further complicates analysis and stability studies.

A significant portion of the chapter is devoted to characterization of the final formulation of DNase (sold as Pulmozyme®), with attention to the deamidation reaction that occurs in aqueous solution over time. A means of reducing the rate of deamidation of DNase was achieved by packaging the protein in single-use plastic ampoules (rather than glass vials) because of the more constant pH afforded in plastic upon standing. The authors also describe the requirements for an isotonic solution that is amenable to aerosolization.

We trust that the reader finds the presentation of these case histories a useful guide in his or her own work. Clearly, the rapid growth of therapeutic agents from biotechnology has forced researchers to solve ever more challenging problems of stability and formulation development. We believe that this book gives adequate examples of these novel approaches and the techniques used to address stability problems of protein drugs. We would like to extend our thanks and appreciation to all of the authors who have contributed to this volume. In many instances, they have included primary data from their own laboratories, and this has helped provide relevance and timeliness of this book.

RODNEY PEARLMAN
Y. JOHN WANG

Contents

Chapter 1

A Compendium and Hydropathy/Flexibility Analysis of Common Reactive Sites in Proteins: Reactivity at Asn, Asp, Gln, and Met Motifs in Neutral pH Solution

Michael F. Powell

1. Introduction 1
2. Prediction of Protein Chemical Reactivity Based on Amino Acid
   Sequence Analysis 3
   2.1. Common Chemical Degradation Pathways in Proteins 4
   2.2. Calculation of Protein Hydropathy and Flexibility 9
3. Summary of Protein Stability in Aqueous Solution 11
   Adrenocorticotropin (ACTH) 12
   Agglutinin 13
   Aldolase 14
   Amylin Antagonist 15
   Amyloid-Related Serum Protein (ARSP) 16
   Angiogenin 17
   Anti-HER-2 Heavy Chain 18
   Anti-HER-2 Light Chain 20
   Antibody 4D5 Heavy Chain 21
   Antibody 4D5 Light Chain 23
   Antibody 17-1A Heavy Chain 24
   Antibody 17-1A Light Chain 26
   Antibody E25 Light Chain 27
   Antibody E25 Heavy Chain 28
   Antibody Light Chain-κ (mouse) 30
   Antibody OKT3 Heavy Chain 31
   Antibody OKT3 Light Chain 32
   Antibody OKT4a Heavy Chain (humanized) 34
   Antibody OKT4a Light Chain (humanized) 35

Atrial Natriuretic Peptide (ANP) (human) 36
Brain-Derived Neurotrophic Factor (BDNF) (human) 37
Calbindin (bovine) 38
Calmodulin 39
Carbonic Anhydrase C 40
CD4 (human) 42
CD4-IgG 43
CD4-PE40 45
Chloroperoxidase (*Caldariomyces fumago*) 48
Cholera B Subunit Protein (*Vibrio cholerae*) 49
Ciliary Neurotrophic Factor (CNTF) (human) 50
Crystallin-A (chicken) 51
Cytochrome *c* 53
DNase (human) 55
Epidermal Growth Factor (EGF 1-48) (human) 56
Epidermal Growth Factor (murine) 57
Erythrocyte Protein 4.1 (human) 58
Fibroblast Growth Factor, Acidic (human) (aFGF) 59
Fibroblast Growth Factor, Basic (human) (bFGF) 61
Glucagon 62
Granulocyte-Colony Stimulating Factor (G-CSF) (human) 63
Growth Hormone (bovine) 64
Growth Hormone (human) 66
Growth Hormone (porcine) 68
Growth Hormone Releasing Factor (GHRF) Variant (human) 69
Hemoglobin (human) 70
Hirudin 71
Histone 73
Hypoxanthine-Guanine Phosphoribosyltransferase (HXGT) 74
Insulin (human) 75
Insulin-like Growth Factor-I (IGF-I) 76
Insulinotropin 78
Interferon-alpha-2b (human) (IFN-α-2b) 79
Interferon-beta (IFN-β) 80
Interferon-gamma (human) (γ-IFN) 81
Interleukin-1 Receptor Antagonist (IL-1RA) 82
Interleukin-1α (IL-1α) 84
Interleukin-1β (human) (IL-1β) 85
Interleukin-1β (murine) 86
Interleukin-2 (IL-2) 88
Interleukin-11 (human) 90
Lung Surfactant SP-C (human) 91
Lysozyme (hen egg white) 92

Myelin Basic Protein (MBP) 93
Neocarzinostatin 94
Nerve Growth Factor (human) (NGF) 95
Parathyroid Hormone 97
Relaxin 98
Ribonuclease A (RNase A) 99
Ribonuclease U2 (RNase U2) (*Ustilago sphaerogena*) 100
Secretin 101
Serine Hydroxymethyltransferase (SHMT) (rabbit) 102
Tissue Factor-243 104
TGF-Beta 106
Thrombopoietin (TPO) 107
Tissue Plasminogen Activator (human) (t-PA) 108
Trypsin (bovine) 109
VEGF 111
4. Statistical Analysis of Protein Degradation Sites in Aqueous Solution .. 112
5. General Conclusions Regarding Protein Degradation in Aqueous
   Solution 118
   References 134

Chapter 2

Characterization, Stability, and Formulations of Basic Fibroblast Growth Factor

Y. John Wang, Zahra Shahrokh, Sriram Vemuri, Gert Eberlein,
Irina Beylin, and Mark Busch

1. Introduction 141
2. Physicochemical Characterization and Analysis 144
   2.1. Structure and the Conformation 144
   2.2. UV Spectroscopy 145
   2.3. Fluorescence Spectroscopy 146
   2.4. Circular Dichroism (CD) and Fourier-Transform Infrared
        Spectroscopy (FTIR) 148
   2.5. Reverse-Phase HPLC (RP-HPLC) 149
   2.6. Ion-Exchange HPLC (HPIEC) 149
   2.7. Affinity HPLC Methods 150
   2.8. Size-Exclusion HPLC (HP-SEC) 150
3. Biological Methods of Evaluation 151
   3.1. Cell Proliferation Assays 151
   3.2. *In Vivo* Animal Models 151
4. Thermal Stability 153

4.1. Use of a Differential Scanning Calorimeter 153
4.2. Thermal Stability as a Function of pH 153
4.3. Effect of Sulfated Ligand 154
4.4. Thermal Stability Determined by Circular Dichroism 155
5. Oxidation of Cysteines 156
    5.1. Disulfide Formation 156
    5.2. Prevention of Cysteine Oxidation 158
    5.3. Sites of Cysteine Oxidation 158
6. Covalent Bond Modification Detected by HPIEC 159
    6.1. Monomer–Multimer Distribution 159
    6.2. Identification of Asp^{28}-Pro Cleaved and Asp^{15}-Gly Cleaved
         bFGF 160
    6.3. Identification of Succinimide at Aspartate^{15} 163
7. Aggregation Determined by UV Spectrometry 164
    7.1. Effect of pH and Buffer Type 164
    7.2. Effect of Excipients 165
    7.3. Effect of Sulfated Ligands 167
8. Characterization of bFGF Aggregates and Precipitates 167
    8.1. Absence of Soluble Aggregates 167
    8.2. Quantitation of Insoluble Aggregates/Precipitates 168
    8.3. Mass Balance 169
    8.4. Characterization of Precipitates 169
    8.5. Aggregation in the Presence of Glycosaminoglycan 170
9. Formulations 173
    9.1. Aqueous Solution 173
    9.2. Freeze-Dried Formulation 173
    9.3. Powder Formulation 174
    9.4. Microspheres 174
    9.5. Gel Formation 175
    9.6. Target to FGF Receptor 176
10. Conclusion 176
    References 177

Chapter 3

**The Characterization, Stabilization, and Formulation of Acidic
Fibroblast Growth Factor**

David B. Volkin and C. Russell Middaugh

1. Introduction 181
2. Nature of the Interaction of aFGF with Heparin 183

2.1. Conformational Stability: Thermal- and Denaturant-Induced
     Unfolding of aFGF in the Presence and Absence of Heparin 184
2.2. Size and Charge Requirements of Heparin Required to Stabilize
     aFGF 188
2.3. Stoichiometry and Affinity of the aFGF–Heparin Interaction 189
3. Nature of the aFGF Polyanion Binding Site 192
   3.1. Specificity of the aFGF Polyanion Binding Site 192
   3.2. Interaction of aFGF with Other Selected Polyanions: Suramin,
        Sucrose Octasulfate, Nucleotides, and Chromatography Resins ... 194
   3.3. Structure of the aFGF Polyanion Binding Site 198
4. Formulation and Delivery of aFGF as a Wound-Healing Agent 200
   4.1. *In Vitro* Stability Considerations: Conformational and Chemical
        Integrity of aFGF 200
   4.2. Delivery of aFGF as a Topical Agent 205
   4.3. *In Vivo* Mouse Model Studies to Support Formulation
        Development 212
5. Conclusions 213
   References 214

Chapter 4

**Stability, Characterization, Formulation, and Delivery System
Development for Transforming Growth Factor-Beta$_1$**

*Wayne R. Gombotz, Susan C. Pankey, Lisa S. Bouchard, Duke H. Phan,
and Alan P. MacKenzie*

1. Introduction 219
   1.1. The TGF-β Family of Proteins 219
   1.2. *In Vitro* Activities of TGF-β 220
   1.3. *In Vivo* Activities of TGF-β 221
   1.4. Potential Clinical Applications 221
2. Structure and Properties of TGF-β$_1$ 222
   2.1. The TGF-β Superfamily 222
   2.2. Structure 223
   2.3. Latency 224
3. Analytical Characterization 225
   3.1. Reversed-Phase High-Performance Liquid Chromatography
        (RP-HPLC) 225
   3.2. Sodium Dodecylsulfate Polyacrylamide Gel Electrophoresis
        (SDS-PAGE), Native PAGE, and Western Blot Analysis 225
   3.3. Enzyme-Linked Immunosorbent Assay (ELISA) 227
   3.4. Cell Growth Inhibition Assay (GIA) 228

3.5. Cell Proliferation Assay 228
4. Stability of TGF-β_1 228
  4.1. Stability in Solution 228
  4.2. Prelyophilization Stability Studies 231
  4.3. Container Adsorption Study 233
  4.4. Stability in the Lyophilized State 234
5. Use of TGF-β_1 in Controlled Release Systems 239
  5.1. Bone Regeneration 239
  5.2. Dermal Wound Healing 240
  5.3. Localized Delivery to Gastrointestinal Tract 240
6. Conclusions 241
  References 241

Chapter 5

Stability and Characterization of Recombinant Human Relaxin

Tue H. Nguyen and Steven J. Shire

1. Background 247
  1.1. Isolation and Purification of Human Relaxin 247
  1.2. Pharmacology and Pharmacokinetics of Relaxin 248
2. Structure and Properties of Recombinant Human Relaxin 252
  2.1. Primary Structure—Peptide Map 252
  2.2. Secondary and Tertiary Structures 254
  2.3. Dimerization of Recombinant Human Relaxin 254
  2.4. Solubility 258
3. Stability Characterization 259
  3.1. Assay Methodology 259
  3.2. Stability in Solution 261
  3.3. Stability in Methylcellulose Gel 265
4. Conclusions 270
  References 271

Chapter 6

Interferon-β-1b (Betaseron®): A Model for Hydrophobic Therapeutic Proteins

Leo S. Lin, Michael G. Kunitani, and Maninder S. Hora

1. Introduction 275
2. Molecular Biology and Protein Chemistry 276
3. Preclinical and Clinical Applications of IFN-β 277

3.1. Preclinical Studies 277
3.2. Clinical Studies 280
4. Physicochemical Characteristics of IFN-β 280
    4.1. Primary Structure 280
    4.2. Secondary and Tertiary Structures 284
5. Analytical Methods for Evaluation of Protein Purity 286
    5.1. SDS-PAGE 286
    5.2. Isoelectric Focusing (IEF) 287
    5.3. RP-HPLC 288
6. *In Vitro* Biological Activity of IFN-β 289
    6.1. Antiviral Yield Reduction Assay 289
    6.2. Cytopathic Effect Bioassay 289
7. Formulation Studies 290
    7.1. Solubility Aspects 291
    7.2. Parenteral Formulations of IFN-β_{ser17} 294
    7.3. Long-Acting Formulations of IFN-β_{ser17} 294
8. Stability of IFN-β 295
    8.1. Stability-Indicating Assays 295
    8.2. Stability of IFN-β_{ser17} 296
9. Conclusions 297
    References 299

Chapter 7

**Characterization, Formulation, and Stability of Neupogen®
(Filgrastim), a Recombinant Human Granulocyte-Colony Stimulating
Factor**

Alan C. Herman, Thomas C. Boone, and Hsieng S. Lu

1. Introduction 303
    1.1. Clinical Uses of Granulocyte-Colony Stimulating Factor 303
    1.2. Molecular and Biological Characterization 304
    1.3. Chemical–Physical Characterization 306
    1.4. Glycosylated versus Nonglycosylated G-CSF 310
2. Structural Analysis 311
    2.1. Sequence Analysis and Peptide Mapping 311
    2.2. Biophysical Analysis 315
    2.3. Biochemical Analysis 316
    2.4. Analysis of the Free Cysteine Residue 321
3. Formulation 322
    3.1. Requirements for Nonglycosylated G-CSF 322
    3.2. Sensitivity to Freezing—Packaging Solution 322

3.3. Sensitivity to Freezing—Reformulation Solution 323
4. Stability and Stability-Indicating Assays 323
    4.1. Aggregation Analysis 323
    4.2. Oxidation and Detergent Effects 324
    4.3. Glutamine Deamidation 325
    4.4. Other Stability Issues 325
5. Conclusions 325
    References 326

Chapter 8

Development and Shelf-Life Determination of Recombinant Human Granulocyte–Macrophage Colony-Stimulating Factor (LEUKINE®, GM-CSF)

John Geigert and Barbara F. D. Ghrist

1. The Human GM-CSF Molecule 329
2. The LEUKINE® Manufacturing Process 331
    2.1. Fermentation and Purification 331
    2.2. Formulation, Fill, and Finish 331
3. Structural Studies of GM-CSF 331
4. LEUKINE® Stability 332
    4.1. LEUKINE® Stability Program 332
    4.2. Potency by TF-1 Cell Proliferation Bioassay 333
    4.3. Protein Integrity by SDS-PAGE Silver Stain 334
    4.4. Protein Integrity by RP-HPLC 334
    4.5. Protein Aggregation by SE-HPLC 335
    4.6. General Product Quality Parameters 340
5. Conclusion 341
    References 341

Chapter 9

Formulation Development of an Antifibrin Monoclonal Antibody Radiopharmaceutical

Madhav S. Kamat, Glen L. Tolman, and John M. Brown

1. Introduction 343
2. Background on Murine Tc-99m–Antifibrin Fab′ Fragment 344
    2.1. The Antifibrin Murine MAb Fab′ Fragment 344
    2.2. Technetium-99m Labeling Chemistry 345
3. Antifibrin Fab′ Production, Purification, and Analytical Characterization   347

3.1. Production and Purification of Antifibrin Fab′ (T2G1s) 347
3.2. Preparation of Antifibrin Fab′ Formulations 347
3.3. Analytical Characterization 348
4. Preformulation Studies: Determination of Critical Factors 350
4.1. Antifibrin T2G1s Fab′ 350
4.2. Stannous Ion [Sn(II)] 353
4.3. Effect of Moisture 354
5. Formulation Studies 355
5.1. Excipient Screening 356
5.2. Stability Studies and Shelf-Life Determination 361
6. Summary 362
References 363

Chapter 10

Biophysical Characterization and Formulation of TP40: A Chimeric Protein that Requires a pH-Dependent Conformational Change for Its Biological Activity

Gautam Sanyal, Dorothy Marquis-Omer, and C. Russell Middaugh

1. Introduction 365
1.1. Rationale behind Designing a Recombinant Chimeric Protein Containing Transforming Growth Factor-α and a Fragment of *Pseudomonas* Exotoxin (PE) 365
1.2. *In Vitro* Cytotoxic Activity of TGF-α-PE40 against Carcinoma Cell Lines Rich in Epidermal Growth Factor Receptors (EGFr) .. 366
1.3. Development of TP40, a Mutant Form of TGF-α-PE40, as a Potential Chemotherapeutic Agent 367
1.4. Expression and Purification of TP40 367
2. Structure–Function Correlation 368
2.1. Structural Characterization of TP40 Employing Biophysical Techniques 368
2.2. pH-Dependent Structural Changes of TP40 371
2.3. Speculations on the TP40 Translocation Mechanism 378
2.4. Equilibrium Unfolding Induced by Guanidine Hydrochloride: Evidence for the Presence of a Molten Globule Intermediate 379
2.5. Kinetics of Refolding 385
2.6. Thermal Unfolding 385
3. Formulation of TP40 for Clinical Administration into the Human Urinary Bladder 387
3.1. Considerations in Designing a Stable and Biologically Active Formulation 387

3.2. Selection of a Formulation for Intravesical Dosing in the Clinic .. 388
3.3. Formulation Summary 389
4. Conclusion 390
References 390

Chapter 11

**Stability Characterization and Formulation Development of
Recombinant Human Deoxyribonuclease I [Pulmozyme® (Dornase
Alpha)]**

Steven J. Shire

1. Background 393
1.1. Cystic Fibrosis 394
1.2. Bovine DNase I as Treatment for Cystic Fibrosis 394
1.3. Human DNase I as Treatment for Cystic Fibrosis 395
2. Structure and Properties of DNase I 397
2.1. Primary Structure of rhDNase and Homology with bDNase 397
2.2. Secondary and Tertiary Structure 400
2.3. Physical and Chemical Properties 401
3. Analytical Characterization 403
3.1. Analysis of Molecular Size 403
3.2. Analysis of Charge Heterogeneity 403
3.3. Analysis of Nuclease Activity 405
4. Formulation Development 406
4.1. Aerosol Delivery of rhDNase: Characterization of DNase Aerosols 406
4.2. Choice of Formulation Components 408
4.3. Solution Stability 410
4.4. Choice of Container Closure 416
5. Summary and Conclusions 420
References 422

Index 427

1

A Compendium and Hydropathy/ Flexibility Analysis of Common Reactive Sites in Proteins: Reactivity at Asn, Asp, Gln, and Met Motifs in Neutral pH Solution

Michael F. Powell

*with Godfrey Amphlett, Jerry Cacia, William Callahan,
Eleanor Cannova-Davis, Byeong Chang, Jeffrey L. Cleland,
Todd Darrington, Linda DeYoung, Bhim Dhingra, Rich Everett,
Linda Foster, John Frenz, Anne Garcia, David Giltinan, Gerry Gitlin,
Wayne Gombotz, Michael Hageman, Reed Harris, Debra Heller,
Alan Herman, Susan Hershenson, Maninder Hora, Rebecca Ingram,
Susan Janes, Madav Kamat, Dan Kroon, Rodney G. Keck,
Ed Luedke, Leonard Maneri, Carl March, Louise McCrossin,
Tue Nguyen, Suman Patel, Hong Qi, Michael Rohde,
Barry Rosenblatt, Nancy Sahakian, Zahra Shahrokh, Steve Shire,
Cynthia Stevenson, Kenneth Stoney, Suzanne Thompson,
Glen Tolman, David Volkin, Y. John Wang, Nicholas Warne,
Colin Watanabe*

Michael F. Powell • Department of Pharmaceutical Research and Development, Genentech, Inc., South San Francisco, California 94080.

Formulation, Characterization, and Stability of Protein Drugs, Rodney Pearlman and Y. John Wang, eds., Plenum Press, New York, 1996.

1. INTRODUCTION

The accurate prediction of protein stability under pharmaceutical formulation conditions is one of the more challenging goals in protein formulation. Almost all protein and peptide liquid formulations are designed to be at or near the pH of maximum stability of the protein, usually between pH 4.5 and 7.5. The reactions that most proteins undergo within this pH range are also narrowly defined; there are several reactions that may occur at high or low pH, but are negligible in the pH 4.5–7.5 range. Within this window of "neutral" pH, the major degradation reactions are deamidation, cyclic imide formation, iso-Asp formation, and oxidation. Other chemical reactions, including backbone cleavage (such as at the reactive Asp-Pro site), racemization, pyroglutamic acid formation, diketopiperazine formation, disulfide exchange, and others, occur predominantly at high or low pHs (Scheme 1).

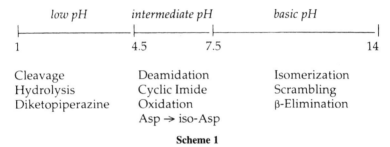

Scheme 1

The goal of this compilation on the chemical reactivity of proteins is to establish boundaries for the reactivity of Asn, Asp, Gln, and possibly Met, in the context of neighboring amino acid sequence, hydrophobicity and backbone flexibility. Given a particular primary amino acid sequence, is it possible to predict with some certainty the likelihood of a particular deamidation or oxidation reaction under conditions of a liquid pharmaceutical formulation? To answer this question, we surveyed the literature for protein degradation under "typical" formulation conditions (aqueous solution, pH 4.5–7.5, 2–37°C). Our goal was to address several questions:

1. What are the predominant site(s) of chemical degradation, either deamidation or oxidation, in the proteins reported so far? Are there many exceptions to the rules already in place for predicting reactivity of proteins in aqueous solution at neutral pH?

2. Are these predominant sites of reactivity in a protein predictable, based on the primary amino acid sequences, and the regional hydropathy and flexibility near the reaction site? What percentage of reactive sites are not predictable based solely on sequence or hydrophobicity calculations?

3. Does the absolute local protein conformation play an overriding role in determining the reactivity of individual Asn, Gln, Asp and Met such that prediction of reaction "hot spots" based on primary sequence and hydrophobicity is a shot in the dark? Or is it just a subtle variable in the background, and other factors are predominant most of the time? There are examples in the literature where the local

conformation and flexibility bring potential catalytic residues from distant regions in the sequence into close proximity of the deamidating amide side chain (Wright, 1991a). Alternatively, constraints on the backbone conformation may inhibit the deamidation of particular Asn residues (Kossiakoff, 1988). Further, potential catalytic side groups may be prevented from participating in the deamidation reaction because of hydrogen bonding or interactions with cofactors or ligands (Wright, 1991b). How much do these effects complicate the prediction of protein chemical reactivity?

4. Is this rate of chemical reaction fast enough to compromise a 2-year shelf life at 2–8°C and at pH 4.5–7.5? Although the kinetics of protein degradation are not addressed specifically in this report, it should be realized that all amino acids will degrade if followed long enough at sufficiently high temperatures, and the reader should be aware of this when reading the protein degradation literature (there are numerous examples of protein degradation at elevated temperatures and high or low pH, and these may not be representative of protein degradation in typical protein formulations).

2. PREDICTION OF PROTEIN CHEMICAL REACTIVITY BASED ON AMINO ACID SEQUENCE ANALYSIS

Although it has been known for years that certain amino acid sequences are prone to hydrolytic degradation (such as deamidation, cyclic imide formation, and iso-Asp formation at Asn, deamidation at Gln, or cyclic imide and iso-Asp formation at Asp), it has been argued that the neighboring substituent effects and conformational aspects are too complicated to allow routine prediction of chemical reactivity based on amino acid sequence and hydrophobicity/flexibility calculations. The same is believed to be true for Met oxidation; there is little correlation of reactivity and neighboring substituent effect (also called the sequence effect). To date, however, there does not exist a systematic analysis of protein reactivity in solution, such that a comparison of these studies is easily made. This chapter attempts to fill this need in formulation science, with the goal of attaining a better understanding of protein chemical reactivity in aqueous solution.

It is appropriate at this point to introduce the caveats in this analysis, lest the unwary reader be led astray from the main focus of this paper:

1. Proteins degrade by different pathways, both chemical and physical. The data and calculations herein do not address all protein degradation pathways, but only the chemical degradation pathways of deamidation, hydrolysis (cleavage), and oxidation. Degradation by other pathways including aggregation, precipitation, conformational denaturation, transamination, disulfide scrambling, reduction, enzymatic degradation, racemization, and other common routes are not part of this analysis. Further, there is no correction made for potential glycosylation at Asn (possible in the hot-spot motifs, -XNGS-, -XNGT-, -XNSS-, or -XNST-) which eliminates reaction at these potential hot spots.

2. There are several protein purification reports in which the isolated and purified protein is heterogeneous at a particular site, often Asn. The heterogeneity is usually caused by deamidation, giving Asp and iso-Asp. Many of these papers describe deamidation under extreme conditions that are not applicable to the long-term storage of protein formulations, including heating to 100°C, or acetic acid exposure during isolation. Further, these proteins are isolated from a biological milieu containing enzymes that may cause deamidation. There is sufficient evidence in the literature to suggest that deamidation can be significantly faster in a cellular or plasma medium than in aqueous solution of comparable pH and temperature (Nyberg *et al.*, 1985; O'Kelley *et al.*, 1985). Further, it is possible that the enzymatic deamidation pathway is different than the nonenzymatic pathway, so data generated under "work-up" conditions must be viewed cautiously.

3. Some proteins are quite small, such as secretin (27 amino acids) or insulin, and are close to the limit of being described as "large peptides." A few of these have been included in this analysis to thoroughly represent pharmaceutically relevant peptides and proteins, as well as to show that the data presented herein are directly applicable to smaller polypeptides as well.

4. Much of the literature on protein degradation focuses on determining the detailed mechanism of degradation and the factors that affect the reaction pathway(s). For example, the mechanistic distinctions in deamidation pathways have been studied in detail, in which deamidation occurs by cyclic imide formation, giving Asp or iso-Asp, or by deamidation of Asn, directly giving Asp without cyclic imide formation. This chapter does not attempt to review the excellent work in this area, but rather attempts to capitalize on it with the goal of addressing the sites of probable reaction and their likelihood of compromising the stability of a liquid protein formulation stored at 2–8°C for 1.5 years or more.

5. The "quality" of the different reports of protein degradation vary widely. Some studies are fairly extensive, for example, when conducted as part of a pharmaceutical drug development program. Others are short reports in the biochemical literature more than 20 years ago when the techniques for detecting protein degradation were not nearly as sophisticated as they are today. For example, detecting iso-Asp formation from Asp has been problematic by most chromatographic methods, and may be underreported in the protein degradation literature. The detection of other species, such as succinimide formation or a particular oxidized isoform, is also often difficult to detect and so may be underreported in older literature reports.

2.1. Common Chemical Degradation Pathways in Proteins

Much of our understanding of protein deamidation comes from the study of deamidation in small peptides. Several reviews on deamidation have been published (Robinson and Rudd, 1974; Wright, 1991b; Cleland *et al.*, 1993) and should be consulted if more detail is required. In general, deamidation is catalyzed by base, heat, and ionic strength and is retarded by the addition of organic solvents (Capasso *et al.*, 1991). The rate of deamidation (as well as the detailed mechanism) is dictated by the pH and the adjacent amino acid(s). The deamidation rate for Asn is usually greater than for Gln, and is greatest when Asn or Gln are adjacent to Gly (-Asn-Gly- or -Gln-Gly-) (Robinson *et al.*, 1973a). The higher reactivity of the -Asn-Gly- bond compared to -Asn-X- (where X ≠ Gly) is shown by the degradation of Val-Tyr-Pro-Asn-X-Ala at pH 7.4 and 37°C. The half-lives for these peptides are X = Gly, 1.1; Ser, 8; Ala, 20; Leu, 70; Pro, 106 days, respectively. Hydrophobic or bulky amino acids in the sequence -Asn-X- appear to slow the deamidation rate considerably. At the preceding position, there are conflicting reports as to the nature of the substituent effect. Inspection of the rate data for peptides containing the -XNA- or the -XQA-motif shows that polar amino acids in the position -X-Asn- or -X-Gln- accelerate the deamidation rate, and bulky or hydrophobic residues tend to retard the deamidation rate. Figure 1 shows the substituent effect for the -X-Asn- and -X-Gln- motifs. In contrast, deamidation of peptides at pH 7.3 and 60°C containing the -XNS- motif showed no substituent effect (Tyler-Cross and Schirch, 1991). In this study, it is possible that any subtle substituent effect may be masked at the higher temperature of this reaction.

The model peptide containing the -GNA- motif was found to degrade exclusively via the cyclic imide intermediate from pH 5–12, and via direct hydrolysis of the amide side chain at acidic pH to give the Asp-hexapeptide (Patel and Borchardt, 1990). Under similar conditions, the deamidation half-lives for a series of penta-peptides yield values ranging from 6 days (Gly-Ser-Asn-His-Gly) to 3400 days (Gly-Thr-Gln-Ala-Gly) (Robinson *et al.*, 1973a; McKerrow and Robinson, 1974). At pH

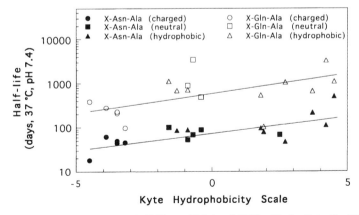

Figure 1. Correlation of deamidation half-life at pH 7.4 and 37°C with the Kyte–Doolittle hydrophobicity parameter. These data are from Robinson and Rudd (1974) and are determined by using a series of peptides defined by Gly-X-Asn-Ala-Gly. Inspection of the data show that, for both Asn and Gln, polar and charged amino acids adjacent to the reaction site accelerate the reaction rate, whereas hydrophobic or bulky residues decrease the rate of deamidation.

7.4 and 37°C, the rate of -Asn-Gly- bond cleavage was found to be 30- to 40-fold faster than for -Asp-Gly- (see below). A summary mechanism for Asn deamidation is shown in Scheme 2, including direct hydrolysis of the amide side chain and cyclic

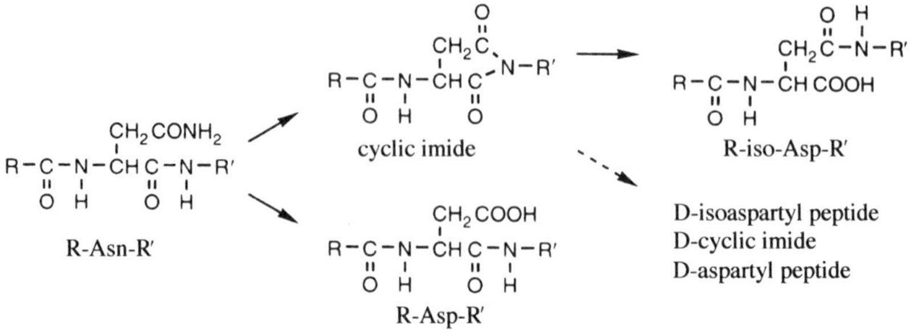

Scheme 2

imide formation. This reaction may also result in racemization, thus forming the D-amino acid analogues.

The -Asp-Gly- bond is also fairly reactive at neutral pH, yielding reversible isomerization between the Asp and iso-Asp forms via the cyclic imide intermediate (Scheme 3). Several Asp-containing peptides also yield detectable amounts of this

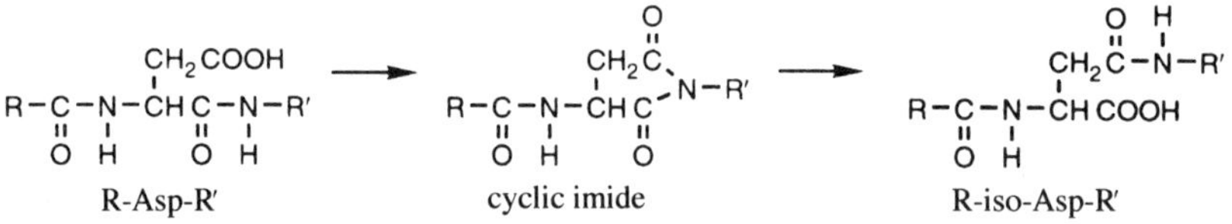

Scheme 3

intermediate (Bodansky et al., 1967). The higher reactivity of the -Asp-Gly- bond is observed in the degradation of Val-Tyr-Pro-Asp-X-Ala at pH 7.4 and 37°C. The half-lives for these peptides are X = Gly, 41; Ser, 168; Ala, 266 days (Stephenson and Clarke, 1989). Iso-Asp also forms from Asp when Asp is adjacent to sterically hindered groups, such as in glucagon (-Asp-Tyr-) (Ota et al., 1987) and calmodulin (-Asp-Gln-, -Asp-Thr-) (Ota and Clarke, 1989). Oliyai et al. (Oliyai and Borchardt, 1993) determined the effect of pH on the degradation of a model hexapeptide, in which the rate constant for -Asp-Gly- hydrolysis below pH 3 at 37°C was 7.5×10^{-4} $M^{-1}s^{-1}$, corresponding to a shelf life at pH 5 of approximately 0.5 year.

Asp is also reactive under acid conditions if the adjacent amino acid is proline, as in -Asp-Pro- (Schultz, 1967). For example, the reaction half-life of the -Asp-X-peptide bond in 0.015 N HCl at 110°C is much more rapid for Pro than for other amino acids: X = Pro, 11; Leu, 84; Ser, 108; Phe, 130; Lys, 228 min. The enhanced rate of this hydrolytic reaction is due to the increased leaving-group ability of the protonated proline due to the higher basicity of the proline nitrogen (Scheme 4). Model peptide studies suggest that this reaction is not sufficiently rapid at pH 5–7 and 2–8°C to compromise an aqueous-based protein formulation, but one should pay attention to

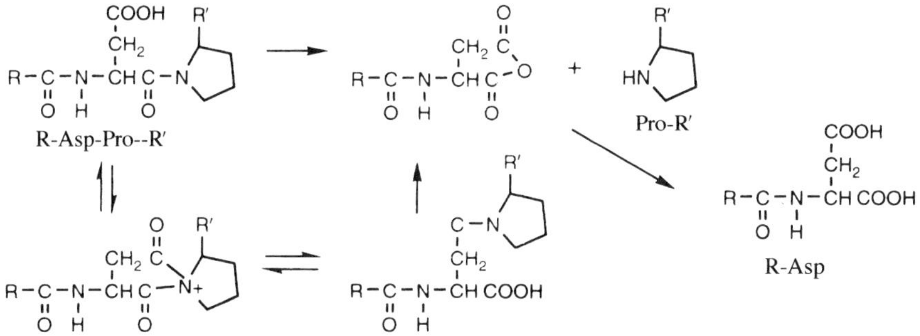

Scheme 4

this degradation reaction as it is unlikely that the clipped fragments of the parent are biologically active.

There are other hydrolytic reactions that may compromise protein shelf life at pH 5–7, such as diketopiperazine (DKP) and pyroglutamic acid formation (Steinberg and Bada, 1983). Peptides containing glycine as the third amino acid from the N-termini undergo DKP formation much more easily than peptides with other amino acids in the third position (Sepetov et al., 1991). Further, DKP formation is enhanced by incorporation of Pro or Gly into positions 1 or 2, whereas cyclization is completely prevented by blocking the α-amino group. Unfortunately, there is a paucity of data for this reaction, especially at 2–8°C, making a stability prediction difficult. It has been shown that there is a modest substituent effect at position 1 for DKP formation; reaction of X-Pro-Ala-Arg-Ser-Pro-Ser-Thr at 55°C and pH 7.0 for 3 days showed variable amounts of N-terminal degradation for X = Ala (83%), X = Val (35%), and X = Ser (89%) (Patel and Gitlin, 1995). In the same study it was shown that the pH of maximum stability for DKP formation of the Ala-Pro-Ala- peptide was approximately pH 4.5. The mechanism of DKP formation involves the nucleophilic attack of the N-terminal nitrogen on the amide carbonyl between the second and third amino acids (Scheme 5).

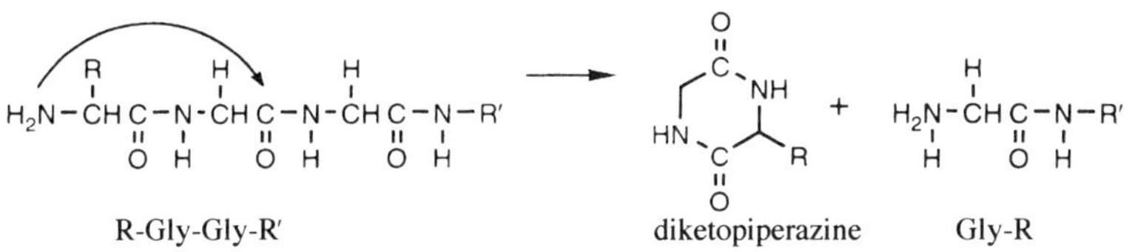

Scheme 5

The reaction of N-terminal Gln is faster than predicted based on other amino acids, including Asn (Blomback, 1967). In this case, the Gln-amide undergoes nucleophilic attack by the N-terminal amino group, giving pyroglutamic acid (Scheme 6). Fukawa has shown that Gln-Gly reacts much faster than the other similar peptides studied, including Pro-Gln-Gly and Leu-Gln-Gly (Fukawa, 1967). Again, there are several kinetic studies of pyroglutamic acid formation at higher tempera-

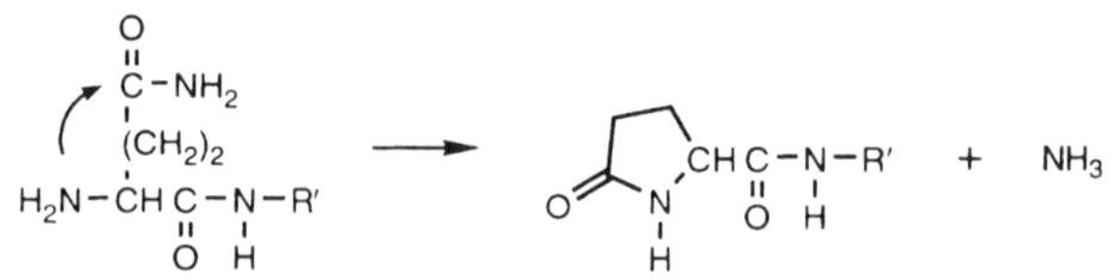

Scheme 6

tures, but few at 2–8°C. The available data in small peptides however, may model the reaction rates of pyroglutamic acid seen in proteins with the Gln-X-Gly- N-terminal sequence, in that proteins often show flexible and disordered N-terminal sequences with little secondary structure. Another interesting reaction of glutamate has been observed for the chimeric Fab antibody fragment, ReoPro, wherein incubation of this protein at 37°C and pH 7.2 gives pyroglutamate, as identified by IEF and hydrophobic interaction chromatography (Everett *et al.*, 1995). The formation of pyroglutamic acid should not be universally considered a "degradation product," as nature has protected several proteins from aminopeptidase attack by this modification.

Another major degradation route for proteins in liquid formulations is thermal oxidation. The terminology "thermal" protein oxidation is actually a misnomer, as the degradation rate is often governed by trace amounts of peroxide, metal ions, light, base, and free-radical initiators (Johnson and Gu, 1988). Although there are several reactive amino acids that are known to oxidize (Met, Cys, cystine, His, Trp, and Tyr), a review of the literature shows that, under mild oxidative conditions at pH 5–7, Met is the predominant amino acid that oxidizes (Stadtman, 1990). Met oxidizes by both chemical and photochemical pathways to give methionine sulfoxide and, under extremely oxidative conditions (rarely found in protein pharmaceutical formulations), methionine sulfone (Scheme 7).

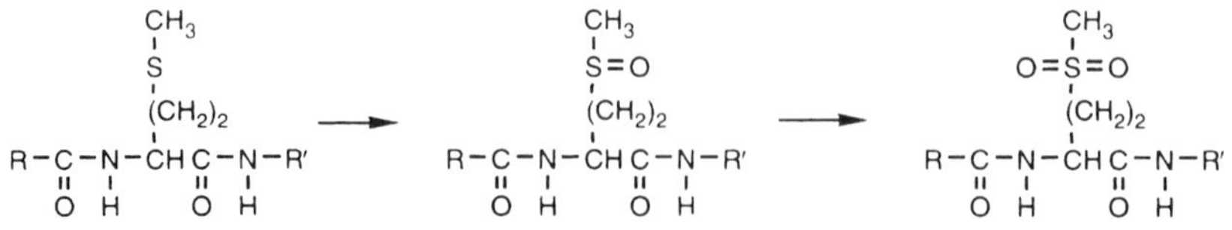

methionyl peptide   sulfoxide peptide   sulfone peptide
(R-Met-R')

Scheme 7

Even though a great deal is known about reactive oxygen species, the presence (or absence) of these initiators makes the prediction of autooxidation in parenteral formulations imprecise. For example, free-radical oxidation involves the separate effects of initiation, propagation, and termination. Further, there are several reactive oxygen species including singlet oxygen $^1O_2$, superoxide radical O_2^-, alkyl or hydrogen peroxide ROOH or H_2O_2, hydroxyl radicals (HO· or HOO·), and halide oxygen complexes (ClO$^-$) (Halliwell and Gutteridge, 1990). There is limited published data on the oxidation of proteins in pharmaceutical formulations because only a few of the proteins developed thus far have shown significant amounts of oxidation. Methionine residues in polypeptides show widely varying reactivity, as some Met residues are protected from oxidation by steric effects or inaccessibility, being buried in the hydrophobic core of the protein (Teh *et al.*, 1987). The second-order rate constants ($M^{-1}s^{-1}$) of Met oxidation by hydrogen peroxide have been determined at room temperature for Met free amino acid (0.93), Ac-Ser-Trp-Met-Glu-Glu-CONH$_2$ (1.07), Ac-CysNH$_2$-S-S-AcCys-Gly-Met-Ser-Thr-CONH$_2$ (1.0), and the Met in re-laxin B chain at positions 25 and 4 (Met B^{25}, 0.85; Met B^4, 0.34) (Nguyen *et al.*, 1993a). This study shows that the peroxide-catalyzed degradation of Met has little temperature dependence ($\Delta H \sim 10$–12 kcal/mol) and is negligibly effected by pH or ionic strength. The amount of peroxide in some excipients such as polyethylene glycols and surfactants varies widely (Hamburger *et al.*, 1975; McGinity *et al.*, 1975) and should be used cautiously in the formulation of Met-containing proteins. Using the data of Nguyen *et al.* (1993a), it is estimated that 1 nM peroxide in a Met-containing formulation would shorten the shelf life to less than 2 years.

2.2. Calculation of Protein Hydropathy and Flexibility

The general literature, and Genentech's GenBank data base, were surveyed for proteins that exhibit deamidation, hydrolysis, cyclization, or oxidation. Also in-cluded are a few unpublished observations from reliable laboratories. The protein sequences were scanned for the reactive residues, Asn, Asp, Gln, and Met, and the motifs surrounding these residues were tabulated as "reactive sites," although it is recognized that not all Asn, Asp, Gln, or Met are predicted to be reactive. To aid the reader, only the highly reactive motifs were labeled on the hydroflex plots (see below), and these included Asn-Gly, Asn-Ser, Asp-Gly, Gln-Gly, Asp-Pro, and Met.

The primary amino acid sequences were then used to construct "hydroflex" plots, consisting of the calculated hydropathy of the amino acid sequence, as well as its flexibility (see below). Hydropathy has been used to calculate antigenic determi-nants, as well as the surface characteristic of proteins (Hopp and Woods, 1981, 1983; Hopp, 1985, 1986). The hydropathy plot was constructed using the "hydro" program that scans the protein (or actually the individual hydropathy values assigned to each amino acid in the protein) with a window of specified size and computes the average hydrophobicity of each window (Watanabe, 1991). For example, a model protein shown in Scheme 8 is subjected to a window size of six amino acids, and the average hydropathy (ϕ) calculated.

Using this nomenclature, a hydropathy plot is simply a plot of ϕ versus amino acid number for the entire amino acid sequence. A window of 6 was chosen for several reasons: a window size of approximately 7–10 is believed to be optimal for searching for interior hydrophobic and exterior hydrophilic regions. A window size of 6–7 is believed to be optimal for searching for antigenic regions. Windows of sizes 5, 6, 7, and 10 amino acids were tested for several proteins with little visual difference

```
_____ϕ1        (ϕ1 = hydropathy average of ASDFGH, plotted at position 3)
_____ϕ2        (ϕ2 = hydropathy average of SDFGHC, plotted at position 4)
_____ϕ3        (ϕ3 = hydropathy average of DFGHCM, plotted at position 5)
_____ϕ4        (ϕ4 = hydropathy average of FGHCMN, plotted at position 6)
_____ϕ5        (ϕ5 = hydropathy average of GHCMNQ, plotted at position 7)
ASDFGHCMNQW...
123456789...
```

Scheme 8

in the hydropathy plots (data not shown). The optimal window size for the flexibility plot calculations is approximately 5 (see below), and so a window size of 6 amino acids was selected as a compromise between the methods for consistency. We chose the Kyte–Doolittle scale for our analysis of the various proteins. The individual amino acid hydropathy values used (Kyte–Doolittle parameters) are shown in Table I along with several other hydropathy scales for comparison.

For our purposes, the absolute values of the hydropathy values ϕ shown in the plots do not have significance; only the relative scale is important. Large positive values of ϕ denote regions of predicted high hydrophobicity; large negative values of ϕ denote regions of hydrophilicity. Although it is likely that hydrophobic regions tend to be found near the core of the protein, this is only a generalization and cannot be held as absolute from a simple calculation (the X-ray crystal, or NMR solution structure are the definitive indicators which amino acids are found in the core and which are found on the exterior of the protein).

The flexibility plots were calculated in a similar fashion using the parameters of hydrophobicity and side-chain volume according to Ragone *et al.* (1989). In this case, the relative flexibility scales gave values ranging from 1000 to 3000 and required normalization to plot with the hydrophobicity values. The mean value of zero for the flexibility plots was determined by computing the average flexibility of all of the proteins in the GenBank database, and included a statistical correction for the relative amino acids available in nature. The individual amino acid flexibility values are shown in Table I. Again, the absolute flexibility values do not have significance, but only the relative position on the plot. In the normalized plots, regions of flexibility have values less than zero; constrained regions have large positive values.

Hydropathy plots were calculated for several proteins using the Kyte, Hopp, Engleman, and Eisenberg hydropathy scales; all gave similar plots regardless of the hydropathy scale used (data not shown). The flexibility plots were often quite different than the hydropathy plots, largely because they are the cross product of hydropathy and amino acid side-chain volume (a correlate of "flexibility). So as to contrast the two major ways to analyze primary sequence analysis, the Kyte hydropathy plot and the flexibility plot are shown together to compare and contrast these methods. Conveniently, these plots provide at a single glance a visual picture of the protein. Reactive regions are typically found in large negative values, and stable regions found in large positive values of both hydropathy and flexibility (using either scale).

Table I. Summary of Hydropathy and Flexibility
Values for Individual Amino Acids[a]

AA	Kyte	Hopp	Engelman	Eisenberg	Ragoné[b]
A (Ala)	1.8	0.5	1.6	0.62	−0.91
C (Cys)	2.5	1.0	2.0	0.29	−0.17
D (Asp)	−3.5	−3.0	−9.2	−9.0	−0.68
E (Glu)	−3.5	−3.0	−8.2	−0.74	−0.68
F (Phe)	2.7	2.5	3.7	1.19	1.37
G (Gly)	−0.4	0.0	1.0	0.48	−1.40
H (His)	−3.2	0.5	−3.0	−0.4	0.25
I (Ile)	4.5	1.8	3.1	1.38	1.09
K (Lys)	−3.9	−3.0	−8.8	1.50	0.13
L (Leu)	3.7	1.8	2.8	1.06	0.89
M (Met)	1.9	1.3	3.4	0.64	0.83
N (Asn)	−3.5	−0.2	−4.8	−0.78	−0.42
P (Pro)	−1.6	0.0	−0.2	0.12	−0.52
Q (Gln)	−3.5	−0.2	−4.1	−0.85	0.06
R (Arg)	−4.5	−3.0	12.3	−2.53	0.71
S (Ser)	−0.9	−0.3	0.6	−0.18	−1.01
T (Thr)	−0.7	0.4	1.2	−0.05	−0.58
V (Val)	4.2	1.5	2.6	1.08	0.52
W (Trp)	−0.9	3.4	1.9	0.81	2.00
Y (Tyr)	−1.3	2.3	−0.7	0.26	1.21

[a]Kyte and Doolittle (1982); Hopp and Woods (1981, 1983); Engelman et al.
(1986); Eisenberg (1984); Ragoné et al. (1989).
[b]Corrected to provide a mean at ≃ 0 and maximum and minimum values over
an average window of six amino acids of approximately +1.0 and −1.0,
respectively.

3. SUMMARY OF PROTEIN STABILITY IN AQUEOUS SOLUTION

The strategy used herein is straightforward: (i) Assemble all of the data on degradation of proteins in pharmaceutical liquid formulations (or in model formulations consisting of aqueous solution of pH ~ 4.5–7.5) where there is evidence for degradation by hydrolysis, cyclization, deamidation, or oxidation. Include salient data obtained from protein purification studies (if controls are available showing reaction in aqueous solution). These data may have some peculiarities due to enzyme catalyzed reactions. (ii) Compile the relevant primary sequence information for these proteins, including a subset analysis of the reactive groups Asn, Asp, Gln, and Met. (iii) Analyze the primary sequence in terms of hydrophobicity and flexibility in order to "guesstimate" regions of preferred chemical reactivity. In this analysis it is assumed that these reactive regions are also hydrophilic, and thus have a higher probability of being on the "outside" of the protein, and should be fairly flexible so as to allow the correct geometry for reaction. The following pages are summaries of these parameters for different proteins. Included in each summary is the primary sequence of the protein, the motifs for all Asn, Asp, Gln, and Met, the calculated hydroflex plot, a short summary of the degradation pathway(s) reported in the literature, and comments on how predictive the primary sequence and the hydroflex plot were for protein degradation in aqueous solution (albeit retrospectively). Further mention is noted as to the reliability of the data for prediction of peptide/protein degradation under neutral pH formulation conditions.

- **Adrenocorticotropin (ACTH) (39 residues)**

SEQUENCE

SYSMEHFRWGKPVGKKRRPVKVYPNGAEDESAEAFPLEF

REACTIVE SITES

.N.(1)	.D.(1)	.M.(1)	.Q.(0)
25 PNG	29 EDE	4 SME	

HYDROFLEX PLOT

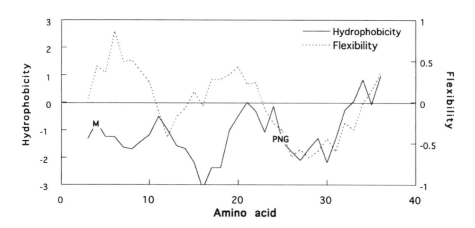

PREDICTED REACTIVITY AND DEGRADATION OF ACTH

ACTH contains only a single site susceptible to hydrolytic degradation, Asn-25, with the -PNG- motif. Further, Asn-25 is located in a region predicted to be fairly flexible and hydrophilic, suggesting that this is the predominant reactive residue. Based on this, ACTH is expected to degrade primarily at Asn-25. Under neutral pH conditions, the 39-mer ACTH peptide underwent deamidation at Asn-25 to give the cyclic imide, and the Asp-25 and iso-Asp-25 ACTH variants (Aswad, 1984; Patel, 1993). The reactivity of Asn-25 was studied extensively in the parent hormone and in smaller peptides of similar motif about Asn (such as the hexapeptide VTPNGA). No oxidation at Met was reported.

Agglutinin (171 residues)

SEQUENCE

QRCGEQGSNMECPNNLCCSQYGYCGMGGDYCGKGCQNGACWTSKRCGSQAGGA-
TCTNNQCCSQYGYCGFGAEYCGAGCQGGPCRADIKCGSQAGGKLCPNNLCCSQW-
GFCGLGSEFCGGGCQSGACSTDKPCGKDAGGRVCTNNYCCSKWGSCGIGPGYCGA-
GCQSGGCDG

REACTIVE SITES

.N.(10)		.D.(5)	.M.(2)	.Q.(11)	
9 SNM	100 PNN	29 GDY	10 NME	6 EQG	79 CQG
14 PNN	101 NNL	86 ADI	26 GMG	20 SQY	92 SQA
15 NNL	143 TNN	129 TDK		36 CQN	106 SQW
37 QNG	144 NNY	135 KDA		49 SQA	122 CQS
57 TNN		170 CDG		59 NQC	165 CQS
58 NNQ				63 SQY	

HYDROFLEX PLOT

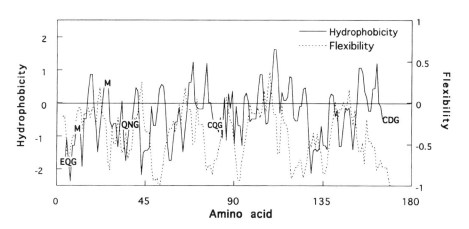

PREDICTED REACTIVITY AND DEGRADATION OF AGGLUTININ

The hydroflex plot shows that there are a few predicted sites of chemical reactivity, notably the Asn-Gly at position 37, and possibly the Asp-Gly at the C-termini. The nucleotide sequence code for agglutinin encodes for Asn at position 37 (within the -QNG- motif), yet amino acid sequence analysis indicated that Asp was the predominant amino acid observed at this site (Wright and Raikhel, 1989). It was not determined if this discrepancy was due to deamidation in the intact protein or in the proteolytically generated peptides used in the sequencing. No oxidation of Met was reported.

- **Aldolase (363 residues)**

SEQUENCE

PHSHPALTPEQKKELSDIAHRIVAPGKGILAADESTGSIAKRLQSIGTENTEENRRFYR-
QLLLTADDRVNPCIGGVILFHETLYQKADDGRPFPQVIKSKGGVVGIKVDKGVVPLA-
GTNGETTTQGLDGLSERCAQYKKDGADFAKWRCVLKIGEHTPSALAIMENANVLA-
RYASICQQNGIVPIVEPEILPDGDHDLKRCQYVTEKVLAAVYKALSDHHIYLEGTLL-
KPNMVTPGHACTQKYSHEEIAMATVTALRRTVPPAVTGVTFLSGGQSEEEASINLNA-
INKCPLLKPWALTFSYGRALQASALKAWGGKKENLKAAQEEYVKRALANSLACQG-
KYTPSGQAGAAASESLFISNHAY

REACTIVE SITES

.N.(14)	.D.(14)	.M.(3)	.Q.(16)
50 ENT	17 SDI	164 IME	11 EQK
54 ENR	33 ADE	232 NMV	44 LQS
70 VNP	66 ADD	250 AMA	60 RQL
119 TNG	67 DDR		85 YQK
166 ENA	88 ADD		95 PQV
168 ANV	89 DDG		125 TQG
180 QNG	109 VDK		136 AQY
231 PNM	128 LDG		178 CQQ
282 INL	148 KDG		179 QQN
284 LNA	143 ADF		202 CQY
287 INK	193 PDG		241 TQK
319 ENL	195 GDH		274 GQS
334 ANS	197 HDL		306 LQA
360 SNH	218 SDH		324 AQE
			339 CQG
			347 GQA

HYDROFLEX PLOT

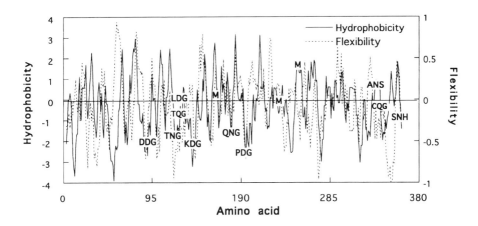

PREDICTED REACTIVITY AND DEGRADATION OF ALDOLASE

This molecule has several predicted degradation sites. Isolation of rabbit muscle aldolase and subsequent amino acid sequencing of the carboxyl-terminal peptide liberated by chymotrypsin hydrolysis shows that Asn undergoes deamidation to give Asp within the motif, -ISNHAY (Midelfort and Mehler, 1972). It has been pointed out that this Asn may be activated by the neighboring His, but otherwise the Asn-Ala motif is usually considered poorly reactive, as based on data obtained from small peptides. In fact, several other proteins have the -XNH- motif, including ARSP, anti-HER-2, 4D5 antibody, 17-1A antibody, CD4-IgG, chloroperoxidase, acidic-FGF, HXGT, IFN-β, OKT-3 antibody, SHMT, and t-PA, and showed no sign of reacting at this site, indicating that -XNH- is not particularly activating unless composed of -SNH-. In this study, no control experiments were carried out to show that the same deamidation reaction occurs in pH 4.5–7.5 buffer, and reaction at this site may be enzymatic in nature. Further, insufficient controls were carried out to determine if deamidation, cyclization, or oxidation occurred at many of the other sites predicted to be labile.

Amylin Antagonist (24 residues)   •

SEQUENCE

Ac-LGRLSQELHRLQTYPRTNTGSNTY-CONH$_2$

REACTIVE SITES

.N.(2)	.D.(0)	.M.(0)	.Q.(2)
18 TNT			6 SQE
22 SNT			12 LQT

HYDROFLEX PLOT

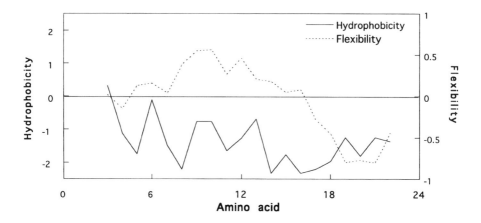

PREDICTED REACTIVITY AND DEGRADATION OF AMYLIN
ANTAGONIST

This peptide is acylated at the N-termini and has the carbamoyl moiety at the C-termini
(no account for these modifications was made in the hydroflex plot). Inspection of the
hydroflex plot shows that this peptide should be quite stable in that it is devoid of the
"traditional" hot spots for chemical degradation. Asn-18 and Asn-22 are adjacent to Thr,
which is reported to activate reactivity at Asn only slightly. The solution stability of this amylin
antagonist was investigated under acidic conditions (pH 2.6–5.0), approaching the desired pH
range for parenteral formulations. Deamidation at Asn-22 was observed, with a rate minimum
at pH 4.3, resulting in the formation of iso-Asp-22 and Asp-22 (3.2:2), consistent with cyclic
imide formation. Deamidation at Asn-18 was not detected (Darrington, 1995).

- **Amyloid-Related Serum Protein (ARSP) (104 residues)**

SEQUENCE

RSFFSFLGEAFDGARDMWRAYSNMREANYIGSDKYFHARGNYDAAKRGPGGAWA-
AEVISNARENIQRFFGHDAENSLADQAANEWGRSGKDPNHFRPAGLPEKY

REACTIVE SITES

.N.(8)		.D.(7)		.M.(2)	.Q.(2)
23 SNM	64 ENI	12 FDG	72 HDA	17 DMW	66 IQR
28 ANY	75 ENS	16 RDM	79 ADQ	24 NMR	80 DQA
41 GNY	83 ANE	33 SDK	91 KDP		
60 SNA	93 PNH	43 YDA			

HYDROFLEX PLOT

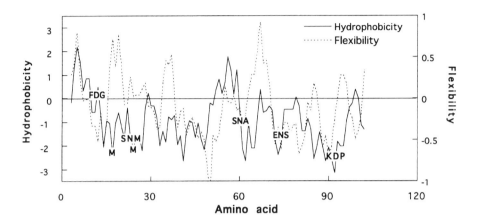

PREDICTED REACTIVITY AND DEGRADATION OF AMYLOID-RELATED SERUM PROTEIN

Isolation of amyloid-related serum protein (ARSP) gives a 104-amino-acid protein that shows microheterogeneity at Asn-23 (-SNM-), Asn-60 (-SNA-), and Asn-75 (-ENS-), where only the later motif (-XNS-) is predicted to be chemically reactive at neutral pH (Sletten *et al.*, 1983). No controls were carried out to determine if this deamidation was due to isolation or differences in protein expression from different patients. Insufficient data was presented to allow the estimation of degradation at pH 4.5–7.5 at 5°C.

Angiogenin (123 residues)

SEQUENCE

EDNSRYTHFLTQHYDAKPQGRDDRYCESIMRRRGLTSPCKDINTFIHGNKRSIKAICE-
NKNGNPHRENLRISKSSFQVTTCKLHGGSPWPPCQYRATAGFRNVVVACENGLPVH-
LDQSIFRRP

REACTIVE SITES

	.N.(9)			.D.(6)	.M.(1)	.Q.(5)	
3	DNS	68	ENL	2 END	30 IMR	12	TQH
43	INT	102	RNV	15 YDA		19	PQG
49	GNK	109	ENG	22 RDD		77	FQV
59	ENK			23 DDR		93	CQY
61	KNG			41 KDI		117	DQS
63	GNP			116 LDQ			

HYDROFLEX PLOT

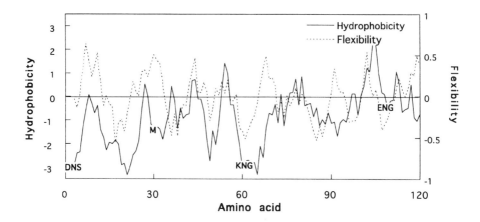

PREDICTED REACTIVITY AND DEGRADATION OF ANGIOGENIN

The hydroflex plot shows that Asn-61 and Asn-109 are likely spots for reactivity, in that they are located adjacent to Gly and are found in moderately flexible regions. A third reactive site could also be Asn-3 in the -DNS- motif. Incubation of angiogenin at pH 8 and 4°C for 2 years resulted in approximately 35% loss of the original molecule (Hallahan *et al.*, 1992). Degradation occurred simultaneously at Asn-61 (-KNG-) and Asn-109 (-ENG-), which likely accounts for their observation of a third (and unidentified) acidic product—the doubly deamidated molecule. Alternatively, deamidation may have occurred at Asn-3, in that the reaction product of this third reaction product was not identified. Deamidation resulted in a dramatic loss in biological activity.

- **Anti-HER-2 Heavy Chain (450 residues)**

SEQUENCE

EVQLVESGGGLVQPGGSLRLSCAASGFNIKDTYIHWVRQAPGKGLEWVARIYPTNG-
YTRYADSVKGRFTISADTSKNTAYLQMNSLRAEDTAVYYCSRWGGDGFYAMDYW-
GQGTLVTVSSASTKGPSVFPLAPSSKSTSGGTAALGCLVKDYFPEPVTVSWNSGALT-
SGVHTFPAVLQSSGLYSLSSVVTVPSSSLGTQTYICNVNHKPSNTKVDKKVEPKSCD-
KTHTCPPCPAPELLGGPSVFLFPPKPKDTLMISRTPEVTCVVVDVSHEDPEVKFNWY-
VDGVEVHNAKTKPREEQYNSTYRVVSVLTVLHQDWLNGKEYKCKVSNKALPAPIE-
KTISKAKGQPREPQVYTLPPSREEMTKNQVSLTCLVKGFYPSDIAVEWESNGQPEN-
NYKTTPPVLDSDGSFFLYSKLTVDKSRWQQGNVFSCSVMHEALHNHYTQKSLSLS-
PGK

REACTIVE SITES

.N.(19)	.D.(18)	.M.(5)	.Q.(16)
28 FNI	31 KDT	83 QMN	3 VQL
55 TNG	62 ADS	107 AMD	13 VQP
77 KNT	73 ADT	255 LMI	39 RQA
84 MNS	90 EDT	361 EMT	82 LQM
162 WNS	102 GDG	431 VMH	112 GQG
204 CNV	108 MDY		178 LQS
206 VNH	151 KDY		199 TQT
211 SNT	215 VDK		298 EQY
279 FNW	224 CDK		314 HQD
289 HNA	252 KDT		345 GQP
300 YNS	268 VDV		350 PQV
318 LNG	273 EDP		365 NQV
328 SNK	283 VDG		389 GQP
364 KNQ	315 QDW		421 WQQ
387 SNG	379 SDI		422 QQG
392 ENN	402 LDS		441 TQK
393 NNY	404 SDG		
424 GNV	416 VDK		
437 HNH			

HYDROFLEX PLOT

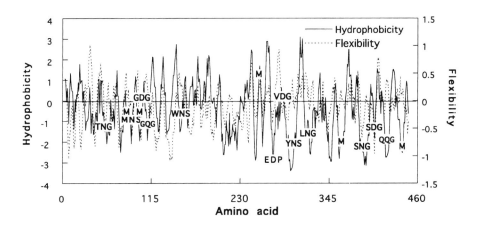

PREDICTED REACTIVITY AND DEGRADATION OF ANTI-HER-2 ANTIBODY HEAVY CHAIN

Inspection of the amino acid sequence for the anti-HER-2 heavy chain shows that there are several reactive sites, including predicted deamidation at Asn-318 in the -LNG- motif, Asn-387 in the -SNG- motif, iso-Asp formation at Asn-55 in the -TNG- motif, at Asp-102 in the

-GDG- motif, at Asp-283 in the -VDG- motif, and Asp-404 in the -SDG- motif. This antibody is formulated as a liquid in 5 mM isotonic acetate, pH 5.0, 0.01% Polysorbate 20. After 1.5 years at 2–8°C storage, it was shown using an ion-exchange assay the formation of cyclic imide at Asp-102 (located in the CDR3 region); this identification of succinimide intermediate was done also carried out by HIC after alkaline hydroxylamine cleavage (Kwong and Harris, 1985). This degradation product, as well as the iso-Asp product (Harris *et al.*, 1995), has been isolated and shown to retain full biological activity. All other assays were virtually unchanged after storage at 2–8°C. Although this protein did not show oxidation under formulation conditions at 2–8°C, rapid oxidation of Met-255 and Met-431 was catalyzed by *t*-butylhydroperoxide (Shen *et al.*, 1996).

- **Anti-HER-2 Light Chain (214 residues)**

SEQUENCE

DIQMTQSPSSLSASVGDRVTITCRASQDVNTAVAWYQQKPGKAPKLLIYSASFLYSG-
VPSRFSGSRSGTDFTLTISSLQPEDFATYYCQQHYTTPPTFGQGTKVEIKRTVAAPSVF-
IFPPSDEQLKSGTASVVCLLNNFYPREAKVQWKVDNALQSGNSQESVTEQDSKDST-
YSLSSTLTLSKADYEKHKVYACEVTHQGLSSPVTKSFNRGEC

REACTIVE SITES

.N.(6)	.D.(9)	.M.(1)	.Q.(15)	
30 VNT	17 GDR	4 QMT	3 IQM	
137 LNN	28 QDV		6 TQS	
138 NNF	70 TDF		27 SQD	
152 DNA	82 EDF		37 YQQ	
158 GNS	122 SDE		38 QQK	
210 FNR	151 VDN		79 LQP	
	167 QDS		89 CQQ	
	170 KDS		90 QQH	
	185 ADY		100 GQG	
			124 EQL	
			147 VQW	
			155 LQS	
			160 SQE	
			166 EQD	
			199 HQG	

HYDROFLEX PLOT

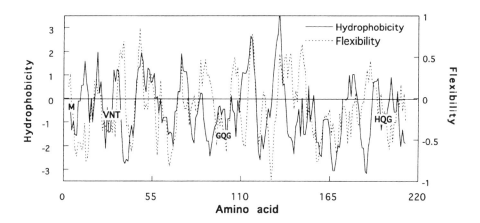

PREDICTED REACTIVITY AND DEGRADATION OF ANTI-HER-2 ANTIBODY LIGHT CHAIN

Inspection of the amino acid sequence for the anti-HER-2 light chain shows that there are few reactive sites, perhaps the most reactive being the single Met. Gln-Gly appears in the HER-2 light chain, but is the least reactive of the traditional (Asn-Gly, Asn-Ser, Asp-Gly, Asp-Pro, Met, and Gln-Gly) hot spots. This absence of hot spots suggests that the light chain of anti-HER-2 should be fairly stable compared to the heavy chain. Some deamidation of the light chain has been observed at Asn-30 in CDR1 of the light chain during the cell culture process, typically 10–12%. Deamidation of Asn-30 in one chain resulted in an ~18% decrease in activity as measured in the ECD plate binding assay (Harris, 1995; Shire, 1995), but little has been observed at pH 5. This residue is not a traditional hot spot, but is predicted to be in a flexible hydrophilic region. All other assays are virtually unchanged at 2–8°C storage.

Antibody 4D5 Heavy Chain (450 residues)

SEQUENCE

EVQLVESGGGLVQPGGSLRLSCAASGFNIKDTYIHWVRQAPGKGLEWVARIYPTNG-
YTRYADSVKRFTISADTSKNTAYLQMNSLRAEDTAVYYCSRWGGDGFYAMDYWG-
QGTLVTVSSASTKGPSVFPLAPSSKSTSGGTAALGCLVKDYFPEPVTVSWNSGALTS-
GVHTFPAVLQSSGLYSLSSVVTVPSSSLGTQTYICNVNHKPSNTKVDKKVEPKSCDK-
THTCPPCPAPELLGGPSVFLFPPKPKDTLMISRTPEVTCVVVDVSHEDPEVKFNWYV-
DGVEVHNAKTKPREEQYNSTYRVVSVLTVLHQDWLNGKEYKCKVSNKALPAPIEK-
TISKAKGQPREPQVYTLPPSREEMTKNQVSLTCLVKGFYPSDIAVEWESNGQPENNY-
KTTPPVLDSDGSFFLYSKLTVDKSRWQQGNVFSCSVMHEALHNHYTQKSLSLSPGK

REACTIVE SITES

.N.(19)	.D.(18)	.M.(5)	.Q.(16)
28 FNI	31 KDT	83 QMN	3 VQL
55 TNG	62 ADS	107 AMD	13 VQP
77 KNT	73 ADT	255 LMI	39 RQA
84 MNS	90 EDT	361 EMT	82 LQM
162 WNS	102 GDG	431 VMH	112 GQG
204 CNV	108 MDY		178 LQS
206 VNH	151 KDY		199 TQT
211 SNT	215 VDK		298 EQY
279 FNW	224 CDK		314 HQD
289 HNA	252 KDT		345 GQP
300 YNS	268 VDV		350 PQV
318 LNG	273 EDP		365 NQV
328 SNK	283 VDG		389 GQP
364 KNQ	315 QDW		421 WQQ
387 SNG	379 SDI		422 QQG
392 ENN	402 LDS		441 TQK
393 NNY	404 SDG		
424 GNV	416 VDK		
437 HNH			

HYDROFLEX PLOT

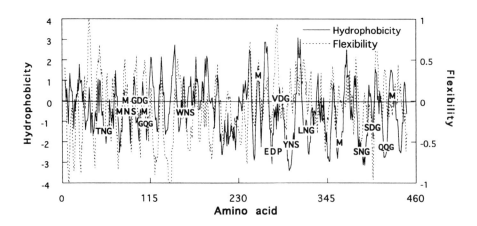

PREDICTED REACTIVITY AND DEGRADATION OF 4D5 ANTIBODY HEAVY CHAIN

There are a number of predicted potentially reactive deamidation and isomerization sites in the 4D5 heavy chain. Inspection of the primary amino acid sequence for the 4D5 heavy chain shows that the most reactive is predicted to be Asn-55 within the -TNG- motif in the

CDR2 domain, Asn-318 within the -LNG- motif, Asn-387 within the -SNG- motif. All reside in a region predicted to be hydrophilic and flexible. There are several other hot spots, including several Asp-Gly (that may isomerize to form iso-Asp-Gly), and three Met residues. The Asp-Gly within the -GNG- motif may be particularly labile, as aspartic acid residues adjacent to C-terminal glycine residues are very susceptible to imide formation and subsequent isomerization (Cleland *et al.*, 1993). This antibody was found to be stable for more than 12 months at 2–8°C by all methods tested, and showed some loss in activity at 25°C and 40°C (Harris, 1995; Shire, 1995). Decrease in activity did not correlate with formation of aggregates, but appears related to alterations in the protein which result in the generation of acidic bands as detected by IEF. No conclusive identification of the reactive site in the heavy chain (if at all) was made.

Antibody 4D5 Light Chain (214 residues)   ●

SEQUENCE

DIQMTQSPSSLSASVGDRVTITCRASQDVNTAVAWYQQKPGKAPKLLIYSASFLYSG-
VPSRFSGSRSGTDFTLTISSLQPEDFATYYCQQHYTTPPTFGQGTKVEIKRTVAAPSVF-
IFPPSDEQLKSGTASVVCLLNNFYPREAKVQWKVDNALQSGNSQESVTEQDSKDST-
YSLSSTLTLSKADYEKHKVYACEVTHQGLSSPVTKSFNRGEC

REACTIVE SITES

.N.(6)	.D.(9)	.M.(1)	.Q.(15)
30 VNT	17 GDR	4 QMT	3 IQM
137 LNN	28 QDV		6 TQS
138 NNF	70 TDF		27 SQD
152 DNA	82 EDF		37 YQQ
158 GNS	122 SDE		38 QQK
210 FNR	151 VDN		79 LQP
	167 QDS		89 CQQ
	170 KDS		90 QQH
	185 ADY		100 GQG
			124 EQL
			147 VQW
			155 LQS
			160 SQE
			166 EQD
			199 HQG

HYDROFLEX PLOT

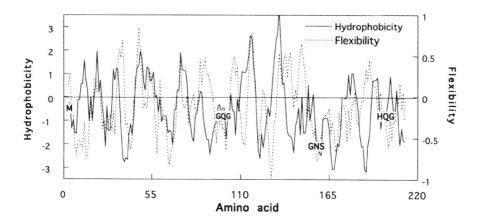

PREDICTED REACTIVITY AND DEGRADATION OF 4D5 ANTIBODY LIGHT CHAIN

Inspection of the primary amino acid sequence for the 4D5 light chain shows that there are few reactive sites, perhaps the most reactive being Asn-158 within the Asn-Ser motif, as it resides in a predicted hydrophilic and flexible region. None of the hot spots reside in the CDR domain. This antibody, formulated as a liquid in isotonic 5 mM acetate at pH 5.0 with 0.01% polysorbate 20, was stable for more than 12 months at 2–8°C (Shire, 1995). At 25°C and 40°C there were decreases in activity (up to 77%). The decrease in activity did not correlate with formation of aggregates, but appeared to be related to alterations in the protein which result in the generation of acidic bands as detected by IEF. No conclusive identification of the reactive site in the light chain (if at all) was made.

● **Antibody 17-1A Heavy Chain (446 residues)**

SEQUENCE

QVQLQQSGAELVRPGTSVKVSCKASGYAFTNYLIEWVKQRPGQGLEWIGVINPGSG-
GTNYNEKFKGKATLTADKSSSTAYMQLSSLTSDDSAVYFCARDGPWFAYWGQGTLV-
TVSAAKTTAPSVYPLAPVCGDTTGSSVTLGCLVKGYFPEPVTLTWNSGSLSSGVHTF-
PAVLQSDLYTLSSSVTVTSSTWPSQSITCNVAHPASSTKVDKKIEPRGPTIKPCPPCKC-
PAPNLLGGPSVFIFPPKIKDVLMISLSPIVTCVVDVSEDDPDVQISWFVNNVEVHTAQ-
TQTHREDYNSTLRVVSALPIQHQDWMSGKEFKCKVNNKDLPAPIERTISKPKGSVR-
APQVYVLPPPEEEMTKKQVTLTCMVTDFMPEDIYVEWTNNGKTELNYKNTEPVLD-
SDGSYFMYSKLRVEKKNWVERNSYSCSVVHEGLHNHHTTKSFSRTPGK

REACTIVE SITES

.N.(19)		.D.(19)		.M.(7)		.Q.(16)	
31 TNY	323 VNN	73 ADK	269 DDP	81 YMQ	357 EMT	3 VQL	287 AQT
52 INP	324 NNK	89 SDD	271 PDV	251 LMI	367 CMV	5 LQQ	289 TQT
59 TNY	382 TNN	90 DDS	294 EDY	313 WMS	372 FMP	6 QQS	308 IQH
61 YNE	383 NNG	99 RDG	311 QDW	357 EMT	405 FMY	39 KQR	310 HQD
159 WNS	389 LNY	133 GDT	326 KDL	367 CMV		43 GQG	346 PQV
199 CNV	392 KNT	176 SDL	370 TDF	372 FMP		82 MQL	361 KQV
232 PNL	415 KNW	210 VDK	375 EDI	405 FMY		108 GQG	
279 VNN	420 RNS	248 KDV	398 LDS			174 LQS	
280 NNV	433 HNH	264 VDV	400 SDG			194 SQS	
296 YNS		268 EDD				273 VQI	

HYDROFLEX PLOT

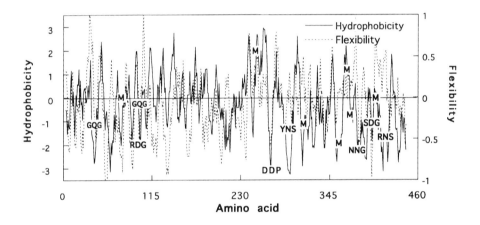

PREDICTED REACTIVITY AND DEGRADATION OF 17-1A ANTIBODY HEAVY CHAIN

The primary amino acid sequence for the 17-1A antibody heavy chain shows that Asn-383 should be very reactive in that it resides within the -NNG- motif, located in a hydrophilic and flexible region. There are several other reactive sites, including Asp-Pro, Asp-Gly, and Met. The observed reaction of the 17-1A antibody occurred largely at the C-terminus, with loss of Lys in a nonenzymatic process (enzyme inhibitors had no effect on this process, and there was no C-terminal reaction of other antibodies sensitive to C-terminal clipping when incubated with 17-1A antibody). This reaction pathway was found to be stabilized at acid pH. It is likely that this novel pathway was not the only reaction pathway for the 17-1A antibody, as numerous IEF bands were observed over time. This protein does, however, represent another example of an "unexpected" protein reaction at a non-hot-spot site.

- **Antibody 17-1A Light Chain (214 residues)**

SEQUENCE

NIVMTQSPKSMSMSVGERVTLTCKASENVVTYVSWYQQKPEQSPKLLIYGASNRYT-
GVPDRFTGSGSATDFTLTISSVQAEDLADYHCGQGYSYPYTFGGGTKLEIKRADAAP-
TVSIFPPSSEQLTSGGASVVCFLNNFYPKDINVKWKIDGSERQNGVLNSWTDQDSK-
DSTYSMSSTLTLTKDEYERHNSYTCEATHKTSTSPIVKSFNRNEC

REACTIVE SITES

.N.(10)		.D.(11)		.M.(4)		.Q.(9)	
28	ENV	60	PDR	4	VMT	6	TQS
53	SNR	70	TDF	11	SMS	37	YQQ
137	LNN	82	EDL	13	SMS	38	QQK
138	NNF	85	ADY	175	SMS	42	EQS
145	INV	110	ADA			79	VQA
157	QNG	143	KDI			90	GQG
161	LNS	151	IDG			124	EQL
190	HNS	165	TDQ			156	RQN
210	FNR	167	QDS			166	DQD
212	RNE	170	KDS				
		184	KDE				

HYDROFLEX PLOT

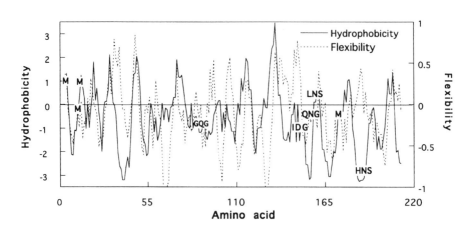

PREDICTED REACTIVITY AND DEGRADATION OF 17-1A ANTIBODY LIGHT CHAIN

The primary amino acid sequence for the 17-1A antibody light chain shows that Asn-157 should be reactive in that it resides within the -QNG- motif, although its motif is located in a region of only modest hydrophilicity and predicted chain flexibility. There are several other reactive sites, including Asp-Gly and Met. The degradation of the 17-1A antibody occurred largely on the heavy chain (see previous entry), although the authors observed that several new IEF bands were found over time, supportive of possible reaction at this Asn-Gly hot spot (Everett, 1995). No oxidation of Met was reported.

Antibody E25 Light Chain (218 residues)   ●

SEQUENCE

DIQLTQSPSSLSASVGDRVTITCRASQSVDYDGDSYMNWYQQKPGKAPKLLIYAAS-
YLESGVPSRFSGSGSGTDFTLTISSLQPEDFATYYCQQSHEDPYTFGQGTKVEIKRTV-
AAPSVFIFPPSDEQLKSGTASVVCLLNNFYPREAKVQWKVDNALQSGNSQESVTEQ-
DSKDSTYSLSSTLTLSKADYEKHKVYACEVTHQGLSSSPVTKSFNRGEC

REACTIVE SITES

.N.(6)	.D.(12)	.M.(1)	.Q.(15)
38 MNW	17 GDR	37 YMN	3 IQL
141 LNN	30 VDY		6 TQS
142 NNF	32 YDG		27 SQS
156 DNA	34 GDS		41 YQQ
162 GNS	74 TDF		42 QQK
214 FNR	86 EDF		83 LQP
	98 EDP		93 CQQ
	126 SDE		94 QQS
	155 VDN		104 GQG
	171 QDS		128 EQL
	174 KDS		151 VQW
	189 ADY		159 LQS
			164 SQE
			170 EQD
			203 HQG

HYDROFLEX PLOT

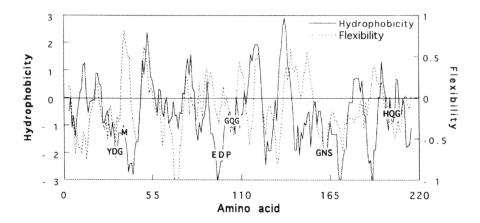

PREDICTED REACTIVITY AND DEGRADATION OF ANTIBODY E25
LIGHT CHAIN

The E25 antibody is a humanized monoclonal antibody that binds to human IgE and is under development for the treatment of asthma and other allergic diseases. The light chain has several reactive sites, including Asn-Gly, Asp-Gly, Asp-Pro, a single Met and Gln-Gly that may show chemical instability in aqueous solution. Recent studies have demonstrated the lability of the Asp-32 (in the YDG motif) towards isomerization, forming both cyclic imide and iso-Asp variants upon storage at pH 5.2 at room temperature (Cacia *et al.*, 1996). The Asp-32 residue also converts to the iso-Asp residue upon storage at pH 7.2 at room temperature, presumably through a cyclic imide intermediate. Both iso-Asp-32 and the cyclic imide variants show reduced binding to IgE. No other significant degradation products have been detected.

- **Antibody E25 Heavy Chain (451 residues)**

SEQUENCE

EVQLVESGGGLVQPGGSLRLSCAVSGYSITSGYSWNWIRQAPGKGLEWVASITYDG-
STNYNPSVKGRITISRDDSKNTFYLQMNSLRAEDTAVYYCARGSHYFGHWHFAVW-
GQGTLVTVSSASTKGPSVFPLAPSSKSTSGGTAALGCLVKDYFPEPVTVSWNSGALT-
SGVHTFPAVLQSSGLYSLSSVVTVPSSSLGTQTYICNVNHKPSNTKVDKKVEPKSCD-
KTHTCPPCPAPELLGGPSVFLFPPKPKDTLMISRTPEVTCVVVDVSHEDPEVKFNWY-
VDGVEVHNAKTKPREEQYNSTYRVVSVLTVLHQDWLNGKEYKCKVSNKALPA-
PIEKTISKAKGQPREPQVYTLPPSREEMTKNQVSLTCLVKGFYPSDIAVEWESNGQPE-
NNYKTTPPVLDSDGSFFLYSKLTVDKSRWQQGNVFSCSVMHEALHNHYTQKSL-
SLSPGK

REACTIVE SITES

.N.(20)	.D.(16)	.M.(4)	.Q.(16)
36 WNW	55 YDG	83 QMN	3 VQL
59 TNY	73 RDD	256 LMI	13 VQP
61 YNP	74 DDS	362 EMT	40 RQA
77 KNT	90 EDT	432 VMH	82 LQM
84 MNS	152 KDY		113 GQM
163 WNS	216 VDK		179 LQS
205 CNV	225 CDK		200 TQT
207 VNH	253 KDT		299 EQY
212 SNT	269 VDV		315 HQD
280 FNW	274 EDP		346 GQP
290 HNA	284 VDG		351 PQV
301 YNS	316 QDW		366 NQV
319 LNG	380 SDI		390 GQP
329 SNK	403 LDS		422 WQQ
365 KNQ	405 SDG		423 QQG
388 SNG	417 VDK		442 TQK
393 ENN			
394 NNY			
425 GNV			
438 HNH			

HYDROFLEX PLOT

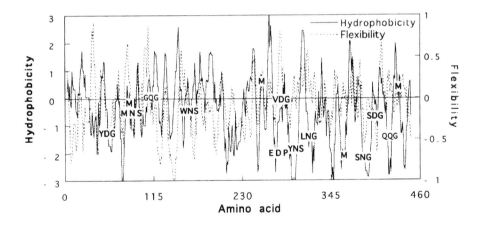

PREDICTED REACTIVITY AND DEGRADATION OF ANTIBODY E25 HEAVY CHAIN

The E25 antibody is an anti-IgE antibody under development for the treatment of asthma and other allergic diseases (Presta *et al.*, 1993). This protein has several reactive sites, including

Asn-Gly, Asn-Ser, Asp-Gly, Asp-Pro, Met and Gln-Gly that may show chemical instability in
aqueous solution. Recent studies have shown no significant degradation under mild conditions.
In particular, Asp-55 (in the YDG motif) did not show evidence of isomerization, even though
a similar Asp-Gly motif in the E25 light chain did show isomerization (see E25 light chain)
(Cacia *et al.*, 1996). This variation in reactivity for Asp-Gly further illustrates the dependence
of reactivity on tertiary structure, as well as on sequence motifs (Kossiakoff *et al.*, 1988).

- **Antibody Light Chain-κ (mouse) (214 residues)**

SEQUENCE

NIVMTQSPKSMSMSVGERVTLTCKASENVVTYVSWYQQKPEQSPKLLIYGASNRYT-
GVPDRFTGSGSATDFTLTISSVQAEDLADTHCGQGYSYPYTFGGGTKLEIKRADAAP-
TVSIFPPSSEQLTSGGASVVCFLNNFYPKDINVKWKIDGSERQNGVLBSBTXWBSKD-
STTSMSSTLTLTKDEYERHNSYTCEATHKTSTSPIVKSFNRNEC

REACTIVE SITES

	.N.(12)		.D.(12)		.M.(4)		.Q.(8)
28 ENV	167 WBS	60 PDR	163 SBT	4 VMT	6 TQS
53 SNR	190 HNS	70 TDF	167 WBS	11 SMS	37 YQQ
137 LNN	210 FNR	82 EDL	170 KDS	13 SMS	38 QQK
138 NNF	212 RNE	85 ADT	184 KDE	175 SMS	42 EQS
145 INV		110 ADA			79 VQA
157 QNG		143 KDI			90 GQG
161 LBS		151 IDG			124 EQL
163 SBT		161 LBS			156 RQN

HYDROFLEX PLOT

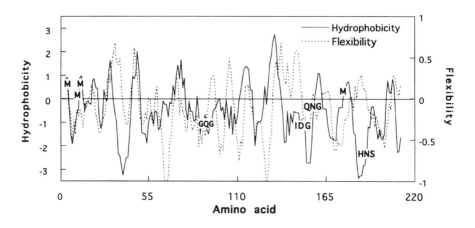

PREDICTED REACTIVITY AND DEGRADATION OF KAPPA LIGHT CHAIN

The hydroflex plot for kappa light chain shows that there are only a few predicted reactive sites for degradation. These include Asn-157 within the -QNG- motif and several Met amino acids. Isolation and complete sequencing of the mouse kappa light chain was carried out over two decades ago, where it was found that the isolated product showed some micro-heterogeneity, likely due to deamidation at Asn-157 (Svanti and Milstein, 1972). The paper chromatography methods used make the assignment of this Asn rather ambiguous but plausible, considering the lack of other hot spots for deamidation in the same tryptic peptide.

Antibody OKT3 Heavy Chain (449 residues)   ●

SEQUENCE

QVQLQQSGAELARPGASVKMSCKASGYTFTRYTMHWVKQRPGQGLEWIGYINPSR-
GYTNYNQKFKDKATLTTDKSSSTAYMQLSSLTSEDSAVYYCARYYDDHYCLDYWG-
QGTTLTVSSAKTTAPSVYPLAPVCGDTTGSSVTLGCLVKGYFPEPVTLTWNSGSLSS-
GVHTFPAVLQSDLYTLSSSVTVTSSTWPSQSITCNVAHPASSTKVDKKIEPRGPTIKPC-
PPCKCPAPNLLGGPSVFIFPPKIKDVLMISLSPIVTCVVDVSEDDPDVQISWFVNNVE-
VHTAQVQTHREDYNSTLRVVSALPIQHQDWMSGKEFKCKVNNKDLPAPIERTISKP-
KGSVRAPQVYVLPPPEEEMTKKQVTLTCMVTDFMPEDIYVEWTNNGKTELNYKNT-
EPVLDSDGSYFMYSKLRVEKKNWVERNSYSCSVVHEGLHNHHTTKSFSRTPGK

REACTIVE SITES

.N.(18)		.D.(21)		.M.(9)	.Q.(17)	
52 INP	66 KDK	378 EDI		20 KMS	3 VQL	
59 TNY	73 TDK	401 LDS		34 TMH	5 LQQ	
61 YNQ	90 EDS	403 SDG		81 YMQ	6 QQS	
161 WNS	101 YDD			254 LMI	39 KQR	
202 CNV	102 DDH			316 WMS	43 GQG	
235 PNL	107 LDY			360 EMT	62 NQK	
282 VNN	136 GDT			370 CMV	82 MQL	
283 NNV	179 SDL			375 FMP	111 GQG	
299 YNS	213 VDK			408 FMY	177 LQS	
326 VNN	251 KDV				197 SQS	
327 NNK	267 VDV				276 VQI	
385 TNN	271 EDD				290 AQT	
386 NNG	272 DDP				292 TQT	
392 LNY	274 PDV				311 IQH	
395 KNT	297 EDY				313 HQD	
418 KNW	314 QDW				349 PQV	
423 RNS	329 KDL				364 KQV	
436 HNH	373 TDF					

HYDROFLEX PLOT

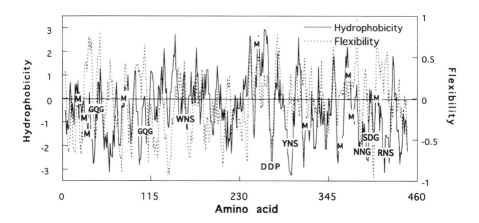

PREDICTED REACTIVITY AND DEGRADATION OF OKT3 HEAVY CHAIN

The larger size of the OKT3 heavy chain makes it more likely that this is the more reactive chain, especially considering the large number of moderately reactive hot spots. This protein is predicted to react predominantly at Asn-386 (-NNG-) and possibly at some of the less reactive Asn-Ser sites. Further, this heavy chain has numerous Met residues, and so some oxidation might be expected. The major degradation pathway for this protein (as a part of the entire OKT3 complex) is at Asn-386 as predicted (Kroon *et al.*, 1992). Additionally, oxidation was observed at Met-34, Met-316, Met-360, and Met-408, most of which are found in fairly hydrophilic regions as predicted by hydropathy analysis. Sufficient oxidation of Met-34 was observed that the first OKT3 product formulation was eventually reformulated to include an inert headspace to reduce oxidation. A minor amount of deamidation was also found at Asn-423 (-RNS-), which is in a hydrophilic region of poor flexibility.

● **Antibody OKT3 Light Chain (213 residues)**

SEQUENCE

QIVLTQSPAIMSASPGEKVTMTCSASSSVSYMNWYQQKSGTSPKRWIYDTSKLASG-
VPAHFRGSGSGTSYSLTISGMEAEDAATYYCQQWSSNPFTFGSGTKLEINRADTAPT-
VSIFPPSSEQLTSGGASVVCFLNNFYPKDINVKWKIDGSERQNGVLNSWTDQDSKDS-
TYSMSSTLTLTKDEYERHNSYTCEATHKTSTSPIVKSFNRNEC

REACTIVE SITES

.N.(11)	.D.(9)	.M.(5)	.Q.(8)
33 MNW	49 YDT	11 IMS	6 RQS
93 SNP	81 EDA	21 TMT	36 YQQ
106 INR	109 ADT	32 YMN	37 QQK
136 LNN	142 KDI	77 GME	88 CQQ
137 NNF	150 IDG	174 SMS	89 QQW
144 INV	164 TDQ		123 EQL
156 QNG	166 QDS		155 RQN
160 LNS	169 KDS		165 DQD
189 HNS	183 KDE		
209 FNR			
211 RNE			

HYDROFLEX PLOT

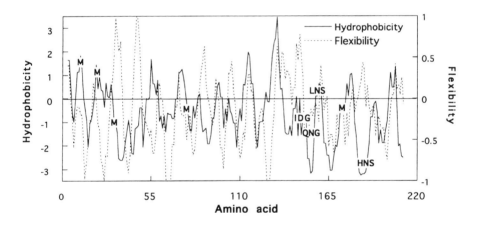

PREDICTED REACTIVITY AND DEGRADATION OF OKT3 LIGHT CHAIN

The OKT3 antibody is a murine IgG2a antibody capable of binding CD3 and is used to clinically reverse rejections of human kidney transplants. Inspection of the hydroflex plot shows that the OKT3 light chain has several hot spots, of which the predominant site is predicted to be Asn-156, possibly followed by Asn-189, found in a hydrophilic region of predicted poor flexibility. The major degradation pathway for this protein (as a part of the entire OKT3 complex) in pH 7 PBS was at Asn-156 as predicted. A small amount of oxidative degradation occurred at Met-174, found in a region of intermediate hydropathy and flexibility. No other significant degradation was observed for the other potential hot spots (Kroon et al., 1992).

● **Antibody OKT4a Heavy Chain (humanized) (447 residues)**

SEQUENCE

QVQLVESGGGVVQPGRSLRLSCSASGFTFSNYAMSWVRQAPGKGLEWVAAISDHST-
NTYYPDSVKGRFTISRDNSKNTLFLQMDSLRPEDTGVYFCARKYGGDYDPFDYWG-
QGTPVTVSSASTKGPSVFPLAPCSRSTSESTAALGCLVKDYFPEPVTVSWNSGALTSG-
VHTFPAVLQSSGLYSLSSVVTVPSSSLGTKTYTCNVDHKPSNTKVDKRVESKYGPP-
CPSCPAPEFLGGPSVFLFPPKPKDTLMISRTPEVTCVVDVSQEDPEVQFNWYVDGVE-
VHNAKTKPREEQFNSTYRVVSVLTVLHQDWLNGKEYKCKVSNKGPSSIEKTISKAK-
GQPREPQVYTLLPPSQEEMTKNQVSLTCLVKGFYPSDIAVEWESNGQPENNYKTTP-
PVLDSDGSFFLYSRLTVDKSRWQEGNVFSCSVMHEALHNHYTQKSLSLSLGK

REACTIVE SITES

.N.(18)		.D.(20)		.M.(5)	.Q.(17)	
31 SNY	315 LNG	53 SDH	215 VDK	34 AMS	3 VQL	342 GQP
57 TNT	325 SNK	62 PDS	249 KDT	83 QMD	13 VQP	347 PQV
74 DNS	361 KNQ	73 RDN	265 VDV	252 LMI	39 RQA	355 SQE
77 KNT	384 SNG	84 MDS	270 EDP	358 EMT	82 LQM	362 NQV
162 WNS	389 ENN	90 EDT	280 VDG	428 VMH	112 GQG	386 GQP
204 CNV	390 NNY	103 GDY	312 QDW		178 LQS	418 WQE
211 SNT	421 GNV	105 YDP	376 SDI		268 SQE	438 TQK
276 FNW	434 HNH	108 FDY	399 LDS		274 VQF	
286 HNA		151 KDY	401 SDG		295 EQF	
297 FNS		206 VDH	413 VDK		311 HQD	

HYDROFLEX PLOT

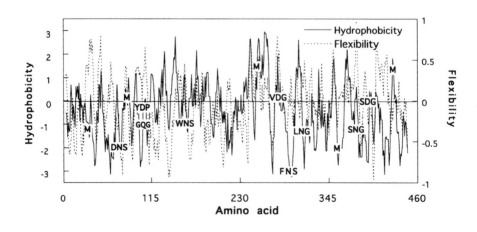

PREDICTED REACTIVITY AND DEGRADATION OF OKT4a HEAVY CHAIN

The larger size of the OKT4a heavy chain makes it the likely reactive chain, especially considering the large number of moderately reactive hot spots. This protein is predicted to react predominantly at Asn-315 (-LNG-) and Asn-384 (-SNG-), and possibly at some of the less reactive Asn-Ser sites. Reaction is also predicted at Asp-Gly to give iso-Asp-Gly (although this is often difficult to detect experimentally), as well as at Asp-Pro at lower pHs. This heavy chain has numerous Met residues, and thus some oxidation might be expected. The major degradation pathway for OKT4 heavy chain (as a part of the entire OKT4a complex) at pH's less than 6.5 was cleavage at Asp-270 within the -EDP- motif (Kroon, 1994). Interestingly, no cleavage was found at Asp-105 within the -YDF- motif. A minor amount of cleavage was observed at bonds N-terminal to several Ser and Thr residues, including Ser-220, Thr-250, Thr-335, and Thr-350. Deamidation was found to be slow for this protein below neutral pH; however, the exact sites of deamidation were not determined, and deamidation was identified only by an acidic shift in the IEF pattern.

Antibody OKT4a Light Chain (humanized) (214 residues)   •

SEQUENCE

DIQMTQSPSSLSASVGDRVTITCKASQDINNYIAWYQQTPGKAPKLLIHYTSTLQPG-
VPSRFSGSGSGTDYTFTISSLQPEDIATYYCLQYDNLLFTFGQGTKLQITRTVAAPSVF-
IFPPSDEQLKSGTASVVCLLNNFYPREAKVQWKVDNALQSGNSQESVTEQDSKDST-
YSLSSTLTLSKADYEKHKVYACEVTHQGLSSPVTKSFNRGEC

REACTIVE SITES

.N.(8)	.D.(10)	.M.(1)	.Q.(16)
30 INN	17 GDR	4 QMT	3 IQM
31 NNY	28 QDI		6 TQS
93 DNL	70 TDY		27 SQD
137 LNN	82 EDI		37 YQQ
138 NNF	92 YDN		38 QQT
152 DNA	122 SDE		55 LQP
158 GNS	151 VDN		79 LQP
210 FNR	167 QDS		90 LQY
	170 KDS		100 GQG
	185 ADY		105 LQI
			124 EQL
			147 VQW
			155 LQS
			160 SQE
			166 EQD
			199 HQG

HYDROFLEX PLOT

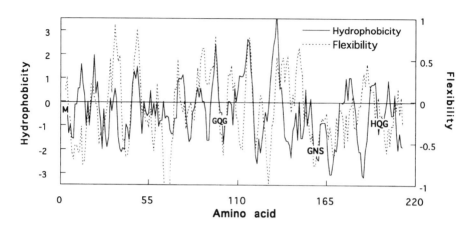

PREDICTED REACTIVITY AND DEGRADATION OF OKT4a LIGHT
CHAIN

This light chain has few reactive sites, suggesting that the OKT4a heavy chain is the major site of chemical degradation. A minor amount of cleavage at Ser-203 was found as a trace reaction. No oxidation of Met-4 was reported (Kroon, 1994).

- **Atrial Natriuretic Peptide (ANP) (human) (28 residues)**

SEQUENCE

SLRRSSCFGGRMDRIGAQSGLGCNSFRY

REACTIVE SITES

.N.(1)	.D.(1)	.M.(1)	.Q.(1)
24 CNS	13 MDR	12 RMD	18 AQS

HYDROFLEX PLOT

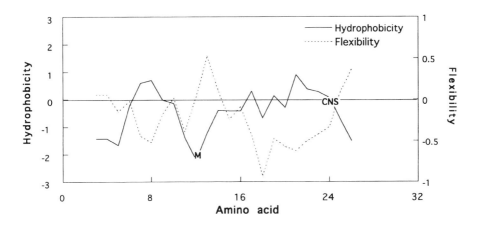

PREDICTED REACTIVITY AND DEGRADATION OF ANP

The primary amino acid sequence for ANP shows that this peptide has only one of the traditional hydrolytic hot spots, Asn-Ser, and lacks the Asn-Gly, Asp-Gly, and Gln-Gly hot spots. Asn-24 resides within the -CNS- motif and is expected to be reactive based on its primary amino acid sequence. It does have, however, a single Met that is capable of being oxidized. Two degradation pathways have been observed for this cyclic peptide, deamidation of Asn-24 and oxidation of Met-12 (Wang, 1995).

Brain-Derived Neurotrophic Factor (BDNF) (human) (120 residues)   ●

SEQUENCE

MHSDPARRGELSVCDSISEWVTAADKKTAVDMSGGTVTVLEKVPVSKGQLKQYFY-
ETKCNPMGYTKEGCRGIDKRHWNSQCRTTQSYVRALTMDSKKRIGWRFIRIDTSCV-
CTLTIKRGR

REACTIVE SITES

.N.(2)	.D.(7)		.M.(4)	.Q.(4)
60 CNP	4 SDP	73 IDK	1 MH	49 GQL
78 WNS	15 CDS	94 MDS	32 DMS	52 KQY
	25 ADK	107 IDT	62 PMG	80 SQC
	31 VDM		93 TMD	85 TQS

HYDROFLEX PLOT

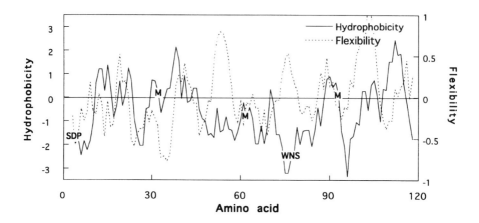

PREDICTED REACTIVITY AND DEGRADATION OF BDNF

This protein is relatively free of activated hot spots, except for Met and the acid-sensitive Asp-Pro motive. Some degradation studies have been carried out in the neutral pH range, where it was found that the primary degradation pathways were cleavage at His-2–Ser-3 and between Asp-4–Pro-5 (Hershensen *et al.*, 1995). Oxidation at Met-1 and Met-62 was also observed, with minor amounts of oxidation at Met-32. Other minor degradation pathways included cleavage at Val-45–Ser-46, Lys-47–Gly-48, and Asn-60–Pro-61 (reaction conditions not specified).

- **Calbindin (bovine) (76 residues)**

SEQUENCE

MKSPEELKGIFEKYAAKEGDPNQLSKEELKLLLQTEFPSLLKGPSTLDELFEELDKN-
GDGEVSFEEFQVLVKKISQ

REACTIVE SITES

.N.(2)	.D.(4)	.M.(0)	.Q.(4)
22 PNQ	20 GDP		23 NQL
57 KNG	48 LDE		34 LQT
	55 LDK		68 FQV
	59 GDG		76 SQ

HYDROFLEX PLOT

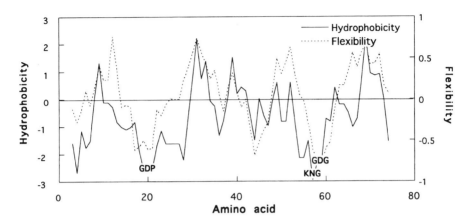

PREDICTED REACTIVITY AND DEGRADATION OF CALBINDIN

The hydroflex plot for calbindin shows that this protein contains the reactive Asn-Gly hot spot within a region that is predicted to be fairly hydrophilic and flexible. An Asp-Gly motive is also found nearby in this hydrophilic region. Preparations of recombinant bovine calbindin D9k have been shown to be heterogeneous by IEF, due to deamidation of Asn-57 within the -KNG- motif (Chazin *et al.*, 1989). Calbindin also contains an Asp-Gly in the same region, but no degradation at the Asp-Gly site or at the acid-labile Asp-Pro site was reported.

Calmodulin (148 residues)

SEQUENCE

ADQLTEEQIAEFKEAFSLFDKDGDGTITTKELGTVMRSLGQNPTEAELQDMINEVDA-
DGNGTIDFPEFLTMMARKMKDTDSEEEIREAFRVFDKDGNGYISAAELRHVMTNLG-
EKLTDEEVDEMIREADIDGDGQVNYEEFVQMMTAK

REACTIVE SITES

.N.(6)		.D.(17)		.M.(9)	.Q.(6)
42 QNP	2 ADQ	80 TDS	36 VMR	3 DQL	
53 INE	20 FDK	93 FDK	51 DMI	8 EQI	
60 GNG	22 KDG	95 KDG	71 TMM	41 GQN	
97 GNG	24 GDG	118 TDE	72 MMA	49 LQD	
111 TNL	50 QDM	122 VDE	76 KMK	135 GQV	
137 VNY	56 VDA	129 ADI	109 VMT	143 VQM	
	58 ADG	131 IDG	124 EMI		
	64 IDF	133 GDG	144 QMM		
	78 KDT		145 MMT		

HYDROFLEX PLOT

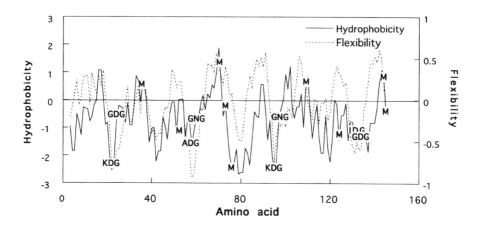

PREDICTED REACTIVITY AND DEGRADATION OF CALMODULIN

Calmodulin contains at least eight sites that may undergo deamidation or cyclization, as well as numerous Met residues. All of the -XDG- and -XNG- reactive motifs lie in moderately hydrophilic regions of good predicted flexibility, further supporting the notion that calmodulin should be particularly susceptible to hydrolytic degradation. Calmodulin has two Asn-Gly sites, which are predicted to be more reactive than the Asp-Gly sites. Measurements of ammonia release and methyl transfer rates showed that calmodulin was extremely reactive towards hydrolytic degradation, giving 0.5 mole of ammonia released per mole calmodulin at pH 7.4 and 37°C after 8–9 days (Johnson et al., 1989a). Comparison measurements of ammonia release and methyl transfer with other proteins showed that calmodulin is much more reactive than the other proteins surveyed. Although the entire degradation profile for calmodulin was not determined, it was believed that the primary sites of deamidation were Asn-60 (-GNG-) and Asn-97 (-GNG-). Calmodulin has numerous methionine residues, and the C-terminal residues are most susceptible to oxidation by peroxynitrite (Hühmer et al., 1996) or by hydrogen peroxide (Yao et al., 1996).

- **Carbonic Anhydrase C (259 residues)**

SEQUENCE

SHHWGYGKHNGPEHWHKDFPIAKGERQSPVDIDTHTAKYDPSLKPLSVSYDQATSL-
RILNNGHAFNVEFDDSEDKAVLKGGPLDGTYRLIQFHFHWGSLDGQGSQHTVDKK-
KYAAELHLVHWNTKYGDFGKAVQQPDGLAVLGIFLKVGSAKPGLQKVVDVLDSIK-
TKGKSADFTNFDPRGLLPESLDYWTYPGSLTTPPLLECVTWIVLKEPISVSSEQVLKF-
RKLNFNGEGEPEELMVDNWRPAQPLKNRQIKASFK

REACTIVE SITES

.N.(10)	.D.(19)	.M.(1)	.Q.(11)
10 HNG	18 KDF	239 LMV	27 RQS
60 LNN	31 VDI		52 DQA
61 NNG	33 IDT		91 IQF
66 FNV	40 YDP		102 GQG
123 WNT	51 YDQ		105 SQH
176 TNF	70 FDD		134 VQQ
228 LNF	71 DDS		135 QQP
230 FNG	74 EDK		156 LQK
242 DNW	84 LDG		220 EQV
251 KNR	100 LDG		247 AQP
	109 VDK		253 RQI
	128 GDF		
	137 PDG		
	160 VDV		
	163 LDS		
	173 ADF		
	178 FDP		
	188 LDY		
	241 VDN		

HYDROFLEX PLOT

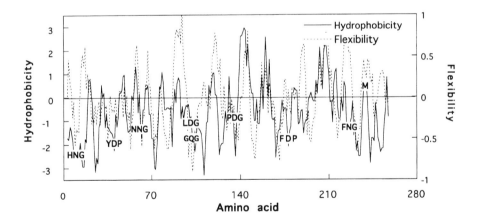

PREDICTED REACTIVITY AND DEGRADATION OF CARBONIC ANHYDRASE C

This protein has several residues predicted to be reactive, including three Asn-Gly motifs. In one of the original papers describing the primary structure of human carbonic anhydrase C it was noted during the sequence analysis work that several residues underwent facile deamidation. All were identified as Asn-Gly sequences (Henderson *et al.*, 1976). It was not determined if the protein was deamidated before isolation, during its purification, or during peptide analysis. Several of the steps used were carried out at elevated temperatures or used strong acid (1 M acetic acid for example), and so it was not possible to determine the origin of the protein microheterogeneity.

- **CD4 (human) (370 residues)**

SEQUENCE

KKVVLGKKGDTVELTCTASQKKSIQFHWKNSNQIKILGNQGSFLTKGPSKLNDRAD-
SRRSLWDQGNFPLIIKNLKIEDSDTYICEVEDQKEEVQLLVFGLTANSDTHLLQGQSL-
TLTLESPPGSSPSVQCRSPRGKNIQGGKTLSVSQLELQDSGTWTCTVLQNQKKVEFK-
IDIVVLAFQKASSIVYKKEGEQVEFSFPLAFTVEKLTGSGELWWQAERASSSKSWITF-
DLKNKEVSVKRVTQDPKLQMGKKLPLHLTLPQALPQYAGSGNLTLALEAKTGKLH-
QEVNLVVMRATQLQKNLTCEVWGPTSPKLMLSLKLENKEAKVSKREKAVWVLNPE-
AGMWQCLLSDSGQVLLESNIKVLPTWSTPVH

REACTIVE SITES

.N.(16)	.D.(13)	.M.(4)	.Q.(27)
30 KNS	10 GDT	249 QMG	20 SQK
32 SNQ	53 NDR	292 VMR	25 IQF
39 GNQ	56 ADS	314 LML	33 NQI
52 LND	63 WDQ	342 GMW	40 NQG
66 GNF	78 EDS		64 DQG
73 KNL	80 SDT		89 DQK
103 ANS	88 EDQ		94 VQL
137 KNI	105 SDT		110 LQG
164 QNQ	153 QDS		112 GQS
233 KNK	173 IDI		129 VQC
271 GNL	230 FDL		139 IQG
288 VNL	244 QDP		148 SQL
300 KNL	349 SDS		152 LQD
321 ENK			163 LQN
337 LNP			165 NQK
358 SNI			180 FQK
			193 EQV
			216 WQA
			243 TQD
			248 LQM
			261 PQA
			265 PQY
			285 HQE
			296 TQL
			298 LQK
			344 WQC
			352 GQV

HYDROFLEX PLOT

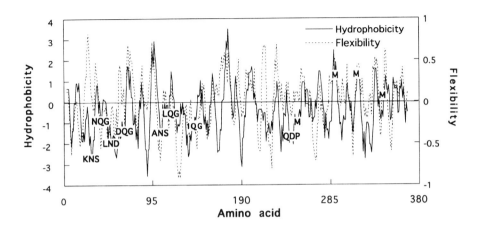

PREDICTED REACTIVITY AND DEGRADATION OF CD4

This protein harbors four Gln-Gly sites and two Asn-Ser sites, all of which are commonly regarded as the potential hot spots for degradation. CD4 also has four Met residues in the C-terminal end of the molecule. An elegant study on the deamidation of soluble CD4 has been reported, wherein it was found that Asn-52 (in the -LND- motif) was the primary degradation site at pH 7.2 and 25°C (Teshima *et al.*, 1991a, 1995a). The -LND- motif is generally thought to be fairly unreactive, and so this is a clear-cut example where deamidation may occur in aqueous formulations at sites other than Asn-Gly or Asn-Ser. It is interesting to note that Asn-52 resides in a region predicted to be moderately hydrophilic and flexible, in good agreement with its crystal structure of the V1 and V2 domains (Wang *et al.*, 1990) and this may contribute to its reactivity. No oxidation at Met was observed.

CD4-IgG (407 residues)

SEQUENCE

KKVVLGKKGDTVELTCTASQKKSIQFHWKNSNQIKILGNQGSFLTKGPSKLNDRAD-
SRRSLWDQGNFPLIIKNLKIEDSDTYICEVEDQKEEVQLLVFGLTANSDTHLLQGQSL-
TLTLESPPGSSPSVQCRSPRGKNIQGGKTLSVSQLELQDSGTWTCTVLQNQKKVEFK-
IDIVVLAFQDKTHTCPPCPAPELLGGPSVFLFPPKPKDTLMISRTPEVTCVVDVSHED-
PEVKFNWYVDGVEVHNAKTKPREEQYNSTYRVVSVLTVLHQDWLNGKEYKCKVS-
NKALPAPIEKTISKAKGQPREPQVYTLPPSREEMTKNQVSLTCLVKGFYPSDIAVEWE-
SNGQPENNYKTTPPVLDSDGSFFLYSKLTVDKSRWQQGNVFSCSVMHEALHNHYT-
QKSLSLSPGK

REACTIVE SITES

.N.(20)		.D.(20)		.M.(3)		.Q.(25)			
30	KNS	10	GDT	212	LMI	20	SQK	322	NQV
32	SNQ	53	NDR	318	EMT	25	IQF	346	GQP
39	GNQ	56	ADS	388	VMH	33	NQI	378	WQQ
52	LND	63	WDQ			40	NQG	379	QQG
66	GNF	78	EDS			64	DQG	398	TQK
73	KNL	80	SDT			89	DQK		
103	ANS	88	EDQ			94	VQL		
137	KNI	105	SDT			110	LQG		
164	QNQ	153	QDS			112	GQS		
236	FNW	173	IDI			129	VQC		
246	HNA	181	QDK			139	IQG		
257	YNS	209	KDT			148	SQL		
275	LNG	225	VDV			152	LQD		
285	SNK	230	EDP			163	LQN		
321	KNQ	240	VDG			165	NQK		
344	SNG	272	QDW			180	FQD		
349	ENN	336	SDI			255	EQY		
350	NNY	259	LDS			271	HQD		
381	GNV	361	SDG			302	GQP		
394	HNH	373	VDK			307	PQV		

HYDROFLEX PLOT

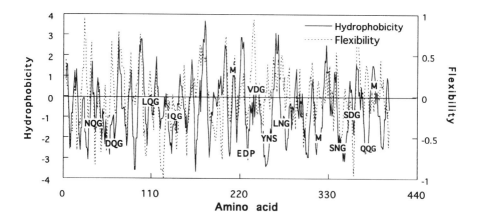

PREDICTED REACTIVITY AND DEGRADATION OF CD4-IgG

This protein has partial identity with CD4 (Harris *et al.*, 1990) and so might be expected to degrade at the same hot spots in this region. This CD4 molecule also has two Asn-Gly and two

Asp-Gly moieties (the two most reactive hot spots) and so is predicted to degrade at these hot spots. The observed degradation pathway of CD4-IgG was found to be similar to CD4, that is, degradation at Asn-52 (in the -LND- motif) (Teshima and Yim, 1995b; Teshima and Wu, 1996). Again, the -LND- motif is generally thought to be fairly unreactive, and so this example illustrates that deamidation may occur in aqueous formulations at sites other than Asn-Gly or Asn-Ser.

CD4-PE40 (545 residues)

SEQUENCE

MKKVVLGKKGDTVELTCTASQKKSIQFHWKNSNQIKILGNQGSFLTKGPSKLNDRA-
DSRRSLWDQGNFPLIIKNLKIEDSDTYICEVEDQKEEVQLLVFGLTANSDTHLLQGQS-
LTLTLESPPGSSPVQCRSPRGKNIQGGKTLSVSQLELQDSGTWTCTVLQNQKKVEFK-
IDIVVLAHMAEEGGSLAALTAHQACHLPLETFTRHRQPRGWEQLEQCGYPVQRLVA-
LYLAARLSWNQVDQVIRNALASPGSGGDLGEAIREQPEQARLALTLAAAESERFVR-
QGTGNDEAGAANADVVSLTCPVAAGECAGPADSGDALLERNYPTGAEFLGDGGDV-
SFSTRGTQNWTVERLLQAHRQLEERGYVFVGYHGTFLEAAQSIVGGVRARSQDL-
DAIWRGFYIAGDPALAYGYAQDQEPDARGRIRNGALLRVYVPRSSLPGFYRTSLTLA-
APEAAGEVERLIGHPLPLRLDAITGPEEEGGRLETILGWPLAERTVVIPSAIPTDPRNV-
GGDLDPSSIPDKEQAISALPDYASQPGKPPREDLK

REACTIVE SITES

.N.(17)		.D.(30)		.M.(1)		.Q.(34)	
31 KNS	11 GDT	338 GDV		181 HMA	21 SQK	215 EQL
33 SNQ	54 NDR	393 QDL			26 IQF	218 EQC
40 GNQ	57 ADS	395 LDA			34 NQI	224 VQR
53 LND	64 WDQ	406 GDP			41 NQG	239 NQV
67 GNF	79 EDS	416 QDQ			65 DQG	242 DQV
74 KNL	81 SDT	420 PDA			90 DQK	264 EQP
104 ANS	89 EDQ	472 LDA			95 VQL	267 EQA
138 KNI	106 SDT	506 TDP			111 LQG	285 RQG
165 QNQ	154 QDS	513 GDL			113 GQS	347 TQN
238 WNQ	174 IDI	515 LDP			130 VQC	356 LQA
246 RNA	241 VDQ	521 PDK			140 IQG	360 RQL
289 GND	256 GDL	531 PDY			149 SQL	380 AQS
296 ANA	290 NDE	543 EDL			153 LQD	392 SQD
325 RNY	298 ADV				164 LQN	415 AQD
348 QNW	316 ADS				166 NQK	417 DQE
427 RNG	319 GDA				195 HQA	524 EQA
509 RNV	335 GDG				209 RQP	535 SQP

HYDROFLEX PLOT

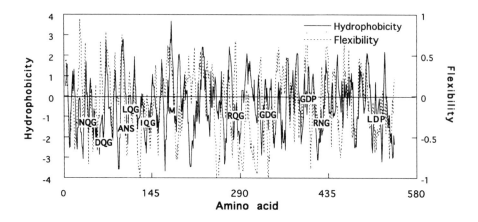

PREDICTED REACTIVITY AND DEGRADATION OF CD4-PE40

The recombinant human CD4-*Pseudomonas* exotoxin hybrid protein shows selective killing of HIV-1 infected cells and thus represents a novel therapeutic agent for the treatment of AIDS (Chaudhary *et al.*, 1988). Comparative analysis of this protein with soluble CD4 (see previous entry) provides additional insight into protein degradation in aqueous solution. CD4-PE40 has a single Asn-Gly site which is predicted to be reactive, as well as a number of lesser reactive sites such as Gln-Gly. This protein also has a single Met near the conjugation site of CD4 and PE40. The major degradation site for this protein in aqueous solution was Met oxidation, with no other clearly detectable degradation pathways noted (Hageman, 1995). Soluble CD4 did not show degradation at Met, because soluble CD4 does not have a Met at this position (see comparison of the soluble CD4 and CD4-PE40 amino acid sequences in Scheme 9). Of note, however, was the lack of degradation at Asn-427 in the RNG motif in CD4-PE40 (a predicted hot spot); this may be due to the conformational nature of the protein about this motif. It is also of interest to note that CD4-PE40 did not show any deamidation at Asn-53 within the -LND- motif, observed to be the major site of degradation of soluble CD4 in aqueous solution (see previous entry). Because the CD4 binding activity of CD4-PE40 is similar to soluble CD4, one must assume that the conformation of the CD4 region in CD4-PE40 is similar to soluble CD4. Thus, this protein provides some contrast to the "unusual" degradation pathway for soluble CD4, in that no degradation was observed at the -LND- motif generally thought to be fairly unreactive. This is likely due to the different methods of analysis used.

```
              10        20        30        40
CD4       KKVVLGKKGDTVELTCTASQKKSIQFHWKNSNQIKILGNQGSFLTKGPS
          ************************************************
CD4-PE40  MKKVVLGKKGDTVELTCTASQKKSIQFHWKNSNQIKILGNQGSFLTKGPS
            10        20        30        40        50


          50        60        70        80        90
CD4       KLNDRADSRRSLWDQGNFPLIIKNLKIEDSDTYICEVEDQKEEVQLLVFG
          ************************************************
CD4-PE40  KLNDRADSRRSLWDQGNFPLIIKNLKIEDSDTYICEVEDQKEEVQLLVFG
            60        70        80        90       100


          100       110       120       130       140
CD4       LTANSDTHLLQGQSLTLTLESPPGSSPSVQCRSPRGKNIQGGKTLSVSQL
          *************************************************
CD4-PE40  LTANSDTHLLQGQSLTLTLESPPGSSPSVQCRSPRGKNIQGGKTLSVSQL
            110       120       130       140       150


          150       160       170       180       190
CD4       ELQDSGTWTCTVLQNQKKVEFKIDIVVLAFQKASSIVYKKEGEQVEFSFP
          ****************************    .         .      *
CD4-PE40  ELQDSGTWTCTVLQNQKKVEFKIDIVVLAHMAEEGGSLAALTAHQACHLP
            160       170       180       190       200


          200       210       220       230       240
CD4       L-AFTVEKLTGSGELWWQAERAS-SSKSWITFDLKNKEVSVKRVTQDPKL
          *  .**  ..      * * *.  .  ...  *   .  .*  ..* *  .
CD4-PE40  LETFTRHRQPRG---WEQLEQCGYPVQRLVALYLAAR-LSWNQVDQVIRN
            210       220       230       240


          250       260       270       280       290
CD4       QMGKKLPLHLTLPQALPQYAGSGNLTLALEAKTGK--LHQEVNLVVMRAT
          ..       .  *.   .    . * * *.   ..       .*       *.
CD4-PE40  ALASPGS-GGDLGEAIREQPEQARLALTLAAAESERFVRQGTGNDEAGAA
            250       260       270       280       290


            300       310       320       330
CD4       QLQ-KNLTCEV-----WGPTSPKLMLSLKLENKEAKVSKREKAVWVLNPE
          . .   .*** .    **.  .  *     .       *     *
CD4-PE40  NADVVSLTCPVAAGECAGPADSGDALLERNYPTGAEFLGDGGDVSFSTRG
            300       310       320       330       340


          340       350       360       370
CD4       AGMWQCLLSDSGQVLLESNIKVLPTWSTPVH
          .  *     ..   **   *.
CD4-PE40  TQNWTVERLLQAHRQLEERGYVFVGYHGTFLEAAQSIVFGGVRARSQDLD
            350       360       370       380       390


CD4-PE40  AIWRGFYIAGDPALAYGYAQDQEPDARGRIRNGALLRVYVPRSSLPGFYR
            400       410       420       430       440


CD4-PE40  TSLTLAAPEAAGEVERLIGHPLPLRLDAITGPEEEGGRLETILGWPLAER
            450       460       470       480       490


CD4-PE40  TVVIPSAIPTDPRNVGGDLDPSSIPDKEQAISALPDYASQPGKPPREDLK
            500       510       520       530       540
```

Scheme 9. Sequence comparison of CD4 and CD4-PE40.

- ## Chloroperoxidase (*Caldariomyces fumago*) (300 residues)

SEQUENCE

EPGSGIGYPYDNNTLPYVAPGPTDSRAPCPALNALANHGYIPHDGRAISRETLQNAF-
LNHMGIANSVIELALTNAFVVCEYVTGSDCGDSLVNLTLLAEPHAFEHDHSFSRKDY-
KQGVANSNDFIDNRNFDAETFQTSLDVVAGKTHFDYADMNEIRLQRESLSNELDFP-
GWFTESKPIQNVESGFIFALVSDFNLPDNDENPLVRIDWWKYWFTNESFPYHLGWH-
PPSPAREIEFVTSASSAVLAASVTSTPSSLPSGAIGPGAEAVPLSFASTMTPFLLATNAP-
YYAQDPTLRPQRQA

REACTIVE SITES

.N.(21)		.D.(19)		.M.(3)	.Q.(8)
12 DNN	129 RNF	11 YDN	152 ADM	61 HMG	54 LQN
13 NNT	154 MNE	24 TDS	168 LDF	153 DMN	116 KQG
33 LNA	165 SNE	44 HDG	193 SDF	276 TMT	136 FQT
37 ANH	181 QNV	86 SDC	198 PDN		159 LQR
55 QNA	195 FNL	89 GDS	200 NDE		180 IQN
59 LNH	199 DND	106 HDH	208 IDW		183 VQS
65 ANS	202 ENP	113 KDY	291 QDP		290 AQD
74 TNA	216 TNE	123 NDF			297 PQR
93 VNL	284 TNA	126 IDN			299 RQA
120 ANS		131 FDA			
122 SND		140 LDV			
127 DNR		149 FDY			

HYDROFLEX PLOT

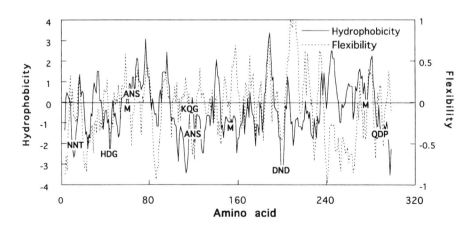

PREDICTED REACTIVITY AND DEGRADATION OF CHLOROPEROXIDASE

This glycoprotein has several sites that may undergo degradation in aqueous solution, including pyroglutamic acid formation at the N-terminus. This was confirmed experimentally, in that approximately two thirds of the protein resisted Edman degradation, indicative of a blocked N-terminus. Purification of chloroperoxidase from the filamentous fungus *Caldario-myces fumago* showed microheterogeneity at Asn-13 (-NNT-), Asn-199 (-DND-), and Gln-183 (converted completely to -VES-) (Kenigsberg *et al.*, 1987), all at sites not thought to be traditional hot spots. Unfortunately the work-up of this protein had a heat-inactivation step (pH >8, 100°C for 2 min), which may account for some of the deamidation observed at these sites. Further, no controls were carried out to show that these chemical modifications were due to enzymatic hydrolysis during the lengthy work-up.

Cholera B Subunit Protein (*Vibrio cholerae*) (103 residues)   •

SEQUENCE

TPQNITDLCAEYHNTQIHTLNNKIFSYTESLAGKREMAIITFKNGATFEVEVPGSQHI-
DSQKKAIERMKNTLRIAYLTEAKVEKLCVWNNKTPHAIAAISMAN

REACTIVE SITES

.N.(9)		.D.(2)	.M.(3)	.Q.(4)
4 QNI	70 KNT	7 TDL	37 EMA	3 PQN
14 HNT	89 WNN	59 IDS	68 RMK	16 TQI
21 LNN	90 NNK		101 SMA	56 SQH
22 NNK	103 AN			61 SQK
44 KNG				

HYDROFLEX PLOT

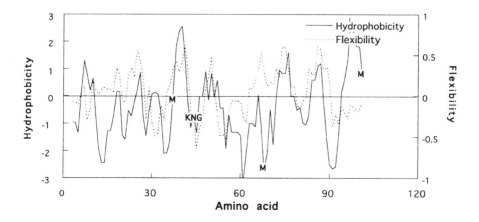

PREDICTED REACTIVITY AND DEGRADATION OF CHOLERA B TOXIN

This subunit protein contains only two different residues predicted to be reactive: Asn-Gly (-KNG-) and Met. Mass spectral analysis and Edman degradation of peptides derived from the B subunit of *Vibrio cholerae* toxin showed microheterogeneity at Asn-44 found within the -KNG- motif (Takao *et al.*, 1985). This is the only site predicted to show hydrolytic reactivity based on primary amino acid sequence and hydroflex analysis. Interestingly, the authors reported Asp instead of Asn at position 22 (-NNK-) and position 70 (-KNT-), even though Asn was found at these positions in some of the earlier cholera B toxin strains (shown in the sequence above). However, the nucleotide sequences encode for both Asp and Asn (depending on the strain), and so Asp for Asn at these sites should not be considered conclusively as microheterogeneity. No indication of Met oxidation in this protein was reported.

● **Ciliary Neurotrophic Factor (CNTF) (human) (199 residues)**

SEQUENCE

AFTEHSPLTPHRRDLCSRSIWLARKIRSDLTALTESYVKHQGLNKNINLDSADGMPV-
ASTDQWSELTEAERLQENLQAYRTFHVLLARLLEDQQVHFTPTEGDFHQAIHTLLL-
QVAAFAYQIEELMILLEYKIPRNEADGMPINVGDGGLFEKKLWGLKVLQELSQWTV-
RSIHDLRFISSHQTGIPARGSHYIANNKKM

REACTIVE SITES

.N.(8)	.D.(10)	.M.(4)	.Q.(12)
44 LNK	14 RDL	55 GMP	41 HQG
46 KNI	29 SDL	126 LMI	62 DQW
48 INL	50 LDS	141 GMP	73 LQE
75 ENL	53 ADG	199 KM	77 LQA
136 RNE	61 TDQ		93 DQQ
144 INV	92 EDQ		94 QQV
195 ANN	103 GDF		106 HQA
196 NNK	139 ADG		114 LQV
	147 GDG		121 YQI
	174 HDL		162 LQE
			166 SQW
			182 HQT

HYDROFLEX PLOT

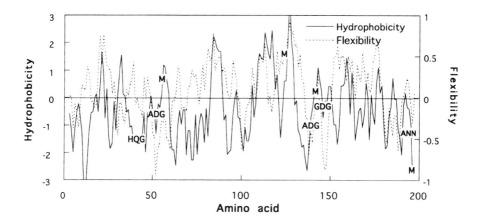

PREDICTED REACTIVITY AND DEGRADATION OF CNTF

Inspection of the hydroflex plot for CNTF shows that this protein has a few moderately reactive hot spots: three Asp-Gly residues and four Mets. None of the Asp-Gly are found in highly hydrophilic regions, and so might be expected to show reduced reactivity (if any at all). The major degradation pathway for CNTF was recently deduced and found not to involve any of the traditional hot spots; deamidation was observed at Asn-195 in the -ANN- motif close to the C-terminus (Maneri, 1994). Although deamidation takes place in the hydrophilic region of the molecule, the -ANN- sequence is not thought to be particularly activating, and so this degradation pathway would not have been predicted.

Crystallin-A (chicken) (173 residues)   ●

SEQUENCE

MDITIQHPWFKRALGPLIPSRLFDQFFGEGLLEYDLLPLFSSTISPYYRQSLFRSVLES-
GISEVRSDRDKFTIMLDVKHFSPEDLSVKIIDDFVEIHGKHSERQDDHGYISREFHRR-
YRLPANVDQSAITCSLSSDGMLTFSGPKVPSNMDPSHSERPIPVSREEKPTSAPSS

REACTIVE SITES

.N.(2)	.D.(14)	.M.(3)	.Q.(5)
123 ANV	2 MDI	74 IML	6 IQH
149 SNM	24 FDQ	138 GML	25 DQF
	35 YDL	150 NMD	50 RQS
	67 SDR		104 RQD
	69 RDK		126 DQS
	76 LDV		
	84 EDL		
	91 IDD		
	92 DDF		
	105 QDD		
	106 DDH		
	125 VDQ		
	136 SDG		
	151 MDP		

HYDROFLEX PLOT

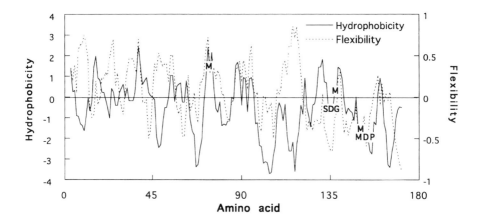

PREDICTED REACTIVITY AND DEGRADATION OF α-CRYSTALLIN-A

This protein has only a few predicted hot spots and may be expected to show degradation at Asp-Gly or Met. This was not observed experimentally, however. Extraction and purification of α-crystallin-A from chicken eye lenses afforded a protein that showed microheterogeneity at position 149 (Voorter *et al.*, 1987) due to deamidation of Asn-149 within the -SNM- motif. This sequence is not predicted to be particularly reactive, in that Asn is not followed by either Gly or Ser. Indeed, the authors pointed out that the deamidation at this site is age-related and that only partial microheterogeneity was observed in 10-year-old chickens, but not observed in young chickens. Crystallin in eye lenses is known to have a negligible turnover rate, indicative that it takes 10 years at physiological temperature for even partial deamidation to occur. That

deamidation did not occur at other Asn residues is not surprising, in that the only other Asn in
α-crystallin-A is located within an even less reactive motif (-ANV-). This protein contains an
Asp that is predicted to show some degradation (Asp-136 within the -SDG- motif), but it is
unlikely that the authors would have seen this with their method of high-voltage paper
electrophoresis. No controls were carried out to show that Asn-149 undergoes deamidation
under formulation conditions (neutral pH at 5–25°C within 2 years).

Cytochrome *c* (140 residues)   ●

SEQUENCE

GDVEKGKKIFVQKCAQCHTVEKGGKHKTGPNLHGLFGRKTGQAPGFSYTDANKN-
KGITWGEETLMEYLENPKKYIPGTKMIFAGIKKKGEREDLIAYLKKATNE

REACTIVE SITES

.N.(5)	.D.(3)	.M.(2)	.Q.(3)
31 PNL	2 GDV	65 LME	12 VQK
52 ANK	50 TDA	80 KMI	16 AQC
54 KNK	93 EDL		42 GQA
70 ENP			
103 TNE			

HYDROFLEX PLOT

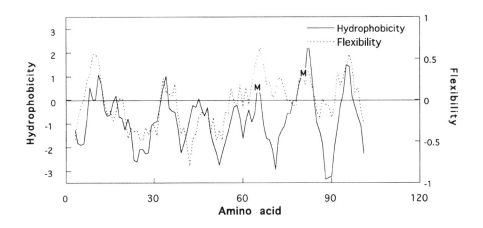

PREDICTED REACTIVITY AND DEGRADATION OF CYTOCHROME c (Cy I)

Inspection of the primary amino acid sequence for cytochrome c shows that it is devoid of traditional hot spots (Asn-Gly, Asn-Ser, Asp-Gly, and Gln-Gly), and so, *a priori*, this protein might be expected to be fairly stable, at least at 2–8°C at neutral pH. One of the earliest studies to detail protein microheterogeneity was reported by Flatmark on the reaction of cytochrome c in aqueous buffers (Flatmark, 1966). This protein showed microheterogeneity at Asn-103 near the C-termini (-TNE) after tryptic mapping. This region of cytochrome c is predicted to be both hydrophilic and flexible, but this Asn is located within a motif not thought to be reactive. Although this early report has some errors in the interpretation of the kinetic data (for example, neglecting pyro-Glu formation in the comparative analysis of Glu and Asn free amino acid reactivity, or the "visual" determination that the rate constant for reaction of Cy I is significantly less than for Cy II for the sequential reaction Cy I → Cy II → Cy III), it was found that the major site of microheterogeneity in Cy I was Asn-103 in the -TNE motif at the C-terminus. (It appears that the Cy II subfraction showing microheterogeneity was obtained by preparative work-up of tissue rather than as the degradation product of Cy I, and so the reaction of Asn-103 is considered a "work-up" deamidation reaction.) Data were reported at both 4 and 37°C and at several pHs ranging from 3 to 11. The pH rate profiles for reaction of Cy I suggest that several reactions may be occurring, in that the slope of these plots in the region of base catalysis has a slope significantly less than unity (when plotted as log k versus pH). Refitting the data to a standard log k–pH rate profile suggests that cytochrome c should exhibit a 2-year shelf life below pH ~7.5. Indeed, use of the kinetic data provided in this chapter to construct a typical log k–pH rate profile suggests that cytochrome c should exhibit a shelf-life in aqueous solution of 20 years or more at pH 6 (Fig. 2). Based on this, the -TNE motif is fairly unreactive, despite its ease of deamidation at high pH and 37°C.

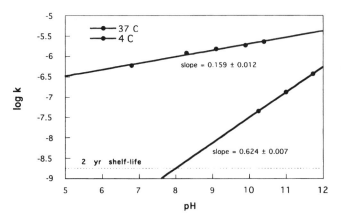

Figure 2.   Log k–pH rate profiles for the reaction of Cy I to Cy II in aqueous buffers at 4° and 37°C. The slopes of values less than unity suggest that degradation may be occurring by several pH-dependent pathways. Linear extrapolation at 4°C suggests that the shelf life (due to deamidation) of cytochrome c will be >20 years at pH 6.

DNase (human) (260 residues)

SEQUENCE

LKIAAFNIQTFGETKMSNATLVSYIVQILSRYDIALVQEVRDSHLTAVGKLLDNLNQ-
DAPDTYHYVVSEPLGRNSYKERYLFVYRPDQVSAVDSYYYDDGCEPCGNDTFNRE-
PAIVRFFSRFTEVREFAIVPLHAAPGDRVAEIDALYDVYLDVQEKWGLEDVMLMGD-
FNAGCSYVRPSQWSSIRLWTSPTFQWLIPDSADTTATPTHCAYDRIVVAGMLLRGA-
VVPDSALPFNFQAAYGLSDQLAQAISDHYPVEVMLK

REACTIVE SITES

.N.(9)	.D.(22)		.M.(5)	.Q.(11)
7 FNI	33 YDI	145 IDA	16 KMS	9 IQT
18 SNA	42 RDS	149 YDV	164 VML	27 VQI
54 DNL	53 LDN	153 LDV	166 LMG	38 VQE
56 LNQ	58 QDA	162 EDV	219 GML	57 NQD
74 RNS	61 PDT	168 GDF	258 VML	88 DQV
106 GND	87 PDQ	198 PDS		155 VQE
110 FNR	93 VDS	201 ADT		180 SQW
170 FNA	98 YDD	212 YDR		193 FQW
234 FNF	99 DDG	228 PDS		236 FQA
	107 NDT	243 SDQ		244 DQL
	139 GDR	251 SDH		247 AQA

HYDROFLEX PLOT

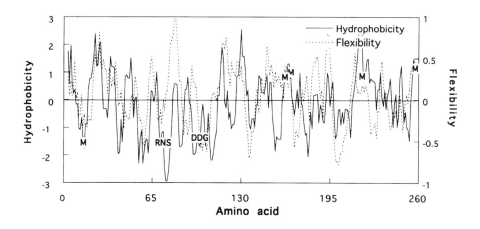

PREDICTED REACTIVITY AND DEGRADATION OF DNase

Deamidation in DNase occurs at the -RNS- motif, where it is expected that this Asn is the likely hot spot due to the presence of Ser on the C-terminal side, as well as the flanking polar

Arg. The hydropathy plot also supports this as the most likely site of deamidation, in that this motif is predicted to exist in a hydrophilic region of intermediate flexibility. There is another motif (-DDG- at Asp-99) that is also predicted to be a hot spot, in that it exists in a hydrophilic flexible region. Reaction at this site, however, has not been observed. The major degradation pathway of DNase at pH 5–8 in aqueous solution was found to be deamidation at Asn-74, giving the Asp and the iso-Asp variants. Modification at this site does not lead to complete inactivity, wherein the deamidated product exhibited ~50% of the original activity (Frenz, 1991; Cipolla *et al.*, 1994). Reaction at this site did not compromise a 2-year shelf life when the product was stored at 2–8°C.

- **Epidermal Growth Factor (EGF 1–48) (human) (48 residues)**

SEQUENCE

NSDSECPLSHDGYCLHDGVCMYIEALDKYACNCVVGYIGERCQYRDLK

REACTIVE SITES

.N.(1)	.D.(5)		.M.(1)	.Q.(1)
1 NS	3 SDS	27 LDK	21 CMY	43 CQY
32 CNC	11 HDG	46 RDL		
	17 HDG			

HYDROFLEX PLOT

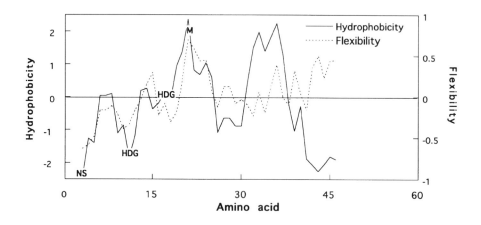

PREDICTED REACTIVITY AND DEGRADATION OF EGF (HUMAN)

The hydroflex plot for EGF shows that there are two reactive hydrolytic sites (Asn-1 in the NS- motif and Asp-11 in the -HDG- motif). Oxidation of Met may also be a likely pathway for degradation. An elegant study on the degradation of EGF showed that succinimide formation at Asp-11 was most prominent below pH 6, whereas deamidation of Asn-1 was the primary degradation pathway above pH 6 (Senderoff *et al.*, 1994). The relative contribution of oxidation was found to increase as the temperature was lowered. This study also included the pH rate profiles for both reactant loss and degradation product formation at both 4 and 30°C. Deamidation as the primary degradation pathway for EGF at neutral pH was recently confirmed in another study showing the effects of buffer ions and surfactants at higher temperatures (Son and Kwon, 1995).

Epidermal Growth Factor (murine) (53 residues)

SEQUENCE

NSYPGCPSSYDGYCLNGGVCMHIESLDSYTCNCVIGYSGDGCQTRDLRWWQLR

REACTIVE SITES

.N.(2)	.D.(4)	.M.(1)	.Q.(2)
1 NS	11 YDG	21 CMH	43 CQT
16 LNG	27 LDS		51 WQL
32 CNC	40 GDG		
	46 RDL		

HYDROFLEX PLOT

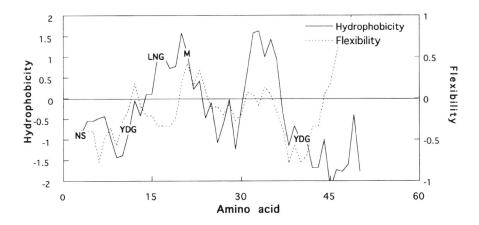

PREDICTED REACTIVITY AND DEGRADATION OF EGF (MURINE)

The hydroflex plot for EGF shows that there are two reactive Asn (Asn-1 in the NS- motif and Asn-16 in the -LNG- motif). Insufficient data exist to predict which of these should react fastest, because of the lack of reactivity data for N-terminal Asn residues. Reaction of murine EGF at pH 9 and 37°C for 48 hr afforded primarily reaction at Asn-1 (NS-), with a small amount of reaction at Asn-16 (-LNG-) (Galletti *et al.*, 1989). Unfolding the protein increased the amount of reaction at Asn-16. A similar reaction was observed at pH 7.4 at 22°C, where the observed half-life was approximately 500 hr (DiAugustine *et al.*, 1987); it was also reported that the half-life at pH ~13 and 22°C was 63 hr, suggesting that the rate of deamidation is not linearly proportional with hydroxide ion concentration (Tyler-Cross and Schirch, 1991). Insufficient experiments were carried out to determine the rate of reaction at pH 4.5–7.5 at 2–8°C.

• Erythrocyte Protein 4.1 (human) (588 residues)

SEQUENCE

MHCKVSLLDDTVYECVVEKHAKGQDLLKRVCEHLNLLEEDYFGLAIWDNATSKT-
WLDSAKEIKKQVRGVPWNFTFNVKFYPPDPAQLTEDITRYYLCLQLRQDIVAGRLPC-
SFATLALLGSYTIQSELGDYDPELHGVDYVSDFKLAPNQTKELEEKVMELHKSYRS-
MTPAQADLEFLENAKKLSMYGVDLHKAKDLEGVDIILGVCSSGLLVYKDKLRINR-
FPWPKVLKISYKRSSFFIKIRPGEQEQYESTIGFKLPSYRAAKKLWKVCVEHHTFFRL-
TSTDTIPKSKFLALGSKFRYSGRTQAQTRQASALIDRPAPHFERTASKRASRSLDGAA-
AVDSADRSPRPTSAPAITQGQVAEGGVLDASAKKTVVPKAQKETVKAEVKKEDEPP-
EQAEPEPTEAWKKKRERLDGENIYIRHSNLMLEDLDKSQEEIKKHHASISELKKNF-
MESVPEPRPSEWDKRLSTHSPFRTLNINGQIPTGEGPPLVKTQTVTISDNANAVKSEI-
PTKDVPIVHTETKTITYEAAQTVKGGISETRIEKRIVITGDADIDHDQVLVQAIKEAK-
EQHPDMSVTKVVVHQETEIADE

REACTIVE SITES

.N.(14)		.D.(37)		.M.(6)		.Q.(25)	
35 LNL	9 LDD	316 IDR	159 VME	24 GQD	493 TQT		
49 DNA	10 DDT	335 LDG	168 SMT	65 KQV	529 AQT		
72 WNF	25 QDL	341 VDS	186 SMY	86 AQL	556 DQV		
76 FNV	40 EDY	344 ADR	425 LML	99 LQL	560 VQA		
149 PNQ	48 WDN	367 LDA	451 FME	102 RQD	568 EQH		
180 ENA	57 LDS	391 EDE	572 DMS	125 IQS	581 HQE		
221 INR	83 PDP	413 LDG		150 NQT			
416 ENI	90 EDI	428 EDL		172 AQA			
423 SNL	103 QDI	430 LDK		247 EQE			
449 KNF	130 GDY	463 WDK		249 EQY			
476 LNI	132 YDP	499 SDN		305 TQA			
478 ING	139 VDY	512 KDV		307 AQT			
500 DNA	143 SDF	549 GDA		310 RQA			
502 ANA	174 ADL	551 ADI		357 TQG			
	190 VDL	533 IDH		359 GQV			
	196 KDL	555 HDQ		379 AQK			
	201 VDI	571 PDM		396 EQA			
	216 KDK	587 ADE		433 SQE			
	284 TDT			480 GQI			

HYDROFLEX PLOT

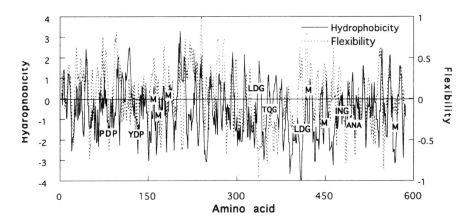

PREDICTED REACTIVITY AND DEGRADATION OF ERYTHROCYTE PROTEIN 4.1

This protein has several hot spots of predicted reactivity, including an Asn-Gly motive. Isolation and purification of this large protein result in the selective deamidation at two sites, Asn-478 and Asn-502 (Inaba *et al.*, 1992). The first is unremarkable in that Asn-478 is adjacent to Gly (-ING-). Asn-502 is flanked by Ala on both sides (-ANA-), yielding an Asn that would be only weakly reactive based on model peptide studies. Indeed, the authors found that reaction of Asn-502 was much slower than at Asn-478, taking months for reaction to occur *in vivo*. No controls were carried out to show that reaction of Asn-502 occurred under formulation conditions in the absence of catalytic enzymes, nor was sufficient kinetic data presented (other than the reaction was slow) to permit an estimation of the reaction rate at 2–8°C.

Fibroblast Growth Factor, Acidic (human) (aFGF) (141 residues)   ●

SEQUENCE

MFNLPPGNYKKPKLLYCSNGGHFLRILPDGTVDGTRDRSDQHIQLQLSAESVGEV-
YIKSTETGQYLAMDTDGLLYGSQTPNEECLFLERLEENHYNTYISKKHAEKNWFV-
GLKKNGSCKRGPRTHYGQKAILFLPLPVSSD

REACTIVE SITES

.N.(8)	.D.(7)	.M.(2)	.Q.(6)
3 FNL	29 PDG	1 MF	41 DQH
8 GNY	33 VDG	68 AMD	44 IQL
19 SNG	37 RDR		46 LQL
81 PNE	40 SDQ		64 GQY
93 ENH	69 MDT		78 SQT
96 YNT	71 TDG		128 GQK
107 KNW	141 SD		
115 KNG			

HYDROFLEX PLOT

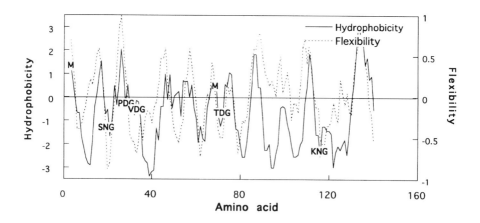

PREDICTED REACTIVITY AND DEGRADATION OF ACIDIC FGF

Acidic FGF contains two Asn-Gly motifs that are predicted to be reactive, as well as a number of Asp-Gly residues. This molecule is known to be fairly reactive in solution, and so elegant formulations have been designed utilizing its stabilizing complexation with heparin to extend shelf life (Volkin and Middaugh, 1996). Some degradation studies have been carried out, wherein it was found that deamidation was one of the major degradation pathways. N-terminal sequence analysis showed that Asn-8 (-GNY-) was deamidated, but that Asn-19 was not (-SNG-). This is somewhat unusual, in that the Asn-Gly sequence is usually much more reactive than the Asn-Tyr sequence. The authors pointed out that Asn-8 is in a hydrophilic flexible region, possibly enhancing its reactivity. Conversely, Asn-19 is located in the heparin binding region for acidic-FGF, and this may contribute to its lack of reactivity. No degradation was reported for the Asn-Gly site near the C-termini, although the methods used (sequence analysis) were not developed to look at this region of the molecule. No oxidation of Met was reported, however oxidation at Cys leads to inactivation of the protein.

Fibroblast Growth Factor, Basic (human) (bFGF) (154 residues)

SEQUENCE

AAGSITTLPALPEDGGSGAFPPGHFKDPKRLYCKNGGFFLRIHPDGRVDGVREKSDP-
HIKLQLQAEERGVVSIKGVCANRYLAMKEDGRLLASKCVTDECFFFERLESNNYNT-
YRSRKYTSWYVALKRTGQYKLGSKTGPGQKAILFLPMSAKS

REACTIVE SITES

.N.(5)		.D.(7)		.M.(2)	.Q.(4)
36 KNG	113 YNT	15 EDG	57 SDP	85 AMK	63 LQL
80 ANR		28 KDP	88 EDG	151 PMS	65 LQA
110 SNN		46 PDG	99 TDE		132 GQY
111 NNY		50 VDG			143 GQK

HYDROFLEX PLOT

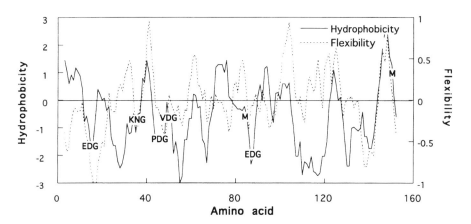

PREDICTED REACTIVITY AND DEGRADATION OF BASIC FGF

Degradation of bFGF occurs at Asp-15 within the -EDG- motif, where it is expected that this Asp is a likely hot spot due to the presence of Gly on the C-terminal side, as well as the flanking polar Glu. The hydropathy plot also supports this as the most likely site of succinimide formation, in that this motif is predicted to exist in a hydrophilic region of moderate flexibility. There also exists a -KNG- motif at Asn-36 that is likely to be a reactive hot spot, particularly at higher pH's. Asn-36 is found in a region of only intermediate hydrophobicity and flexibility, and so may be of reduced reactivity compared with a -KNG- motif found in smaller peptides. There is also another -EDG- motif found at Asp-88, although this Asp is predicted to be of lower reactivity because the regional flexibility is less than at Asp-15. When the stability of bFGF was investigated at pH 6.5, the degradation product eluted sooner than the parent by HP-IEC, indicative of a more acidic deamidated product (although this was not confirmed with product analysis). The major degradation pathway of bFGF at pH 5 in aqueous solution was succinimide formation at Asp-15 (Shahrokh *et al.*, 1994). In addition, two truncated monomer forms were found as minor degradation products, due to cleavage at Asp-28-Pro and Asp-15-Gly. Modification at these sites did not lead to inactivity, where the cleaved or cyclized products remained bioactive in a heparin binding assay and in a cell proliferation assay. No evidence was found for oxidative degradation of Met within 13 weeks at pH 5 at 25°C. The stability of bFGF at 2–8°C was not addressed directly in this chapter, but mention was made that iso-Asp formation was less than 2% in 24 weeks at 4°C, which should be interpreted as a lower limit because the cyclic imide is also formed.

- **Glucagon (29 residues)**

SEQUENCE

HSQGTFTSDYSKYLDSRRAQDFVQWLMNT

REACTIVE SITES

.N.(1)	.D.(3)	.M.(1)	.Q.(3)
28 MNT	9 SDY	27 LMN	3 SQG
	15 LDS		20 AQD
	21 QDF		24 VQW

HYDROFLEX PLOT

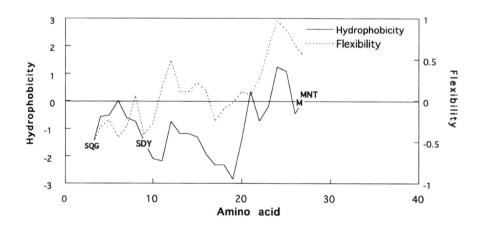

PREDICTED REACTIVITY AND DEGRADATION OF GLUCAGON

This peptide is not predicted to be very reactive, in that it is missing most of the traditional hot spots. Inspection of the hydroflex plot shows a Gln-Gly motive near the N-termini which may be expected to be mildly reactive. Methylation of glucagon to identify iso-Asp residues showed that glucagon contained some iso-Asp at Asp-9 and Asn-28 (Ota *et al.*, 1987). Both of these amino acids are located within motifs that are not expected to be reactive (-SDY- and -MNT-) based on data obtained in synthetic peptides. No control experiments were carried out to determine if the same degradation reaction occurs in pH 4.5–7.5 buffer. Of note, glucagon samples were boiled for a short time before carrying out the enzymatic maps, and the consequence of this preparative step on the degradation of glucagon was undetermined.

Granulocyte-Colony Stimulating Factor (G-CSF) (human) (175 residues)   ●

SEQUENCE

MTPLGPASSLPQSFLLKCLEQVRKIQGDGAALQEKLCATYKLCHPEELVLLGHSLGI-
PWAPLSSCPSQALQLAGCLSQLHSGLFLYQGLLQALEGISPELGPTLDTLQLDVADFA-
TTIWQQMEELGMAPALQPTQGAMPAFASAFQRRAGGVLVASHLQSFLEVSYRVLRH-
LAQP

REACTIVE SITES

.N.(0)	.D.(4)	.M.(3)	.Q.(17)
	28 GDG	122 QME	12 PQS
	105 LDT	127 GMA	21 EQV
	110 LDV	138 AMP	26 IQG
	113 ADF		33 LQE
			68 SQA
			71 LQL
			78 SQL
			87 YQG
			91 LQA
			108 LQL
			120 WQQ
			121 QQM
			132 LQP
			135 TQG
			146 FQR
			159 LQS
			174 AQP

HYDROFLEX PLOT

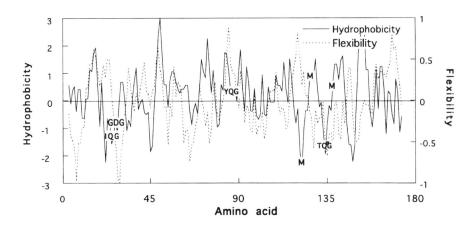

PREDICTED REACTIVITY AND DEGRADATION OF GCSF

This molecule is devoid of Asn and has only a few predicted hot spots such as Asp-Gly (cyclization and iso-Asp formation), Gln-Gly (deamidation), or Met (oxidation). The degradation pathways of GCSF in aqueous solution have been determined, wherein it was found that the predominant site of deamidation was at Gln-21 (in the -EQV- motif), and oxidation at Met-122 and at either Met-127 or Met-138 (these residues are in the same peptide in the tryptic digest and so differentiation has not been made) (Herman *et al.*, 1995). Even though Gln-21 is located in a region of predicted hydrophilicity, deamidation at Gln-21 is unexpected because the -EQV- motif is not a traditional hot spot based on the deamidation of Gln in small peptides.

- **Growth Hormone (bovine) (191 residues)**

SEQUENCE

AFPAMSLSGLFANAVLRAQHLHQLAADTSKEFERTYIPEGQRYSIQNTQVAFCFSET-
MPAPTGKNEAQQKSDLELLRISLLLIQSWLGPLQFLSRVFTNSLVFGTSDRVYEKLK-
DLEEGILALMRELEDGTPRRGQILKQTYDKFDTNMRSDDALLKNYGLLSCFRKDL-
HKTETYLRVMKCRRFGEASCAF

REACTIVE SITES

.N.(6)	.D.(10)		.M.(5)	.Q.(11)	
13 ANA	27 ADT	143 YDK	5 AMS	19 AQH	69 QQK
47 QNT	72 SDL	146 FDT	58 TMP	23 HQL	84 IQS
65 KNE	107 SDR	152 SDD	124 LMR	41 GQR	91 LQF
99 TNS	115 KDL	153 DDA	149 NMR	46 IQN	136 GQI
148 TNM	129 EDG	168 KDL	179 VMK	49 TQV	140 KQT
158 KNY				68 AQQ	

HYDROFLEX PLOT

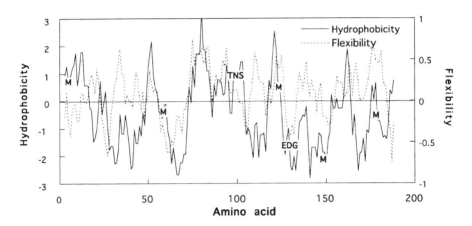

PREDICTED REACTIVITY AND DEGRADATION OF BOVINE GROWTH HORMONE

The primary sequence of bovine growth hormone has two potential hot spots for hydrolytic degradation, where Asn-99 in the -TNS- motif is the most likely. The other hot spot is Asp-129, although it is likely that reactivity at this site at pH 7.4 will be much slower than at Asn-99. [It has been reported that Asp-129 is the predominant site of reaction in porcine somatotropin under acidic conditions giving the cyclic imide (Violand et al., 1992).] Although the Asn-99 site is a predicted hot spot based on primary sequence alone, it is not predicted to be a hot spot based on the hydroflex plot, in that Asn-99 lies in a hydrophobic region of little flexibility. In contrast, Asp-129 lies in a hydrophilic flexible region. It has been shown that the primary site of degradation in bovine (and porcine) growth hormone at pH 7.4 was deamidation at Asn-99 to give predominantly iso-Asp-99 (Violand et al., 1990). The authors pointed out that it is likely that reaction may occur at other sites in bovine growth hormone, but may not be resolvable under their HPLC conditions. These studies were carried out at 37°C, so an estimate of the reaction rate at 2–8°C could not be made from these studies. There is sufficient data on bovine growth hormone showing conclusively that bovine growth hormone undergoes different degradation pathways under "work-up" conditions and under "formulation" conditions, even at the same pH and temperature. For example, the major reaction site in purified pituitary bovine growth hormone in aqueous buffer was Asn-99, but the predominant variants isolated from work-up samples were Asn-13 and Asn-148 in one study (Violand *et al.*, 1990) and Asp-129 in another (Wood *et al.*, 1989). Although reactivity at Asp-129 is not unexpected (see above), neither the Asn-13 (-ANA-) nor Asn-148 (-TNM-) is predicted to reactive based on primary sequence and hydroflex plot analysis. This is another example showing that deamidation or iso-Asp formation under work-up conditions should not be used to predict the site(s) of major degradation in typical pH 5–7 aqueous formulations. The interspecies variation in GH primary amino acid sequence is given in Scheme 10 for reference.

```
GH-b    1 AFPAMSLSGLFANAVLRAQHLHQLAADTSKEFERTYIPEGQRYS-IQNTQ
GH-h    1 -FPTIPLSRLFDNAMLRAHRLHQLAFDTYQEFEEAYIPKEQKYSFLQNPQ
GH-p    1 -FPAMPLSSLFANAVLRAQHLHQLAADTYKEFERTYIPEGQRYS-IQNAQ

GH-b   50 VAFCFSETMPAPTGKNEAQQKSDLELLRISLLLIQSWLGPLQFLSRVFTN
GH-h   50 TSLCFSESIPTPSNREETQQKSNLELLRISLLLIQSWLEPVQFLRSVFAN
GH-p   49 AAFCFSETIPAPTGKDEAQQRSDVELLRISLLLIQSWLGPVQFLSRVFTN

GH-b  100 SLVFGTSD-RVYEKLKDLEEGILALMRELEDGTPRRGQILKQTYDKFDTN
GH-h  100 SLVYGASDSNVYDLLKDLEEGIQTLMGRLEDGSPRTGQIFKQTYSKFDTN
GH-p   99 SLVFGTSD-RVYEKLKDLEEGIQALMRELEDGSPRAGQILKQTYDKFDTN

GH-b  149 MRSDDALLKNYGLLSCFRKDLHKTETYLRVMKCRRFGEASCAF
GH-h  150 SHNDDALLKNYGLLYCFRKDMDKVETFLRIVQCRS-VEGSCGF
GH-p  148 LRSDDALLKNYGLLSCFKKDLHKAETYLRVMKCRRFVESSCAF
```

Scheme 10. Primary amino acid sequences of bovine, human, and porcine growth hormones.

- **Growth Hormone (human) (191 residues)**

SEQUENCE

FPTIPLSRLFDNAMLRAHRLHQLAFDTYQEFEEAYIPKEQKYSFLQNPQTSLCFSESIP-
TPSNREETQQKSNLELLRISLLLIQSWLEPVQFLRSVFANSLVYGASDSNVYDLLKDL-
EEGIQTLMGRLEDGSPRTGQIFKQTYSKFDTNSHNDDALLKNYGLLYCFRKDMDKV-
ETFLRIVQCRSVEGSCGF

REACTIVE SITES

.N.(9)		.D.(11)		.M.(3)	.Q.(13)	
12 DNA	152 HND	11 FDN	153 NDD	14 AML	22 HQL	84 IQS
47 QNP	159 KNY	26 FDT	154 DDA	125 LMG	29 YQE	91 VQF
63 SNR		107 SDS	169 KDM	170 DMD	40 EQK	122 IQT
72 SNL		112 YDL	171 MDK		46 LQN	137 GQI
99 ANS		116 KDL			49 PQT	141 KQT
109 SNV		130 EDG			68 TQQ	181 VQC
149 TNS		147 FDT			69 QQK	

HYDROFLEX PLOT

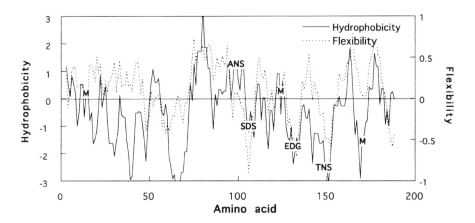

PREDICTED REACTIVITY AND DEGRADATION OF HUMAN GROWTH HORMONE

There are three likely hot spots for hydrolytic degradation in hGH: Asn-99, Asp-130, and Asn 149. Degradation of hGH occurred primarily at Asn-149 and Asp-130, as might be expected in that Asn is next to Ser and Asp is next to Gly. The hydropathy plot also supports this as the most likely site of degradation, in that these motifs exist in a hydrophilic region of good flexibility. Peptide chain flexibility is probably quite important for the deamidation of Asn-149 in human growth hormone (Johnson *et al.*, 1989b). The structure of human growth hormone is likely to be similar to porcine growth hormone, which is poorly ordered in the region of residues 128 to 151 (Abdel-Meguid *et al.*, 1987). Asn-99 has a similar motif (-ANS-) as Asn-149 (-TNS-), and yet Asn-99 does not undergo reaction. An elegant explanation for this has been given by comparing the bovine and human sequences of growth hormone and then rationalizing the decreased reactivity at this site by an unfavorable conformational structure near Asn-99. Often this in-depth explanation is not possible because the 3D structure is unavailable, so it would be useful if this lack of reactivity could be predicted based on primary sequence hydrophobicity calculations. Indeed, inspection of the hydropathy and flexibility plots suggests that Asn-149 should be reactive (in that it exists in a hydrophilic region of good flexibility), whereas the Asn-99 exists in a hydrophobic region of lower flexibility and thus may be removed from the solvent and less available for reaction. The major degradation pathway of hGH at pH 6 in aqueous solution was found to be deamidation at Asn-149, with minor degradation pathways including cyclic imide and iso-Asp formation at Asp-130 (Teshima *et al.*, 1991b), and oxidation at Met-14 and Met-125 (Teshima and Canova-Davis, 1992). None of these reactions, nor their sum, compromised the shelf life of the liquid growth hormone formulation, having a shelf life of at least 18 months at 2–8°C. This formulation contained a preservative, as well as Tween 20. In another study, the degradation products of hGH were also determined after incubation at pH 7.4 and 37°C, giving largely deamidation at Asn-149 to form the iso-Asp and Asp degradation products. A small amount of deamidation was found at Asn-152. Iso-Asp formation at Asp-130 was also observed, but not deamidation at Asn-99, a similar Asn sequence of -ANS-. It has also been reported that hGH forms the N-terminal diketopiperazine product during fermentation and/or work-up, although this is not a degradation product in the final formulation (Battersby *et al.*, 1994).

● **Growth Hormone (porcine) (190 residues)**

SEQUENCE

FPAMPLSSLFANAVLRAQHLHQLAADTYKEFERTYIPEGQRYSIQNAQAAFCFSETIP-
APTGKDEAQQRSDVELLRISLLLIQSWLGPVQFLSRVFTNSLVFGTSDRVYEKLKDL-
EEGIQALMRELEDGSPRAGQILKQTYDKFDTNLRSDDALLKNYGLLSCFKKDLHKA-
ETYLRVMKCRRFVESSCAF

REACTIVE SITES

.N.(5)		.D.(11)		.M.(3)		.Q.(12)	
12 ANA	26 ADT	142 YDK	4 AMP	18 AQH	68 QQR
46 QNA	64 KDE	145 FDT	123 LMR	22 HQL	83 IQS
98 TNS	71 SDV	151 SDD	178 VMK	40 GQR	90 VQF
147 TNL	106 SDR	152 DDA		45 IQN	120 IQA
157 KNY	114 KDL	167 KDL		48 AQA	135 GQI
	128 EDG			67 AQQ	139 KQT

HYDROFLEX PLOT

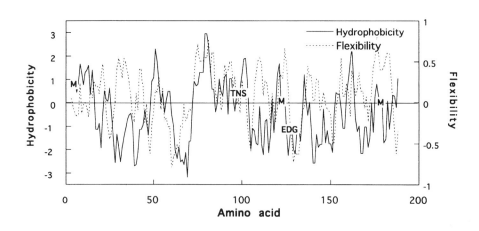

PREDICTED REACTIVITY AND DEGRADATION OF PORCINE GROWTH HORMONE

In contrast to human GH, there are only a few predicted hot spots for hydrolytic degradation in porcine GH, at Asn-98, Asp-128, and the Met residues. Degradation of pGH is predicted to occur primarily at Asn-98, as might be expected in that Asn is next to Ser (Violand *et al.*, 1990). This residue is in a moderately hydrophobic region, and so degradation might be expected to be slower than if it were in a hydrophilic region. The major degradation pathway of pGH in aqueous solution was found to be deamidation at Asn-98, with other degradation pathways at residues Cys-180–Cys-188 and Cys-52–Cys-163 (McCrossin *et al.*, 1994). This study was carried out at pH 9 to effect faster reaction rates, and this higher pH may be the reason that reaction occurred at the Cys-Cys bonds. Under these conditions, reaction at Asn-98 gave iso-Asp-98 and Asp-98 in a 3:1 ratio.

Growth Hormone Releasing Factor (GHRF) Variant (human) (32 residues)   ●

SEQUENCE

YADAIFTNSYRKVLGQLSARKLLQDILSRQQG

REACTIVE SITES

.N.(1)	.D.(2)	.M.(0)	.Q.(4)	
8 TNS	3 ADA		16 GQL	30 RQQ
	25 QDI		24 LQD	31 QQG

HYDROFLEX PLOT

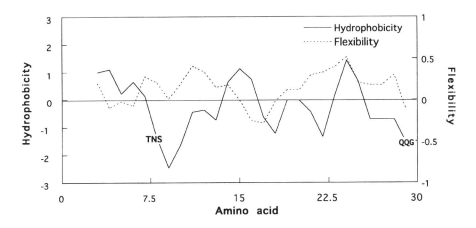

PREDICTED REACTIVITY AND DEGRADATION OF (Leu-27) GHRF (1–32) NH$_2$

The hydroflex plot for this GHRF variant shows that Asn-8 resides in a hydrophilic region or intermediate flexibility (although peptides such as GHRF may show flexibility throughout because of their small size), and thus Asn-8 may be expected to be a reactive site. Of secondary predicted reactivity is the C-terminal Glu, in that Glu-Gly typically reacts somewhat slower than Asn-Ser. Reaction of GHRF in aqueous solution at pH 7.4 and 37°C gave primarily reaction at Asn-8 (-TNS-) (Friedman *et al.*, 1991). Studies have been carried out using modified bovine GHRF analogues (for example, substitution of Gly-15 with Pro-15 or Ala-15 to disrupt the helical structure in the helical region near Asn-8), and these showed altered rates of deamidation (Stevenson *et al.*, 1993). Insufficient experiments were carried out to determine the rate of reaction at pH 4.5–7.5 or at 2–8°C. The parent molecule has Met at position 27, and has been nonenzymatically oxidized to give Met sulfoxide (Campbell *et al.*, 1990).

• Hemoglobin (human) (146 residues)

SEQUENCE

VLSPADKTNVKAAWGKVGAHAGEYGAEALERMFLSFPTTKTYFPHFDLSHGSAQ-
VKGHGKKVADALTNAVAHVDDMPNALSALSDLHAHKLRVDPVNFKLLSHCLLVTL-
AAHLPAEFTPAVHASLDKFLASVSTVLTSNTVKLQPR

REACTIVE SITES

.N.(5)	.D.(8)	.M.(2)	.Q.(2)
9 TNV	6 ADK	32 RMF	54 AQV
68 TNA	47 FDL	76 DMP	144 LQP
78 PNA	64 ADA		
97 VNF	74 VDD		
139 SNT	75 DDM		
	85 SDL		
	94 VDP		
	126 LDK		

HYDROFLEX PLOT

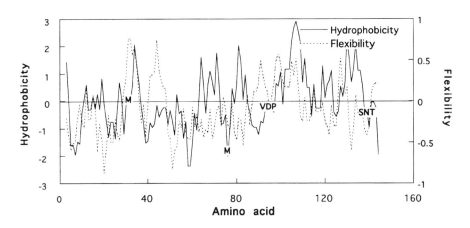

PREDICTED REACTIVITY AND DEGRADATION OF HEMOGLOBIN (WAYNE)

This variant of hemoglobin has few predicted reactive sites, the most likely being cleavage of Asp-Pro (-VDP-) at low pH, or oxidation of Met. Isolation and purification of this alpha-chain variant gives two forms, where the microheterogeneity was found at Asn-139 within the internal sequence -SNT- (Seid-Akhavan *et al.*, 1976). This motif is considered fairly unreactive, based on data obtained in small peptides (Tyler-Cross and Schirch, 1991). No controls were carried out to show that reaction of Asn-139 occurs under formulation conditions (for example, in the absence of catalytic enzymes), nor was sufficient kinetic data presented (other than the reaction was slow) to permit an estimation of the reaction rate at 2–8°C. This is another example of deamidation occurring at site other than Asn-Gly or Asn-Ser, but no evidence showing that the reaction proceeds rapidly by a nonenzymatic reaction.

Hirudin (65 residues)

SEQUENCE

VVYTDCTESGQNLCLCEGSNVCGQGNKCILGSNGEKNQCVTGEGTPKPQSHNNG-
DFEEIP

REACTIVE SITES

.N.(5)	.D.(4)	.M.(0)	.Q.(5)
12 QNL	5 TDC		11 GQN
20 SNV	55 GDF		24 GQG
26 GNK			38 NQC
33 SNG			49 PQS
37 KNQ			65 LQ
52 HND			
53 NNG			

HYDROFLEX PLOT

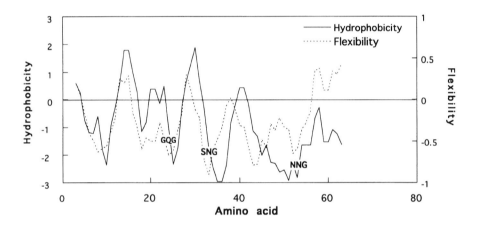

PREDICTED REACTIVITY AND DEGRADATION OF HIRUDIN

Hirudin is a glycoprotein under development as an antithrombotic agent. This small protein contains two Asn-Gly residues in flexible, hydrophilic regions, and may be expected to undergo some cyclization and iso-Asp formation. Mass spectral degradation product studies on hirudin showed that Asn-33 underwent cyclic imide formation to form the Q4 variant with resultant Asp-33 formation, as well as a Q5 variant with Asp-53 (Grossenbacher *et al.*, 1993). These studies were carried out under slightly acidic conditions, which may promote degradation. Further, these product studies were carried out under harsh conditions (180-fold molar excess DTT, followed by pyridylation at pH 8.3 and enzymatic degradation at pH 7.8 at 37°C), making it difficult to determine if these degradation pathways would compromise hirudin shelf-life in a neutral pH aqueous formulation at 2–8°C. Another study of the hirudin variant 2 (rHV-Lys-47) showed that Asn-33 and Asn-53 (again both found within the Asn-Gly motif) were altered, either in the fermentation process or during the work-up (no stability data under formulation conditions were reported); it was determined that the variants were stable succinimide intermediates (Bischoff *et al.*, 1993). Based on these studies, both Asn-33 and Asn-53 in hirudin are very susceptible to cyclic imide formation.

Histone (102 residues)

SEQUENCE

SGRGKGGKGLGKGGAKRHRKVLRDNIQGITKPAIRRLARRGGVKRISGLIYEETRG-
VLKVFLENVIRDAVTYTEHAKRKTVTAMDVVYALKRQGRTLYGFGG

REACTIVE SITES

.N.(2)	.D.(3)	.M.(1)	.Q.(2)
25 DNI	24 RDN	84 AMD	27 IQG
64 ENV	68 RDA		93 RQG
	85 MDV		

HYDROFLEX PLOT

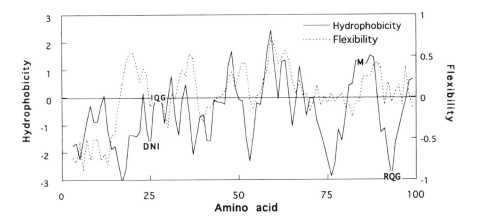

PREDICTED REACTIVITY AND DEGRADATION OF HISTONE

The amino acid sequence of histone from several species was carried out as part of a study on histone evolution (Hayashi *et al.*, 1982). The authors found that histone-H4 (one of the fractionated histones in this study) showed microheterogeneity at Asn-25 after purification, where some Asp-25 was detected. Asn-25 resides within the -DNI- primary sequence motif, one that is thought to be fairly unreactive because of the neighboring Ile. Isolation of histone-H4 was done using several steps that might promote deamidation, including storage of the denatured protein with 2-mercaptoethanol at pH 8 and 40°C, an extraction and separation at pH 2.8, and purification using a pyridine–performic acid gradient at 55°C. No controls were carried out to determine if this unusual deamidation reaction occurred during the work-up or if the deamidation would occur in pH 4.5–7.5 formulation buffer.

- **Hypoxanthine-Guanine Phosphoribosyltransferase (HXGT) (217 residues)**

SEQUENCE

ATRSPGVVISDDEPGYDLDLFCIPNHYAEDLERVFIPHGLIMDRTERLARDVMKEMG-
GHHIVALCVLKGGYKFFADLLDYIKALNRNSDRSIPMTVDFIRLKSYCNDQSTGDIK-
VIGGDDLSTLTGKNVLIVEDIIDTGKTMQTLLSLVRQYNPKMVKVASLLVKRTPRSV-
GYKPDFVGFEIPDKFVVGYALDYNEYFRDLNHVCVISETGKAKYKA

REACTIVE SITES

.N.(8)	.D.(21)		.M.(6)	.Q.(3)
25 PNH	11 SDD	107 NDQ	42 IMD	108 DQS
85 LNR	12 DDE	112 GDI	53 VMK	143 MQT
87 RNS	17 YDL	119 GDD	56 EMG	151 RQY
106 CND	19 LDL	120 DDL	94 PMT	
128 KNV	30 EDL	134 EDI	142 TMQ	
153 YNP	43 MDR	137 IDT	156 KMV	
195 YNE	51 RDV	176 PDF		
202 LNH	76 ADL	184 PDK		
	79 LDY	193 LDY		
	89 SDR	200 RDL		
	97 VDF			

HYDROFLEX PLOT

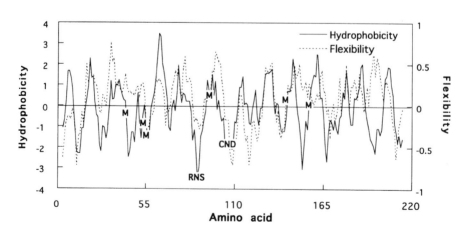

PREDICTED REACTIVITY AND DEGRADATION OF HXGT

This protein has several Met residues, suggesting that this may be one of the predominant degradation pathways. In addition, it has an Asn-Ser motif that may be expected to be mildly reactive. Isolation and purification of HXGT from normal human erythrocytes afforded a tetrameric product that showed heterogeneity after tryptic digestion and peptide mapping (Wilson *et al.*, 1982). The heterogeneity was localized to a peptide spanning Ser-103 to Lys-114, which encompasses Asn-106 within the -CND- motif. Although the work-up used in this paper included strong acid (9% formic acid), sufficient control experiments were carried out to show that this deamidation was not due to the work-up but to *in vivo* deamidation. No control experiments were carried out to show that the same deamidation reaction occurs in pH 4.5–7.5 buffer. No oxidation was reported.

Insulin (human)

SEQUENCE (A CHAIN) (21 residues)

GIVEQCCTSICSLYQIENYCN

SEQUENCE (B CHAIN) (30 residues)

FVNQHLCGSHLVEALYLVCGERGFFYTPKT

REACTIVE SITES (A CHAIN)

.N.(2)	.D.(0)	.M.(0)	.Q.(2)
18 ENY			5 EQC
21 CN			15 YQI

REACTIVE SITES (B CHAIN)

.N.(1)	.D.(0)	.M.(0)	.Q.(1)
3 VNQ			4 NQH

HYDROFLEX PLOT

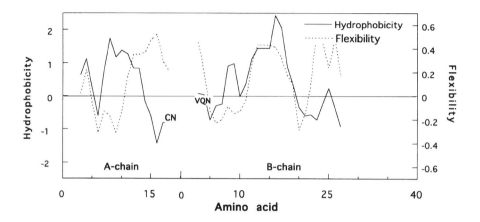

PREDICTED REACTIVITY AND DEGRADATION OF HUMAN INSULIN

Insulin contains three Asn and two Gln that might be available for hydrolytic degradation. None of these residues, however, are predicted to be particularly susceptible to degradation based on their primary sequence, in that the motifs of highest reactivity, -XNG-, -XNS-, -XDG-, and -XQG-, are absent in insulin. Of the three Asn motifs in insulin, the -VNQ- would be predicted to be more reactive than the -ENY- or the -CN motifs, based on the deamidation rates in model peptides (Robinson and Rudd, 1974). Inspection of the hydropathy plots for insulin shows that the Asn-3 residue is in a region of intermediate hydrophobicity and flexibility. The major degradation pathway of insulin at neutral pH was deamidation of an Asn-3 in the B chain (Asn-B3), giving a mixture of Asp-3 and iso-Asp-3 (Brange *et al.*, 1992). The stability data also suggested that this deamidation at neutral pH is fairly slow, where only 0.05% per month was lost, corresponding to a shelf life of several years. Although of limited utility for the prediction of insulin stability at neutral pH, it was also noted that deamidation under acidic conditions occurred predominantly at Asn-21 in the A chain (Asn-A21) (Darrington and Anderson, 1994, 1995), where the reaction proceeded via rate-limiting formation of a cyclic anhydride intermediate.

● **Insulin-like Growth Factor I (IGF-I) (70 residues)**

SEQUENCE

GPETLCGAELVDALQFVCGDRGFYFNKPTGYGSSSRRAPQTGIVDECCFRSCDLRR-
LEMYCAPLKPAKSA

REACTIVE SITES

.N.(1)	.D.(4)	.M.(1)	.Q.(2)
26 FNK	12 VDA	59 EMY	15 LQF
	20 GDR		40 PQT
	45 VDE		
	53 CDL		

HYDROFLEX PLOT

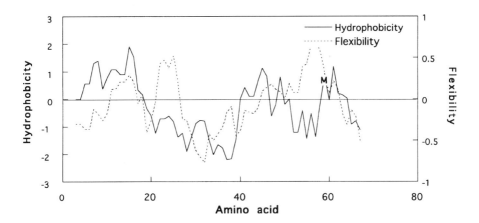

PREDICTED REACTIVITY AND DEGRADATION OF IGF-I

Inspection of the primary sequence shows that IGF-I is missing the traditional hot spots for hydrolytic degradation, in that it is missing Asn-Gly, Asn-Ser, Asp-Gly, Asp-Pro, and Gln-Gly. There is a single Met (Met-59) found in a fairly hydrophobic region of low flexibility. Based on the primary amino acid sequence and the hydroflex plot, IGF-I is predicted to be a stable protein to hydrolytic and oxidative degradation. The major degradation route for IGF-I at pH 6 was found to be oxidation at Met-59; there was also some evidence for minor amounts of the des-Gly-Pro product formed by diketopiperazine formation (which is favored by Pro at position 2) (Poulter *et al.*, 1990). The sum of these degradation products did not compromise the shelf life of the product, where IGF-I was stable for more than 2 years at 2–8°C.

- **Insulinotropin (26 residues)**

SEQUENCE

GTFTSDVSSYLEGQAAKEFIAWLVKG

REACTIVE SITES

.N.(0)	.D.(1)	.M.(0)	.Q.(1)
	6 SDV		14 GQA

HYDROFLEX PLOT

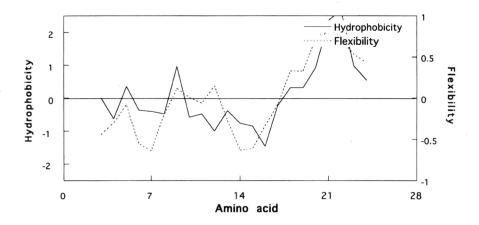

PREDICTED REACTIVITY AND DEGRADATION OF INSULINOTROPIN

Insulinotropin does not have the traditional hot spots and so is predicted to be fairly stable in aqueous solution. As an aside, this peptide has a highly hydrophobic C-terminal region and may be expected to show adsorption to surfaces and filters (Brophy and Lambert, 1994). This peptide is formulated in aqueous solution at pH containing 22.6% dextran to promote once-a-day subcutaneous injection. Under these conditions it was found that this peptide degraded fairly rapidly (t_{90} = ~40 hr at 25°C) giving biphasic kinetics (Heller and Qi, 1994). Excipient and degradation studies suggest that the Trp moiety is the reactive site in this peptide, corroborated by a significant loss in the absorption spectra at 300 nm.

Interferon-alpha-2b (human) (IFN-α-2b) (165 residues)

SEQUENCE

CDLPQTHSLGSRRTLMLLAQMRRISLFSCLKDRHDFGFPQEEFGNQFQKAETIPVLH-
EMIQQIFNLFSTKDSSAAWDETLLDKFYTELYQQLNDLEACVIQGVGVTETPLMKE-
DSILAVRKYFQRITLYLKEKKYSPCAWEVVRAEIMRSFSLSTNLQESLRSKE

REACTIVE SITES

.N.(4)	.D.(8)	.M.(5)	.Q.(12)
45 GNQ	2 CDL	16 LML	5 PQT
65 FNL	32 KDR	21 QMR	20 AQM
93 LND	35 HDF	59 EMI	40 PQE
156 TNL	71 KDS	111 LMK	46 NQF
	77 WDE	148 IMR	48 FQK
	82 LDK		61 IQQ
	94 NDL		62 QQI
	114 EDS		90 YQQ
			91 QQL
			101 IQG
			124 FQR
			158 LQE

HYDROFLEX PLOT

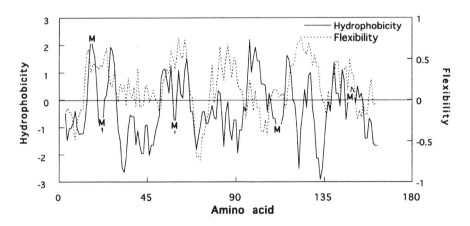

PREDICTED REACTIVITY AND DEGRADATION OF IFN-α-2b

This protein does not have any hydrolytic hot spots, so the main degradation routes (if any) would likely be due to Met oxidation. The Met-111 variant was isolated by RP-HPLC and identified by tryptic mapping and mass spectral studies (Gitlin *et al.*, 1995). The oxidation of Met-111 did not affect the biological activity of this protein. Further, this variant was observed after fermentation and likely was not a formulation degradation product. Upon storage of IFN-α-2b in pH 7.2 phosphate buffer, there was some evidence for deamidation upon high-temperature thermal stress studies, but no extrapolation was made to determine the extent of deamidation at 2–8°C. These thermal stress studies did not increase the rate of Met oxidation at neutral pH.

• Interferon-beta (IFN-β) (166 residues)

SEQUENCE

MSYNLLGFLQRSSNFQCQKLLWQLNGRLEYCLKDRMNFDIPEEIKQLQQFQKEDA-
ALNIYEMLQNIFAIFRQDSSSTGWNETIVENLLANVYHQINHLKTVLEEKLEKEDFT-
RGKLMSSLHLKRYYGRILHYLKAKEYSHCAWTIVRVEILRNFYFINRLTGYLRN

REACTIVE SITES

.N.(13)		.D.(5)	.M.(3)	.Q.(11)	
4 YNL	86 ENL	34 KDR	36 RMN	10 LQR	51 FQK
14 SNF	90 ANV	39 FDI	62 EML	16 FQC	64 LQN
25 LNG	96 INH	54 EDA	117 LMS	18 CQK	72 RQD
37 MNF	153 RNF	73 QDS		23 WQL	94 HQI
58 LNI	158 INR	110 EDF		46 KQL	
65 QNI	166 RN			48 LQQ	
80 WNE				49 QQF	

HYDROFLEX PLOT

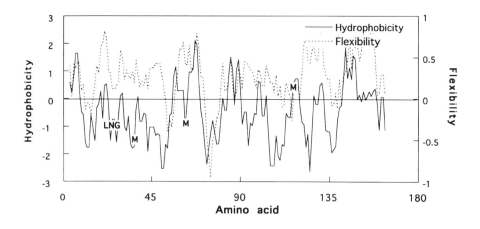

PREDICTED REACTIVITY AND DEGRADATION OF IFN-β

This protein has only a few sites predicted to be reactive, including an Asn-Gly (-LNG-) and three Mets. The Asn-Gly motif is located within a region predicted to be fairly hydrophilic but only moderately flexible. Stability studies of Ser-17-IFN-β at pH 5.5 with 0.1% SDS at 4°C for 1 year showed no detectable degradation of IFN-β by bioassay, SDS-PAGE, or RP-HPLC (Geigert *et al.*, 1988). Unfortunately no methods were used that were specific for detecting charged variants (such as an -LNG- to an -LDG- conversion), so it is uncertain whether the Asn-Gly residue reacts at 4°C. Oxidation of Met-62 was reported in liquid parenteral formulations under "conditions specific for Met oxidation" (Lin *et al.*, 1995). This protein was also found to be unstable in biological media (although the degradation pathway was not determined), indicative that the formulation and *ex vivo* stabilities may be different and depend on the nature of both the protein and the biological fluid (O'Kelley *et al.*, 1985).

Interferon-gamma (human) (γ-IFN) (144 residues)

SEQUENCE

MQDPYVKEAENLKKYFNAGHSDVADNGTLFLGILKNWKEESDRKIMQSQIVSFYF-
KLFKNFKDDQSIQKSVETIKEDMNVKFFNSNKKKRDDFEKLTNYSVTDLNVQRKAI-
HELIQVMAELSPAAKTGKRKRSQMLFRGRRASQ

REACTIVE SITES

.N.(10)		.D.(10)		.M.(4)		.Q.(9)	
11	ENL	3	QDP	46	IMQ	2	MQD
17	FNA	22	SDV	78	DMN	47	MQS
26	DNG	25	ADN	118	VMA	49	SQI
36	KNW	42	SDR	135	QML	65	DQS
60	KNF	63	KDD			68	IQK
79	MNV	64	DDQ			107	VQR
84	FNS	77	EDM			116	IQV
86	SNK	91	RDD			134	SQM
98	TNY	92	DDF			144	SQ
105	LNV	103	TDL				

HYDROFLEX PLOT

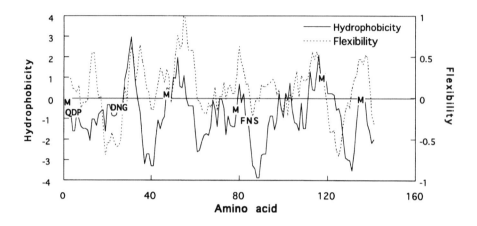

PREDICTED REACTIVITY AND DEGRADATION OF INTERFERON-GAMMA

γ-IFN has only a few sites predicted to undergo hydrolytic degradation (Asn-26, Asn-84). Asn-26 is predicted to be the faster of the two, based on primary amino acid sequence (Asn-26 is adjacent to Gly; Asn-84 is adjacent to Ser). Both Asn are found in regions of similar hydrophobicity, but Asn-26 is in a region of greater flexibility. It is not surprising that reaction at Asp was not observed, in that none of the Asp in γ-IFN are predicted hot spots based on primary sequence (no -XDG-). Similarly, there are nine Gln in γ-IFN, but again none are traditional hot spots (no -XQG-). The major degradation pathway of γ-IFN at neutral pH was found to be deamidation at Asn-26 and Asn-84 (Pearlman and Nguyen, 1992; Keck, 1995). A minor amount of Met oxidation was observed at Met-1 and Met-135. No evidence was found for cleavage at the -QDP- motif, nor reaction at Asp or Gln. At pH 5, the sum of these reaction rates did not compromise shelf life when the product is stored at 2–8°C. Interestingly, the covalent dimerization of γ-IFN has also been reported (Lauren et al., 1993).

- **Interleukin-1 Receptor Antagonist (IL-1RA) (153 residues)**

SEQUENCE

MRPSGRKSSKMQAFRIWDVNQKTFYLRNNQLVAGYLQGPNVNLEEKIDVVPIEPHA-
LFLGIHGGKMCLSCVKSGDETRLQLEAVNITDLSENRKQDKRFAFIRSDSGPTTSFES-
AACPGWFLCTAMEADQPVSLTNMPDEGVNVTKFYFQEDE

REACTIVE SITES

.N.(9)		.D.(9)		.M.(5)		.Q.(8)	
20	VNQ	18	WDV	1	MR	12	MQA
28	RNN	48	IDV	11	KMQ	21	NQK
29	NNQ	75	GDE	66	KMC	30	NQL
40	PNV	88	TDL	126	AME	37	LQG
42	VNL	96	QDK	137	NMP	80	LQL
85	VNI	105	SDS			95	KQD
92	ENR	129	ADQ			130	DQP
136	TNM	139	PDE			150	FQE
143	VNV	152	EDE				

HYDROFLEX PLOT

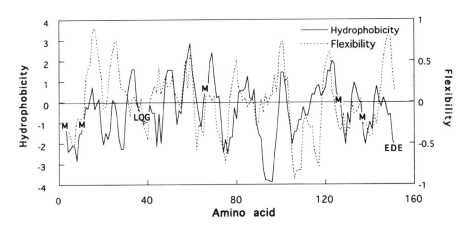

PREDICTED REACTIVITY AND DEGRADATION OF IL-1RA

This protein has few reactive hot spots and is predicted to be fairly stable because the few reactive sites (Met and Gln-Gly) are often not shelf-life-limiting. The degradation of IL-1RA has been studied in some detail, and a number of unusual reaction sites have been observed (Maneri, 1994). IL-1RA formed a stable cyclic imide at Asp-152 (in the -EDE- motif) and underwent disulfide formation at Cys-68–Cys-71, and cyclization between the N- and C-termini of des-Glu-153. Minor degradation pathways were oxidation at the N-terminal Met (Met-1) and deamidation of Asn-136 (in the -TNM- motif). The pH of maximum stability was near pH 6, and aggregation was the primary route of degradation (and so not applicable to this analysis).

- **Interleukin-1α (IL-1α) (155 residues)**

SEQUENCE

SFLSNVKYNFMRIIKYEFILNDALNQSIIRANDQYLTAAALHNLDEAVKFDMGAYKS-
SKDDAKITVILRISKTQLYVTAQDEDQPVLLKEMPEIPKTITGSETNLLFFWETHGTK-
NYFTSVAHPNLFIATKQDYWVCLAGGPPSITDFQILENQA

REACTIVE SITES

.N.(10)	.D.(10)	.M.(3)	.Q.(8)
5 SNV	22 DNA	11 FMR	26 NQS
9 YNF	33 NDQ	52 DMG	34 DQY
21 LND	45 LDE	91 EMP	74 TQL
25 LNQ	51 FDM		80 AQD
32 AND	60 KDD		84 DQP
43 HNL	61 DDA		132 KQD
104 TNL	81 QDE		149 FQI
116 KNY	83 EDQ		154 NQA
125 PNL	133 QDY		
153 ENQ	147 TDF		

HYDROFLEX PLOT

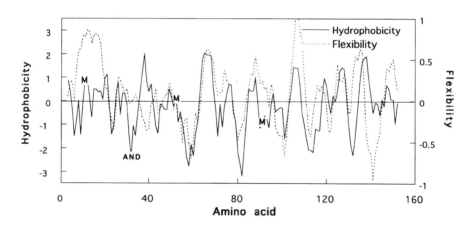

PREDICTED REACTIVITY AND DEGRADATION OF IL-1α

　　IL-1α lacks all of the traditional hydrolysis hot spots: Asn-Gly, Asn-Ser, Asp-Gly, and Gln-Gly. IL-1α contains three Met residues, and all of them are found in regions predicted to be fairly rigid, although it is not known if this should inhibit their oxidation. Based on the hydroflex plot, it is predicted that IL-1α should be fairly stable. The only residue found to degrade was Asn-32 (-AND-) giving a $t_{1/2}$ of approximately 25–30 hr at pH 7.5 and 42°C, considered accelerated reaction conditions. In retrospect, it is perhaps not surprising that reaction was observed at this site, in that it exists in a hydrophilic region of intermediate flexibility. Perhaps even more surprising is that this site is significantly more reactive than would be expected based on the reactivity found in small peptides (Robinson and Rudd, 1974). For example, the peptide GTND (where the TNX sequence is more reactive than the ANX motif) showed a half-life of 380 hr under the similar reaction conditions of pH 7.5 and 37°C, significantly longer than observed for the -AND- motif of IL-1α. The major degradation pathway of IL-1α at both pH 7.5 and pH 10.5 was found to be deamidation at Asn-32 (Wingfield *et al.*, 1987). This is in agreement with deamidation found in recombinant IL-1α purified from *E. coli*, as identified by the appearance of pI bands at 5.45 and 5.20, and by ¹H-NMR. Similar results were observed in another study describing the development of a deamidation-specific ELISA for detection of Asn-32-IL-1α and Asp-32-IL-1α (Sunahara *et al.*, 1989). No evidence was reported for Met oxidation. Unfortunately, the stability data presented in the literature were insufficient to determine whether or not this deamidation reaction proceeds sufficiently fast to compromise product shelf life at 2–8°C. IL-1α provides a clear cut example showing that the prediction of protein reactivity is not straightforward, when basing the prediction on a primary sequence analysis and reactivity in small peptides of similar motif. It is satisfying to find that Asn-32 is harbored in a hydrophilic region of intermediate flexibility. IL-1α also shows that the -XND- motif can be sufficiently reactive in aqueous solution that it may become the dominant site of degradation if other, more reactive sites (such as Asn-Gly, Asn-Ser, Asp-Gly, and Gln-Gly) are not available.

Interleukin-1β (human) (IL-1β) (153 residues)

SEQUENCE

APVRSLNCTLRDSQQKSLVMSGPYELKALHLQGQDMEQQVVFSMSFVQGEESNDK-
IPVALGLKEKNLYLSCVLKDDKPTLQLESVDPKNYPKKKMEKRFVFNKIEINNKLEF-
ESAQFPNWYISTSQAENMPVFLGGTKGGQDITDFTMQFVSS

REACTIVE SITES

.N.(9)	.D.(8)	.M.(6)	.Q.(12)	
7 LNC	12 RDS	20 VMS	14 SQQ	116 AQF
53 SND	35 QDM	36 DME	15 QQK	126 SQA
66 KNL	54 NDK	44 SMS	32 LQG	141 GQD
89 KNY	75 KDD	95 KME	34 GQD	149 MQF
102 FNK	76 DDK	130 NMP	38 EQQ	
107 INN	86 VDP	148 TMQ	39 QQV	
108 NNK	142 QDI		48 VQG	
119 PNW	145 TDF		81 LQL	
129 ENM				

HYDROFLEX PLOT

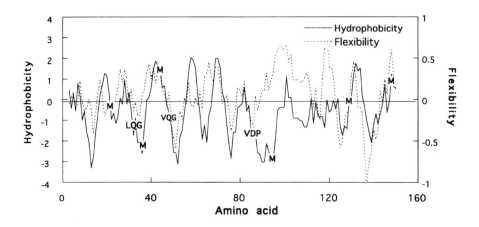

PREDICTED REACTIVITY AND DEGRADATION OF IL-1β

    Inspection of the human sequence suggests that the most likely site for deamidation is
either Gln-32 or Gln-48. Although these Gln are preceded by bulky hydrophobic residues
(-LQG- and -VQG-) that are deactivating, both of these Gln are in regions of moderate
hydrophobicity and flexibility which may allow their reaction. An alternative, but less likely,
reaction site is Asn-53 (-SND-), in that it is activated by the preceding Ser and exists in a region
predicted to be hydrophilic and flexible. The major degradation pathway of IL-1β at neutral
pH and temperatures less than 30°C was reported to be deamidation, although the site of
deamidation was not determined (Gu *et al.*, 1991). It was reported that murine recombinant
IL-1β selectively deamidated at Asn-32 (-LNG-), but this sequence is not found in human
IL-1β, as it is modified to contain Gln (-LQG-) of lower chemical reactivity (Daumy *et al.*,
1991). Modification at this site did not lead to complete inactivity, wherein the deamidated
product had ~50% of the original activity. The reactivity of IL-1β was sufficiently slow at
temperatures less than 5°C that it was predicted that this reaction would not compromise the
formulation shelf life. H_2O_2-catalyzed oxidation has been observed at Met-20, Met-36 or -44,
Met-130, and Met-148 (Foster, 1996).

●   **Interleukin-1β (murine) (152 residues)**

SEQUENCE

VPIRQLHYRLRDEQQKSLVLSDPYELKALHLNGQNINQQVIFSMSFVQGEPSNDKIP-
VALGLKGKNLYLSCVMKDGTPTLQLESVDPKQYPKKKMEKRFVFNKIEVKSKVEF-
ESAEFPNWYISTSQAEHKPVFLGNNSGQDIIDFTMESVSS

REACTIVE SITES

.N.(9)	.D.(7)	.M.(4)	.Q.(11)
32 LNG	12 RDE	44 SMS	5 RQL
35 QNI	22 SDP	73 VMK	14 EQQ
37 INQ	54 NDK	95 KME	15 QQK
53 SND	75 KDG	147 TME	34 GQN
66 KNL	86 VDP		38 NQQ
102 FNK	141 QDI		39 QQV
119 PNW	144 IDF		48 VQG
136 GNN			81 LQL
137 NNS			89 KQY
			126 SQA
			140 GQD

HYDROFLEX PLOT

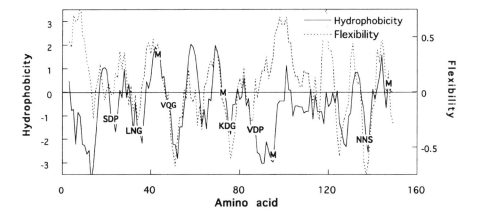

PREDICTED REACTIVITY AND DEGRADATION OF IL-1β (MURINE)

Inspection of the hydroflex plot shows that the -LNG- motif (Asn-32) lies in a hydrophilic region of moderate flexibility and is the most likely reaction site. Interestingly, Asn-137 (-NNS-) also resides in a hydrophilic flexible region and may also react slightly. Comparison of the amino acid sequences for human and murine IL-1β show that neither of these predicted hot spots is available for reaction on human IL-1β, so it is expected that murine and human IL-1β should have different degradation pathways (see comparison of sequences in Scheme 11). Incubation of murine IL-1β in pH 8.5 aqueous solution at 37°C for 35 hr afforded deamidated IL-1β, where deamidation occurred primarily at Asn-32 (original numbering, Asn-149). Although the tryptic maps on IL-1β (murine) were inconclusive for deamidation in several regions of the molecule, they did show that the C-terminal end (containing the -NNS- motif) did not undergo chemical reaction. Insufficient data were reported to predict the shelf life of this molecule at pH 4.5–7.5 or at 2–8°C.

```
                  10        20        30        40        50
IL1h  APVRSLNCTLRDSQQKSLVMSGPYELKALHLQGQDMEQQVVFSMSFVQGE
      *.* *.   *** ****** * ********* **   *** *********
IL1m  VPIRQLHYRLRDEQQKSLVLSDPYELKALHLNGQNINQQVIFSMSFVQGE
                  10        20        30        40        50

                  60        70        80        90       100
IL1h  ESNDKIPVALGLKEKNLYLSCVLKDDKPTLQLESVDPKNYPKKKMEKRFV
      ************ ******** **  *********** .**********
IL1m  PSNDKIPVALGLKGKNLYLSCVMKDGTPTLQLESVDPKQYPKKKMEKRFV
                  60        70        80        90       100

                 110       120       130       140       150
IL1h  FNKIEINNKLEFESAQFPNWYISTSQAENMPVFLGGTKGGQDITDFTMQF
      *****...* ***** ************. **** *  .**** ****.
IL1m  FNKIEVKSKVEFESAEFPNWYISTSQAEHKPVFL-GNNSGQDIIDFTMES
                 110       120       130       140

IL1h  VSS
      ***
IL1m  VSS
         150
```

Scheme 11.   Comparison of amino acid sequences for human and murine IL-1β.

● **Interleukin-2 (IL-2) (133 residues)**

SEQUENCE

APTSSSTKKTQLQLEHLLLDLQMILNGINNYKNPKLTRMLTFKFYMPKKATELKHL-
QCLEEELKPLEEVLNLAQSKNFHLRPRDLISNINVIVLELKGSETTFMCEYADETATIV-
EFLNRWITFCQSIISTLT

REACTIVE SITES

.N.(9)	.D.(3)	.M.(4)	.Q.(6)
26 LNG	20 LDL	23 QMI	11 TQL
29 INN	84 RDL	39 RML	13 LQL
30 NNY	109 ADE	46 YMP	22 LQM
33 KNP		104 FMC	57 LQC
71 LNL			74 AQS
77 KNF			126 CQS
88 SNI			
90 INV			
119 LNR			

HYDROFLEX PLOT

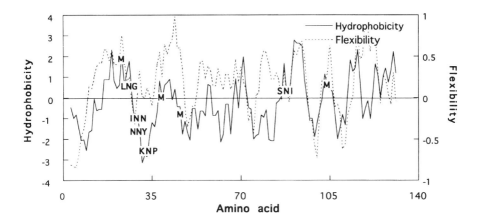

PREDICTED REACTIVITY AND DEGRADATION OF IL-2

The primary amino acid sequence for IL-2 shows one site (Asn-26 in the -LNG- motif) that should be fairly reactive at neutral pH range. The hydroflex plot shows that this is in a fairly hydrophobic and only weakly flexible region which may be expected to reduce its reactivity somewhat. Thus, it was somewhat surprising that Asn-88 was found to be the predominant, albeit very slow, site of reaction. This Asn is harbored within a motif predicted to be fairly unreactive (-SNI-) because of the sterically constrained Ile next to the Asn. Further, this motif is also located in a region not predicted to be hydrophilic or flexible, so it is not expected to show enhanced reactivity due to the nature of its environment. There was little correlation between Met reactivity and predicted hydropathy of the Met-containing motifs; Met-104 is both hydrophobic and fairly inflexible according to the hydroflex calculation. The degradation of IL-2 is not straightforward, in that conflicting results have been obtained from different laboratories. Recombinant IL-2 stored at pH 5.0 and 25°C for several months resulted in deamidation of Asn-88 as assayed by RP-HPLC. The deamidated IL-2 was of similar bioactivity to the parent molecule. It was also noted that this deamidation reaction was fairly slow, and none was found to occur at 5°C over the same time period (Sasaoki *et al.*, 1992). It has also been noted that the primary degradation sites were, in reactive order, Asn-29, Asn-30, Asn-33 and no detectable degradation at Asn-26 or Asn-88 (Hora, 1995). IL-2 also underwent oxidative degradation, predominantly at Met-104, when stored at pH 5 and 25°C over 180 days (Sasaoki *et al.*, 1989). Secondary sites of oxidation were Met-23 and Met-39; no oxidation was found at Met-46.

● **Interleukin-11 (human) (178 residues)**

SEQUENCE

PGPPPGPPRVSPDPRAELDSTVLLTRSLLADTRQLAAQLRDKFPADGDHNLDSLPTL-
AMSAGALGALQLPGVLTRLRADLLSYLRHVQWLRRAGGSSLKTLEPELGTLQARL-
DRLLRRLQLLMSRLALPQPPPDPPAPPLAPPSSAWGGIRAAHAILGGLHLTLDWAVR-
GLLLLKTRL

REACTIVE SITES

.N.(1)	.D.(11)	.M.(2)	.Q.(7)
50 HNL	13 PDP	59 AMS	34 RQL
	19 LDS	123 LMS	38 AQL
	31 ADT		68 LQL
	41 RDK		88 VQW
	46 ADG		109 LQA
	48 GDH		120 LQL
	52 LDS		130 PQP
	79 ADL		
	113 LDR		
	134 PDP		
	165 LDW		

HYDROFLEX PLOT

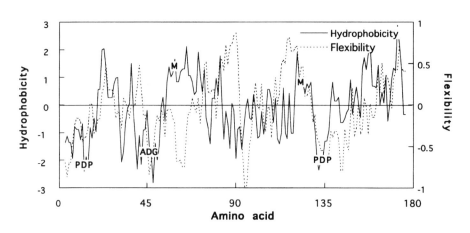

PREDICTED REACTIVITY AND DEGRADATION OF INTERLEUKIN-11

The hydroflex plot for IL-11 shows that there are only a few predicted reactive sites for degradation. These include two Asp-Pro linkages that may be susceptible to acid-catalyzed cleavage: Asp-Gly, which may form iso-Asp-Gly, and Met oxidation. An excellent study on IL-11 degradation by Ingram and Warne (1994) included the effect of pH on the different pathways and degradation due to dimerization and aggregation. Briefly, IL-11 showed cleavage between Asp-13–Pro-14 and Asp-134–Pro-135 under acid conditions, but only minor amounts of cleavage at pH 7.2 after 146 days. IL-11 also showed some deamidation at higher pHs at Asn-50 (6.2%/wk at pH 9.6 and 30°C), but only minor amounts at lower pHs (0.19%/wk at pH 5.5 at 30°C). Based on these rates, it is roughly predicted that deamidation at these sites would not compromise the shelf life at 2–8°C. Some oxidation of Met-59 was also observed, especially at lower pH, but was minor at neutral pH for most of the buffers studied. No degradation of the Asp-Gly site was reported (-ADG-), although it is unknown whether the analytical methods used would have detected this.

Lung Surfactant SP-C (human) (34 residues)   ●

SEQUENCE

GIPSSPVHLKRLLIVVVVVVLIVVVIVGALLMGL

REACTIVE SITES

.N.(0)   .D.(0)   .M.(1)   .Q.(0)
_____
                  32 LMG

HYDROFLEX PLOT

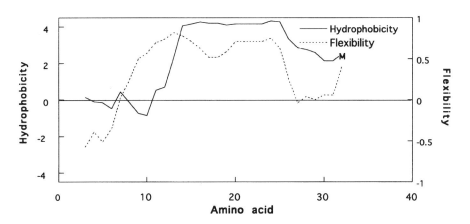

PREDICTED REACTIVITY AND DEGRADATION OF LUNG SURFACTANT

Recombinant human lung surfactant is predicted to be extremely resistant to hydrolytic degradation, notably because of a complete absence of reactive sites. Lung surfactant does have a single Met near its C-termini, although this is in a hydrophobic region that is predicted to be fairly inflexible. Lung surfactant did not show any hydrolysis after reconstitution and storage at 2–8°C after 1 month. This polypeptide was susceptible to oxidation at Met-32, the only site of predominant chemical reactivity.

- **Lysozyme (hen egg white) (129 residues)**

SEQUENCE

KVFGRCELAAAMKRHGLDNYRGYSLGNWVCAAKFESNFNTQATNRNTDGSTDYG-
ILQINSRWWCNDGRTPGSRNLCNIPCSALLSSDITASVNCAKKIVSDGNGMNAWVA-
WRNRCKGTDVQAWIRGCRL

REACTIVE SITES

.N.(14)		.D.(7)		.M.(2)	.Q.(3)
19 DNY	65 CND	18 LDN	12 AMK	41 TQA	
27 GNW	74 RNL	48 TDG	105 GMN	57 LQI	
37 SNF	77 CNI	52 TDY	121 VQA		
39 FNT	93 VNC	66 NDG			
44 TNR	103 GNG	87 SDI			
46 RNT	106 MNA	101 SDG			
59 INS	113 RNR	119 TDV			

HYDROFLEX PLOT

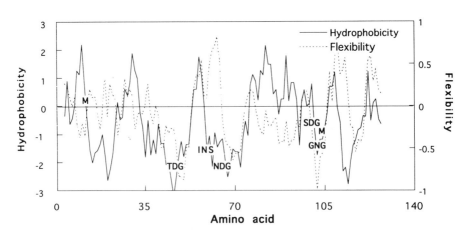

PREDICTED REACTIVITY AND DEGRADATION OF LYSOZYME

Inspection of the primary amino acid sequence for lysozyme shows that there are several reactive residues, including Asn-103 within the -GNG- motif, and several Asp-Gly residues. Based on this, it is anticipated that lysozyme should be fairly unstable in aqueous solution; indeed, anecdotal observations of lysozyme instability likely prompted the seminal peptide model studies of Robinson and colleagues (Robinson and Tedro, 1973b). Unfortunately, the degradation pathways of lysozyme itself were not studied in depth nor monitored using chromatographic techniques where subtle changes such as Asp conversion to iso-Asp would be detected. It was noted that the primary amino acid sequence consisted of Gly-Asp-Gly instead of Gly-Asn-Gly at positions 102–104 (Canfield, 1963), indicating a high propensity for deamidation at this reactive site. There is also another report showing cyclic imide formation of Asp-101 in the -SDG- motif when incubated at 40°C and pH 4 (Tomizawa *et al.*, 1994). This motif is known to be located within a solvent-accessible and flexible region. Interestingly, the -TDG- motif is also located in a region of predicted hydrophilicity and flexibility, and yet the authors did not report cyclic imide formation or iso-Asp formation at this site. No account of lysozyme oxidation was reported in aqueous formulation.

Myelin Basic Protein (MBP) (169 residues)   •

SEQUENCE

AAQKRPSQRSKYLASASTMDHARHGFLPRHRDTGILDSLGRFFGSDRGAPKRGSGK-
DGHHAARTTHYGSLPQKAQGHRPQDENPVVHFFKNIVTPRTPPPSQGKGRGRSLSR-
FSWGAEGQKPGFGYGGRASDYKSAHKGLKGHDAQGTLSKIFKLGGRDSRSGSPM-
ARR

REACTIVE SITES

.N.(2)	.D.(9)	.M.(2)	.Q.(8)
83 ENP	20 MDH	19 TMD	3 AQK
91 KNI	32 RDT	166 PMA	8 SQR
	37 LDS		72 PQK
	46 SDR		75 AQG
	57 KDG		80 PQD
	81 QDE		102 SQG
	132 SDY		120 GQK
	144 HDA		146 AQG
	159 RDS		

HYDROFLEX PLOT

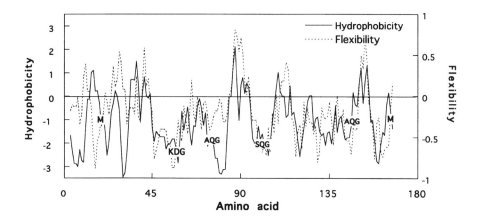

PREDICTED REACTIVITY AND DEGRADATION OF MYELIN BASIC PROTEIN

MBP has a single Asp-Gly (-KDG-) that may undergo cyclization and iso-Asp formation, as well as some Gln-Gly residues or predicted lesser reactivity. Both of these Gln are located in hydrophilic regions of modest flexibility. Isolation of bovine MBP resulted in partial deamidation of the Gln residues at positions 102 and 146 (corrected numbering) (Chou *et al.*, 1976). Unfortunately, it was not possible to distinguish whether the microheterogeneity was present in the original protein or was due to the work-up carried out at pH 10.4. There also exists a reactive Asp-Gly linkage, but it is unlikely that the paper chromatography methods used in this paper would isolate the iso-Asp product.

● **Neocarzinostatin (109 residues)**

SEQUENCE

AAPTATVTPSSGLSDGTVVKVAGAGLQAGTAYDVGQCASVNTGVLWNSVTAAGSA-
CDPANFSLTVRRSFQGFLFDFTRWGTVNCTTAACQVGLSDAAGDGQPGVAISFN

REACTIVE SITES

.N.(5)		.D.(6)		.M.(0)	.Q.(5)	
41 VNT	83 VNC	15 SDG	75 FDF		27 LQA	90 CQV
47 WNS	109 FN	33 YDV	95 SDA		36 GQC	101 GQP
60 ANF		57 CDP	99 GDG		70 FQG	

HYDROFLEX PLOT

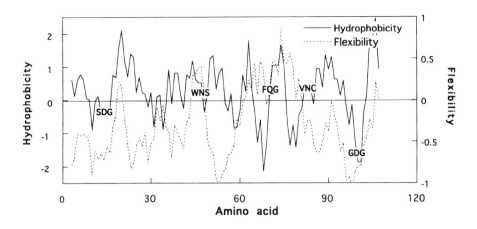

PREDICTED REACTIVITY AND DEGRADATION OF
NEOCARZINOSTATIN

Inspection of the primary amino acid sequence for neocarzinostatin shows that there are several reactive hydrolysis sites, including Asn-47 (-WNS-), Asp-15 (-SDG-), and Asp-99 (-GDG-). The Asn-47 site may be only mildly reactive, in that it is in a region of moderate hydrophobicity. On the other hand, Asp-99 is in a flexible, hydrophilic region and is expected to be reactive. Under weakly acidic conditions at 4°C the major degradation pathway of neocarzinostatin was conversion of Asn-83 to Asp-83 (Maeda and Kuromizu, 1977). No other degradation products were observed during the several-day course of the reaction. Because these experiments were carried out at pH 3.2 (somewhat lower than would likely be used in a protein parenteral liquid formation), the rate data obtained in this paper are of limited utility in determining the preferred pathway at intermediate pH or for estimating whether or not neocarzinostatin would exhibit a shelf life of 2 years between pH 5 and pH 7. This protein shows that reaction in aqueous solution may occur at sites other than the traditional hot spots (or that pH is crucial in making predictions and that data at pH 3 should not be used to predict the major degradation pathways at pH 5–7). From the methods used, it is unlikely that iso-Asp formation would have been detected at Asp-15 or Asp-99, so it is unknown whether or not reaction at these hot spots actually occurred.

Nerve Growth Factor (human) (NGF) (120 residues)   ●

SEQUENCE

SSSHPIFHRGEFSVCDSVSVWVGDKTTATDIKGKEVMVLGEVNINNSVFKQYFFETK-
CRDPNPVDSGCRGIDSKHWNSYCTTTHTFVKALTMDGKQAAWRFIRIDTACVCVLS-
RKAVRRA

REACTIVE SITES

.N.(5)	.D.(8)	.M.(2)	.Q.(2)
43 VNI	16 CDS	37 VMV	51 KQY
45 INN	24 GDK	92 TMD	96 KQA
46 NNS	30 TDI		
62 PNP	60 RDP		
77 WNS	65 VDS		
	72 IDS		
	93 MDG		
	105 IDT		

HYDROFLEX PLOT

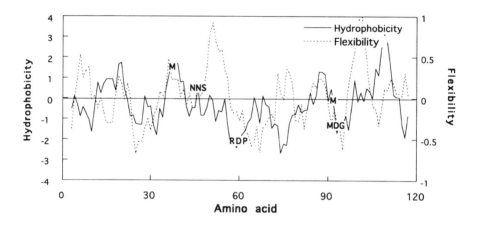

PREDICTED REACTIVITY AND DEGRADATION OF NGF

The primary sequence of NGF indicated that there are three hot spots for hydrolytic degradation: Asn-46 (-NNS-), Asp-93 (-MDG-), and Asp-60 (-RDP-). This last motif is sensitive to acid-catalyzed cleavage only, and is generally stable above pH 5 at 2–8°C. Of the other two motifs, Asp-93 resides in a hydrophilic region that is calculated to be fairly flexible, and so this site might be expected to be reactive. Asn-46 is adjacent to the Ser and is expected to be only moderately activated (as compared to Gly). It resides in a region of intermediate hydrophobicity and flexibility, and so may be expected to be only moderately reactive. Met-37 resides in a hydrophobic, inflexible region. It was shown that the primary degradation site in NGF at pH 5.5 was iso-Asp formation at Asp-93 (-MDG-). Only minor amounts of deamidation were observed at Asn-45 (-INN-), a site not predicted to be normally reactive, and it was believed that this may have occurred in the processing steps at higher pH. Also minor amounts of Met oxidation were found, both at Met-37 and Met-92. The sum of all these hydrolytic and oxidative degradation reactions did not compromise the shelf life of liquid parenteral formulations of NGF at 2–8°C.

Parathyroid Hormone (84 residues)

SEQUENCE

SVSEIQLMHNLGKHLNSMERVEWLRKKLQDVHNFVALGAPLAPRDAGSQRPRKKE-
DNVLVESHEKSLGEADKADVNVLTKAKSQ

REACTIVE SITES

.N.(5)	.D.(5)	.M.(2)	.Q.(4)
10 HNL	30 QDV	8 LMH	6 IQL
16 LNS	45 RDA	18 SME	29 LQD
33 HNF	56 EDN		49 SQR
57 DNV	71 ADK		84 SQ
76 VNV	74 ADV		

HYDROFLEX PLOT

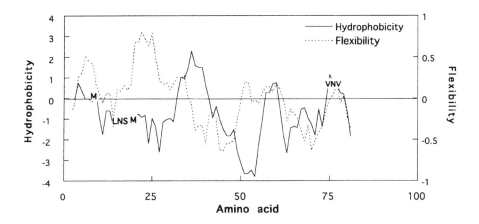

PREDICTED REACTIVITY AND DEGRADATION OF PARATHYROID HORMONE

This protein has only a few hot spots, including Asn-16 in the -LNS- motif and the Met sites. For years it was believed that parathyroid hormone contained Asp at position 76, in that all reports of extracted and purified human, bovine, or porcine parathyroid hormone contained Asp-76 (Keutmann *et al.*, 1978). Later, however, nucleotide sequencing of cloned cDNAs encoding human parathyroid hormone messenger RNA showed that the correct residue was Asn-76 (Hendy *et al.*, 1981). This is another dramatic example of *in vivo* deamidation and so complete that no microheterogeneity was observed at position 76. This reaction occurred at an unlikely site, that is, within the -VNV- motif. Further, this reactive site is in a region that is not particularly hydrophilic or flexible. No control experiments were carried out to show that the same deamidation reaction occurs in pH 4.5–7.5 formulation buffer. The oxidation of para-thyroid hormone has also been studied using H_2O_2 as catalyst. After incubation at pH 10 with 1 mM H_2O_2, both Met-8 and Met-18 were oxidized, giving the two monooxidized products, as well as the dioxidized product. Biological activity was reduced moreso after oxidation at Met-8 than Met-18 (Nabuchi *et al.*, 1995).

- **Relaxin**

SEQUENCE (A CHAIN) (24 residues)

QLYSALANKCCHVGCTKRSLARFC

SEQUENCE (B CHAIN) (29 residues)

DSWMEEVIKLCGRELVRAQIAICGMSTWS

REACTIVE SITES (A CHAIN)

.N.(1)	.D.(0)	.M.(0)	.Q.(0)
8 ANK			

REACTIVE SITES (B CHAIN)

.N.(0)	.D.(1)	.M.(2)	.Q.(1)
	1 DS	4 WME	19 AQI
		25 GMS	

HYDROFLEX PLOT

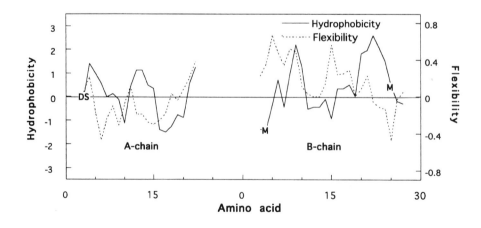

PREDICTED REACTIVITY AND DEGRADATION OF RELAXIN

This small protein has few predicted reactive sites, perhaps the likeliest being oxidation of the Met residues on the relaxin B chain. It was shown that the predominant cleavage pathway for relaxin at pH 3–5 was cleavage of the N-terminal Asp on the B chain (Nguyen *et al.*, 1993a). At pH 5–7, the major degradation pathways were again cleavage of this Asp, and oxidation of Met-4 and Met-25 on the B chain (Cipolla and Shire, 1991), in agreement with hydrogen peroxide-catalyzed oxidation studies (Nguyen *et al.*, 1993a). Disulfide scrambling occurred at higher pHs (Canova-Davis *et al.*, 1990, 1991).

Ribonuclease A (RNase A) (124 residues)   ●

SEQUENCE

KETAAAKFERQHMDSSTSAASSSNYCNQMMKSRNLTKDRCKPVNTFVHESLADV-
QAVCSQKNVACKNGQTNCYQSYSTMSITDCRETGSSKYPNCAYKTTQANKHIIVAC-
EGNPYVPVHFDASV

REACTIVE SITES

.N.(10)		.D.(5)	.M.(4)	.Q.(7)	
24 SNY	67 KNG	14 MDS	13 HMD	11 RQH	74 YQS
27 CNQ	71 TNC	38 KDR	29 QMM	28 NQM	101 TQA
34 RNL	94 PNC	53 ADV	30 MMK	55 VQA	
44 VNT	103 ANK	83 TDC	79 TMS	60 SQK	
62 KNV	113 GNP	121 FDA		69 GQT	

HYDROFLEX PLOT

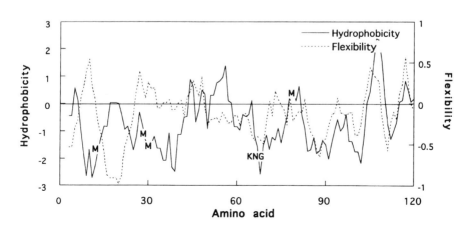

PREDICTED REACTIVITY AND DEGRADATION OF RNase A

Inspection of the primary amino acid sequence, and the hydropathy and flexibility plots for RNase A shows that there is a single site for facile hydrolytic degradation at Asn-67 in the -KNG- motif. Based on this, Asn-67 is the most likely site of degradation. There are also several Met residues found in fairly hydrophilic regions of varying flexibility. This protein degraded primarily at its predicted hot spot (Asn-67) at both low and high pH. Reaction under strong acid conditions at 30°C showed reaction at Asn-67 (Venkatesh and Vithayathil, 1984) as it did at pH 8 and above (Bornstein and Balian, 1970; Wearne and Creighton, 1989). The conformation of this protein played a major role in its rate of deamidation, as shown by deamidation studies of ribonuclease (Bornstein and Balian, 1970; Wearne and Creighton, 1989) where an Asn that ordinarily does not deamidate in the native structure deamidates in the denatured protein. The oxidative degradation pathways of RNase A have not been reported.

● **Ribonuclease U2 (RNase U2) (*Ustilago sphaerogena*) (114 residues)**

SEQUENCE

CDIPQSTNCGGNVYSNDDINTAIQGALDDVANGDRPDNYPHQYYDEASDQITLCC-
GSGPWSEFPLVYNGPYYSSRDNYVSPGPDRVIYQTNTGEFCATVTHTGAASYDGFT-
QCS

REACTIVE SITES

.N.(9)	.D.(12)	.M.(0)	.Q.(6)
8 TNC	2 CDI		5 PQS
12 GNV	17 NDD		24 IQG
16 SND	18 DDI		42 HQY
20 INT	28 LDD		50 DQI
32 ANG	29 DDV		89 YQT
38 DNY	34 GDR		112 TQC
68 YNG	37 PDN		
77 DNY	45 YDE		
91 TNT	49 SDQ		
	76 RDN		
	84 PDR		
	108 YDG		

HYDROFLEX PLOT

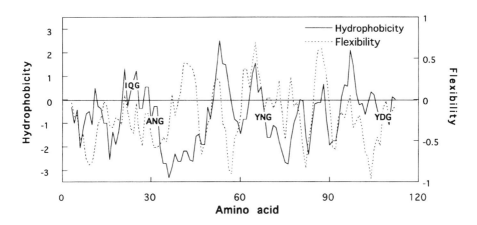

PREDICTED REACTIVITY AND DEGRADATION OF RNase U2

Inspection of the primary amino acid sequence and the hydropathy and flexibility plots for ribonuclease U2 shows that there is a site for facile hydrolytic degradation at Asn-32 in the -ANG- motif and another Asn-Gly in the -YNG- motif. There also exists an Asp-Gly near the C-termini that may be susceptible to iso-Asp formation. Isolation of this protein results in two isoforms, RNase U2-A and RNase U2-B, of which the major difference in these is a change in the protein pI (Kanaya and Uchida, 1986). Degradation of this protein at one of its predicted hot spots (Asn-32) is the cause of the RNase U2-B isoform, where an iso-Asp-Gly linkage was found. The catalyst for this deamidation reaction was not determined but was likely due to simple pH catalysis during work-up (although enzymatic catalysis during fermentation cannot be ruled out based on the conditions used). Of interest, there is also another Asn-Gly motif in RNase U2 (-YNG-) that is surprisingly resistant to hydrolytic modification. Asn-68 is in a region of similar predicted hydrophobicity, and only slightly less flexible than Asn-32, and remained stable as the Asn form.

Secretin (27 residues)   •

SEQUENCE

HSDGTFTSELSRLRDSARLQRLLQGLV

REACTIVE SITES

.N.(0)	.D.(2)	.M.(0)	.Q.(2)
	3 SDG		20 LQR
	15 RDS		24 LQG

HYDROFLEX PLOT

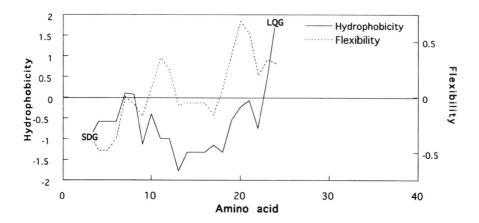

PREDICTED REACTIVITY AND DEGRADATION OF SECRETIN

The amino acid sequence for secretin is short, with a concomitant few number of reactive sites. Nevertheless, the predicted site of reactivity is reaction at Asp-3 (-SDG-), and this should predominate easily over reaction at Gln-24 in the -LQG- motif. The -SDG- motif is also found in a fairly hydrophilic and flexible environment, suggesting that reaction may be possible (this flexibility calculation may be of little value in a peptide of this size which is likely to be highly flexible through its entire length). The major degradation pathway of secretin at neutral pH was reaction at Asp-3 to give the iso-Asp-3 product (Tsuda *et al.*, 1990). In this study, the degradation of secretin was carried out at 60°C, much higher than the 2–30°C likely for storage of an aqueous secretin formulation. This example is still included, however, in that secretin is a small peptide rather than a protein, and data obtained at higher temperatures under accelerated stability conditions are likely to mimic the reaction pathway observed at lower temperatures. Unfortunately, these authors did not carry out their stability kinetics at different temperatures, so it is not possible to estimate the shelf life for secretin at 2–8°C.

● **Serine Hydroxymethyltransferase (SHMT) (rabbit) (483 residues)**

SEQUENCE

ATAVNGAPRDAALWSSHEQMLAQPLKDSDAEVYDIIKKESNRQRVGLELIASENFAS-
RAVLEALGSCLNNKYSEGYPGQRYYGGTEHIDELETLCQKRALQAYGLDPQCWGV-
NVQPYSGSPANFAVYTALVEPHGRIMGLDLPDGGHLTHGFMTDKKKISATSIFFESM-
AYKVNPDTGYIDYDRLEENARLFHPKLIIAGTSCYSRNLDYGRLRKIADENGAYLM-
ADMAHISGLVVAGVVPSPFEHCHVVTTTTHKTLRGCRAGMIFYRRGVRSVDPKTGK-
EILYNLESLINSAVFPGLQGGPHNHAIAGVAVALKQAMTPEFKEYQRQVVANCRAL-
SAALVELGYKIVTGGSDNHLILVDLRSKGTDGGRAEKVLEACSIACNKNTCPGDKS-
ALRPSGLRLGTPALTSRGLLEKDFQKVAHFIHRGIELTVQIQDDTGPRATLKEFKEKL-
AGDEKHQRAVRALRQEVESFAALFPLPGLPGF

REACTIVE SITES

.N.(18)	.D.(24)	.M.(8)	.Q.(17)
5 VNG	10 RDA	20 QML	19 EQM
41 SNR	27 KDS	138 IMG	23 AQP
54 ENF	29 SDA	153 FMT	43 RQR
69 LNN	34 YDI	169 SMA	79 GQR
70 NNK	89 IDE	225 LMA	96 CQK
113 VNV	106 LDP	228 DMA	101 LQA
123 ANF	141 LDL	265 GMI	108 PQC
174 VNP	144 PDG	319 AMT	115 VQP
188 ENA	155 TDK		300 LQG
207 RNL	176 PDT		317 KQA
220 ENG	181 IDY		327 YQR
286 YNL	183 YDR		329 RQV
292 INS	209 LDY		418 FQK
305 HNH	218 ADE		433 VQI
333 ANC	227 ADM		435 IQD
355 DNH	276 VDP		458 HQR
384 CNK	354 SDN		466 RQE
386 KNT	361 VDL		
	368 TDG		
	391 GDK		
	416 KDF		
	436 QDD		
	437 DDT		
	454 GDE		

HYDROFLEX PLOT

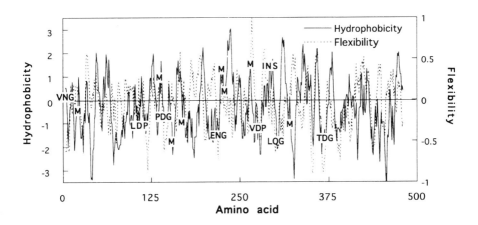

PREDICTED REACTIVITY AND DEGRADATION OF SHMT

There are several sites of potential reactivity in SHMT, including two Asn-Gly sites. The first, Asn-5, is found in a fairly flexible region of intermediate hydrophobicity and might be expected to show deamidation. The second, Asn-220, is found in a motif predicted to be fairly reactive (-ENG-) and is found in a hydrophilic flexible region. Other reactive hot spots include Asp-144 (-PDG-), Asp-368 (-TDG-), and Gln-300 (-LQG-), all of which are found in fairly hydrophilic, flexible regions of the protein. Artigues *et al.* (1990) demonstrated that SHMT deamidated *in vivo* at Asn-5 to give iso-Asp-5. In addition, they carried out a short set of control experiments and showed that this deamidation reaction was not a consequence of the purification work-up, and that deamidation occurred at pH 7.3 and 37°C. They found that the Asn-5 moiety in SHMT disappeared with a half-life of 450 hr, significantly slower than model peptides Ac-VNGA ($t_{1/2}$ = 80 hr) and Ac-ATAVNGAPRDAALW ($t_{1/2}$ = 70 hr) of the identical N-terminal sequence. The work-up procedure (chymotryptic cleavage of the N-terminal 15-mer followed by HPLC analysis) precluded determination of deamidation at other sites in the protein. No analysis was made to determine if Met oxidation occurred upon storage in aqueous solution. The degradation rate constants were determined at only 37°C, so no extrapolation can be made as to the stability at 2–8°C.

- **Tissue Factor-243 (243 residues)**

SEQUENCE

SGTTNTVAAYNLTWKSTNFKTILEWEPKPVNQVYTVQISTKSGDWKSKCFYTTDTE-
CDLTDEIVKDVKQTYLARVFSYPAGNVESTGSAGEPLYENSPEFTPYLETNLGQPTIQ-
SFEQVGTKVNVTVEDERTLVRRNNTFLSLRDVFGKDLIYTLYYWKSSSSGKKTAKT-
NTNEFLIDVDKGENYCFSVQAVIPSRTVNRKSTDSPVECMGQEKGEFREIFYIIGAVV-
FVVIILVIILAISLH

REACTIVE SITES

.N.(14)	.D.(11)	.M.(1)	.Q.(8)
5 TNT	44 GDW	210 CMG	32 NQV
11 YNL	54 TDT		37 VQI
18 TNF	58 CDL		69 KQT
31 VNQ	61 TDE		110 GQP
82 GNV	66 KDV		114 IQS
96 ENS	129 EDE		118 EQV
107 TNL	145 RDV		190 VQA
124 VNV	150 KDL		212 GQE
137 RNN	178 IDV		
138 NNT	180 VDK		
171 TNT	204 TDS		
173 TNE			
184 ENY			
199 VNR			

HYDROFLEX PLOT

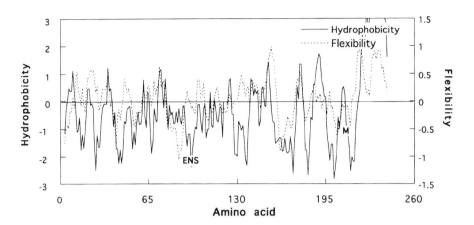

PREDICTED REACTIVITY AND DEGRADATION OF TISSUE FACTOR-243

Tissue factor is a blood coagulation protein cofactor which exists as a glycosylated integral membrane protein. A truncated form of tissue factor that includes the transmembrane domain (amino acids 1–243) has been developed, and some stability data exist for this truncated form. Inspection of the amino acid sequence of TF-243 shows that, even though there are a large number of Asn, Asp, and Gln, only one residue (Asn-96) in the -ENS- motif is a predicted hot spot. This motif containing Ser rather than Gly adjacent to Asn is predicted to be only moderately reactive. Note, however, that Asn-96 resides in a hydrophilic region, but of only intermediate flexibility. Formulation of the truncated form of tissue factor at 0.1 mg/ml and pH 7.3 in 10 mM isotonic pH 7.3 sodium phosphate and 0.8% octylglucoside showed no signs of degradation by several different methods when stored for 0.5 year at 2–8°C (Shire, 1995). No alterations in tissue factor were detected by SDS PAGE, size-exclusion chromatography, ELISA, chromogenic and clotting activity assays after 54 weeks at 2–8°C and at 25°C, when compared to a sample stored at −70°C. In the starting material stored at −70°C there were two bands at approximately pI 5.3, and after 54 weeks at 2–8°C another band was formed at ~pI of 5.2. At 25°C, the band at pI 5.2 was more intense than the doublet of bands at pI 5.3, and there was also an additional band at pI 5.0, whereas the original doublet at pI 5.3 was barely visible. The generation of acidic components suggests that deamidation occurred during storage, but was not conclusively proven. The activity of tissue factor as determined by a chromogenic assay remained unaltered after 54 weeks at 2–8°C but decreased by 33% during storage at 25°C. Extrapolation of these data suggest that TF-243 is sufficiently stable to permit storage at 2–8°C for at least 18 months.

• TGF-Beta (112 residues)

SEQUENCE

ALDTNYCFSSTEKNCCVRQLYIDFRKDLGWKWIHEPKGYHANFCLGPCPYIWSLDT-
QYSKVLALYNQHNPGASAAPCCVPQALEPLPIVYYVGRKPKVEQLSNMIVRSCKCS

REACTIVE SITES

.N.(6)		.D.(4)		.M.(1)	.Q.(5)	
5 TNY	66 YNQ	3 LDT	55 LDT	104 NMI	19 RQL	81 PQA
14 KNC	69 HNP	23 IDF			57 TQY	100 EQL
42 ANF	103 SNM	27 KDL			67 NQH	

HYDROFLEX PLOT

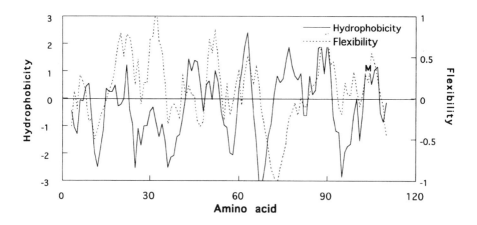

PREDICTED REACTIVITY AND DEGRADATION OF TGF-β

Inspection of the primary amino acid sequence reveals that TGF-β does not have any of the traditional hot spots for hydrolytic reactivity at neutral pH, in that Asn-Gly, Asn-Ser, Asp-Gly, and Asp-Pro are absent. TGF-β does have a single Met, and this is found in a region of predicted high hydrophobicity and decreased flexibility, possibly rendering this Met only weakly susceptible to oxidation. Recombinant TGF-β was remarkably stable and did not undergo noticeable chemical degradation in 0.1–1.0 mg/ml liquid formulations at pH 5 when stored for at least 1 year at 2–8°C. This is in good agreement with its hydroflex plot analysis, in that there are no traditional sites of reaction (except for a single Met in a nonflexible, hydrophobic environment).

Thrombopoietin (TPO) (332 residues)

●

SEQUENCE

SPAPPACDLRVLSKLLRDSHVLHSRLSQCPEVHPLPTPVLLPAVDFSLGEWKTQMEE-
TKAQDILGAVTLLEGVMAARGQLGPTCLSSLLGQLSGQVRLLLGALQSLLGTQLP-
PQGRTTAHKDPNAIFLSFQHLLRGKVRFLMLVGGSTLCVRRAPPTTAVPSRTSLVLTL-
NELPNRTSGLLETNFTASARTTGSGLLKWQQGFRAKIPGLLNQTSRSLDQIPGYLNRI-
HELLNGTRGLFPGPSRRTLGAPDISSGTSDTGSLPPNLQPGYSPSPTHPPTGQYTLFP-
LPPTLPTPVVQLHPLLPDPSAPTPTPTSPLLNTSYTHSQNLSQEG

REACTIVE SITES

.N.(10)		.D.(9)		.M.(3)		.Q.(19)			
125	PNA	8	CDL	55	QME	28	SQC	201	WQQ
172	LNE	18	RDS	75	VMA	54	TQM	202	QQG
176	PNR	45	VDF	143	LML	61	AQD	214	NQT
185	TNF	62	QDI			80	GQL	221	DQI
213	LNQ	123	KDP			92	GQL	268	LQP
227	LNR	220	LDQ			96	GQV	282	GQY
234	LNG	252	PDI			105	LQS	298	VQL
266	PNL	259	SDT			111	TQL	326	SQN
319	LNT	305	PDP			115	PQG	330	SQE
327	QNL					132	FQH		

HYDROFLEX PLOT

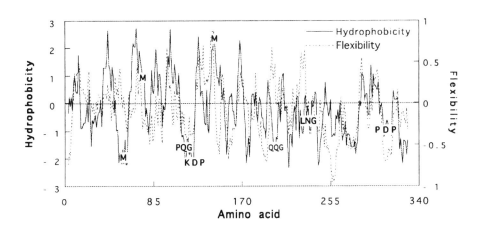

PREDICTED REACTIVITY AND DEGRADATION OF THROMBOPOIETIN

There are several forms of TPO, including the natural full length sequence shown above (produced in either *E. coli* or CHO cells), as well as a number or truncated forms, some of which have also been pegylated. A preliminary stability analysis has been carried out on the full length "natural" molecule under physiological conditions (pH 7.4) (Lim *et al.*, 1996). Inspection of the primary amino acid sequence for TPO shows that the most reactive is predicted to be Asn-234 within the -LNG- motif, Asp-123 within the -KDP- motif, Asn-305 within the -PDP- motif, and Gln-115 within the -PQG- motif. The first of these, Asn-234, showed N-linked glycosylation in the CHO-derived molecule studied, and so this site was unavailable for reaction. All reside in a region predicted to be hydrophilic and flexible. The chemical stability of TPO was monitored by SEC and tryptic mapping. TPO deamidated at Asn-227 (in the -LNR- motif) and formed iso-Asp at Asp-220 (in the -LDQ- motif). Reaction at these sites did not alter TPO activity, nor did diketopiperazine formation at Ala-3 (des-Ser-Pro). Further, it was found that TPO aggregates, as well as oxidized TPO (using hydrogen peroxide), had little or no biological activity. The time required to achieve 90% rhTPO monomer (t_{90} shelf life) was determined to be greater than 2 years at 2–8°C.

- **Tissue Plasminogen Activator (human) (t-PA) (527 residues)**

SEQUENCE

SYQVICRDEKTQMIYQQHQSWLRPVLRSNRVEYCWCNSGRAQCHSVPVKSCSEPR-
CFNGGTCQQALYFSDFVCQCPEGFAGKCCEIDTRATCYEDQGISYRGTWSTAESGAE-
CTNWNSSALAQKPYSGRRPDAIRLGLGNHNYCRNPDRDSKPWCYVFKAGKYSSE-
FCSTPACSEGNSDCYFGNGSAYRGTHSLTESGASCLPWNSMILIGKVYTAQNPSAQ-
ALGLGKHNYCRNPDGDAKPWCHMLKNRRLTWEYCDVPSCSTCGLRQYSQPQFR-
IKGGLFADIASHPWQAAIFAKHRRSPGERFLCGGILISSCWILSAAHCFQERFPPHHLT-
VILGRTYRVVPGEEEQKFEVEKYIVHKEFDDDTYDNDNALLQLKSDSSRCAQESS-
VVRTVCLPPADLQLPDWTECELSGYGKHEALSPFYSERLKEAHVRLYPSSRCTSQH-
LLNRTVTDNMLCAGDTRSGGPQANLHDACQGDSGGPLVCLNDGRMTLVGIISWGL-
GCGQKDVPGVYTKVTNYLDWIRDNMRP

REACTIVE SITES

.N.(23)		.D.(28)		.M.(6)		.Q.(26)	
29 SNR	248 KNR	8 RDE	366 DDT	13 QMI	3 YQV	271 SQP
37 CNS	370 DND	70 SDF	369 YDN	207 SMI	12 TQM	273 PQF
58 FNG	372 DNA	87 IDT	371 NDN	245 HML	16 YQQ	290 WQA
115 TNW	448 LNR	95 EDQ	380 SDS	455 NML	17 QQH	325 FQE
117 WNS	454 DNM	132 PDA	400 ADL	490 RMT	19 HQS	350 EQK
140 GNH	469 ANL	148 PDR	405 PDW	525 NMR	42 AQC	376 LQL
142 HNY	486 LND	150 RDS	453 TDN		63 CQQ	386 AQE
146 RNP	516 TNY	179 SDC	460 GDT		64 QQA	402 LQL
177 GNS	524 DNM	236 PDG	472 HDA		74 CQC	444 SQH
184 GNG		238 GDA	477 GDS		96 DQG	467 PQA
205 WNS		257 CDV	487 NDG		123 AQK	475 CQG
218 QNP		283 ADI	506 KDV		217 AQN	504 GQK
230 HNY		364 FDD	519 LDW		222 AQA	
234 RNP		365 DDD	523 RDN		268 RQY	

HYDROFLEX PLOT

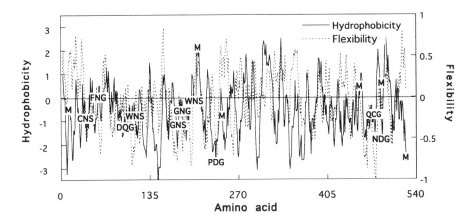

PREDICTED REACTIVITY AND DEGRADATION OF t-PA

This serine protease is predicted to have several sites of possible degradation, notably deamidation at Asn-58 in the sequence -FNG, Asn-184 in the -GNG- sequence, Asn-177 in the sequence -GNS-, Asn-37 in the -CNS- motif, and Asn-117 in the -WNS- motif. Reaction was observed at most of these sites, including iso-Asp formation via deamidation of Asn-37 in the sequence -CNS- (Paranandi *et al.*, 1994). The Asn-Gly motifs are predicted to be reactive at neutral pH; the Asn-Ser motifs are also predicted to be reactive at 37°C based on synthetic peptide studies. When incubated at pH 7.3, 37°C, human recombinant t-PA accumulated 0.77 mol of iso-Asp per mol of t-PA over a 14-day period. All three sites appeared to be on the surface of the protein, and all three occurred in regions of the protein predicted to have higher than average chain mobility. It is interesting to note that Asn-184 within the -GNGS- motif was not susceptible to deamidation. The reason for this is straightforward; this Asn is glycosylated in t-PA expressed in CHO cells and so is unavailable for reaction. This protein is also glycosylated at Asn-117, possibly accounting for its lack of reaction at this motif (although the -WNS- is not necessarily reactive). Although this molecule has numerous Mets, no reports of Met oxidation were reported. These hydrolysis reactions did not limit the shelf life in that this molecule is subject to another, more rapid, degradation pathway (Nguyen and Ward, 1993b). This molecule is a serine protease and so is subject to autocatalytic degradation; because of this, it is formulated as a lyophilized powder and reconstituted before use.

Trypsin (bovine) (223 residues)

SEQUENCE

IVGGYTCGANTVPYQVSLNSGYHFCGGSLINSQWVVSAAHCYKSGIQVRLGEDN-
INVVEGNEQFISASKSIVHPSYNSNTLNNDIMLIKLKSAASLNSRVASISLPTSCASAG-
TQCLISGWGNTKSSGTSYPDVLKCLKAPILSDSSCKSAYPGQITSNMFCAGYLEGG-
KDSCQGDSGGPVVCSGKLQGIVSWGSGCAQKNKPGVYTKVCNYVSWIKQTIASN

REACTIVE SITES

.N.(16)		.D.(6)	.M.(2)	.Q.(10)	
10 ANT	82 LNN	53 EDN	86 IML	15 YQV	199 AQK
19 LNS	83 NND	84 NDI	160 NMF	33 SQW	218 KQT
31 INS	97 LNS	133 PDV		47 IQV	
54 DNI	123 GNT	145 SDS		63 EQF	
56 INV	159 SNM	171 KDS		115 TQC	
61 GNE	201 KNK	176 GDS		155 GQI	
77 YNS	211 CNY			174 CQG	
79 SNT	223 SN			188 LQG	

HYDROFLEX PLOT

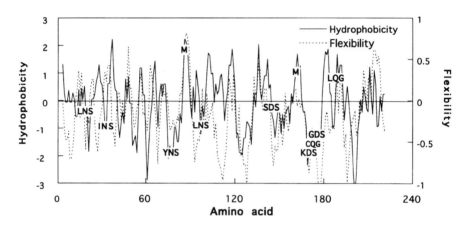

PREDICTED REACTIVITY AND DEGRADATION OF TRYPSIN

Inspection of the amino acid sequence of trypsin shows that there are several Asn-Ser motifs, all located in hydrophilic, flexible regions. Trypsin also contains two Met residues, both located in hydrophobic, inflexible regions. Based on this, it is likely that trypsin may show deamidation or cyclic imide formation at any (or all) of the -XNS- motifs. Interestingly, Gln-174 is found in a region that is fairly flexible and hydrophilic, although this motif contains a cysteine that, when forming a disulfide bridge, may reduce the local flexibility dramatically, rendering it fairly unreactive. An elegant NMR study showed that three residues were prone to microheterogeneity (in the form of a deamidated product): Asn -31 (-INS), Asn-77 (-YNS-), and Asn-97 (-LNS) (revised numbering system to make the N-termini start at 1) (Kossiakoff, 1988). None of the other 13 Asn residues showed reactivity under the experimental conditions used. Of note, Asn-19 (-LNS-) did not show microheterogeneity, even though it has the same motif as Asn-97. This is another clear-cut demonstration that conformational aspects are crucial for deamidation in proteins. In this study, it was not determined if deamidation occurred prior to crystallization or if it occurred during the 1-year period of crystal growth and data collection. Nevertheless, these data show that trypsin does not degrade at sites other than the predicted hot spots.

Vascular Endothelial Growth Factor (VEGF) (165 residues) ●

SEQUENCE

APMAEGGGQNHHEVVKFMDVYQRSYCHPIETLVDIFQEYPDEIEYIFKPSCVPLMR-
CGGCCNDEGLECVPTEESNITMQIMRIKPHQGQHIGEMSFLQHNKCECRPKKDRA-
RQENPCGPCSERRKHLFVQDPQTCKCSCKNTDSRCKARQLELNERTCRCDKPRR

REACTIVE SITES

.N.(7)	.D.(8)	.M.(6)	.Q.(11)
10 QNH	19 MDV	3 PMA	9 GQN
62 CND	34 VDI	18 FMD	22 YQR
75 SNI	41 PDE	55 LMR	37 FQE
100 HNK	63 NDE	78 TMQ	79 MQI
115 ENP	109 KDR	81 IMR	87 HQG
141 KNT	131 QDP	94 EMS	89 GQH
154 LNE	143 TDS		98 LQH
	161 CDK		113 RQE
			130 VQD
			133 PQT
			150 RQL

HYDROFLEX PLOT

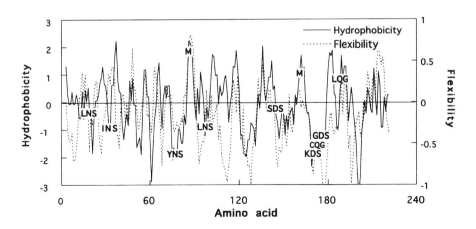

PREDICTED REACTIVITY AND DEGRADATION OF VEGF

Inspection of the amino acid sequence of VEGF shows that there are few hot-spot motifs, and the two that exist (Gln-Gly and Asp-Pro) are not predicted to be as reactive as Asn-Gly or Asn-Ser. VEGF has a Pro at position 2 (APM ...), suggesting that this molecule might undergo diketopiperazine formation. It also has several Met residues that may oxidize. The degradation of VEGF in aqueous solutions from pH 5 to 7 has been determined (Keyt and Cleland, 1995). From pH 5 to 6, the major degradation route at accelerated conditions of 40°C was deamidation at Asn-10 in the -QNH- motif to give a variety of products, as yet to be determined. At higher pH, proteolysis and additional deamidation were observed but not fully characterized. At or above pH 6.5, some diketopiperazine formation was observed under accelerated conditions of 40°C for 4 weeks, giving the expected reaction product, des-Ala-Pro VEGF.

4. STATISTICAL ANALYSIS OF PROTEIN DEGRADATION SITES IN AQUEOUS SOLUTION

These data show that the primary reaction of proteins at pH 4.5–7.5 occurs largely at Asn and Asp within these motifs: -Asn-Gly-, -Asn-Ser-, -Asp-Gly-, and to a lesser extent -Gln-Gly-, -Asp-Pro-, and -Met-. A few proteins, however, react at sites other than these and are exceptions to the rule. These proteins react at sites that are deemed "unreactive" sites (such as at Asn 52 in the -LND- motif in CD4), based largely upon data obtained in small model peptides. There are several reasons why proteins may show unusually high reactivity at these non-hot-spot sites:

(i)   The motif is in the "correct" conformation for reaction to occur.
(ii) Reaction may be due to enzymatic catalysis (traces of unwanted proteases in the purified protein product).
(iii) The protein degrades under the harsh conditions of isolation and work-up.
(iv) The DNA encodes for both the parent and the product forms (such as encoding for Asn and Asp in cholera B subunit, depending on the strain studied), so both isoforms are expressed.

The first reason that the reactive motif is held conformationally in a geometry that facilitates reaction is an often-touted explanation for "non-hot-spot" protein reactivity. But is it the only reason? For example, some proteins deamidate faster under work-up conditions than in pH 7.4 buffer at 37°C, suggesting that enzyme catalysis [point (ii)] is operational. Enzymatic catalysis may not only cause an acceleration in the rate of deamidation, but may also promote deamidation at motifs that would have otherwise been unreactive at pH 7.4 and 37°C. There are also numerous examples in the literature (see below) of non-hot-spot protein degradation coming from publications where the work-up of the protein was carried out under fairly harsh conditions and often without controls. Finally, a few concrete examples of protein microheterogeneity due to different DNA coding have been reported and provide an elegant rationale for apparent non-hot-spot protein degradation.

To sort through this, we have constructed a table summarizing protein reactivity in aqueous solution, based on whether or not the primary degradation pathway was observed to be at one or more of the predicted hot spots (Table II). This table contains information on the degradation behavior of 73 proteins, including information on the frequency of hot spots of each type. Most of these proteins show degradation, and this degradation information is available as to whether it has been observed to occur at a hot spot, at some other motif, or through oxidation. Information on 54 of the 73 proteins was obtained under formulation conditions (i.e., carefully controlled formulation-type studies where the reaction catalyst and the degradation kinetics are fairly well understood and not complicated by the initial protein quality or enzymatic degradation); for 21 proteins, degradation information pertains to behavior determined under "work-up" conditions (where degradation may also occur due to the work-up process, enzymatic catalysis in a biological milieu, or to fermentation degradation before isolation). Two proteins, calmodulin and interleukin 2, have been studied under both formulation and work-up conditions and so are included in both data sets. An additional column was added to address oxidation as the primary degradation pathway (under either formulation or work-up conditions), and no distinction between formulation and work-up was made as few proteins undergo oxidation as the primary degradation pathway in aqueous solution. A final column summarizes those proteins that react as predicted, based on the hypothesis that the primary degradation pathway occurs at one of the predicted hot spots for reaction.

Inspection of the data in Table II shows that there are several proteins that react at non-hot-spots; these are traditionally thought to be exceptions to the rule of protein reactivity. For example, of the 54 proteins that were studied under formulation conditions, 32 (~60%) showed primary reaction at hot-spot sites and 22 (~40%) showed reaction at non-hot-spot sites. Of the 21 proteins that were studied under work-up conditions, 10 (~48%) showed primary reaction at hot-spot sites and 11 (~52%) show reaction at non-hot-spot sites. Closer scrutiny of the data, however, shows that some of these differences arise because many proteins are devoid (or have very few) of the traditional hot spots, so when degradation is observed it is ultimately at a non-hot-spot site of degradation. To account for this, a column in the table called "predicted reactivity" was added. An absence of an X in the last column indicates proteins that are the truly unusual cases of protein degradation (i.e., proteins that degrade at non-hot-spots, even though there are traditional hot spots which remain unreactive). Inspection of the table shows that there is a slightly higher tendency to observe non-hot-spot protein degradation when studied under work-up conditions, although this may not be statistically valid (i.e., $p < 0.05$) because of the limited data subset size. In several of these cases, these exceptions are found under conditions where work-up reaction may occur, or where harsh conditions of protein isolation may account for some of the observed degradation. From a formulator's point of view, reaction of proteins at 37°C at pH 7.4 in a biological milieu containing enzymes

Table II. Statistical Analysis of Protein Degradation Pathways[a]

Protein	# NG	# NS	# DG	# DP	# QG	# M	Hot-spot formul.	Other formul	Hot-spot work-up	Other work-up	Oxidation	Pred reac
Adrenocorticotropin	1					1	X					X
Agglutinin	1				2	2			X			X
Aldolase	2	1	4		2	3				X		
Amylin antagonist								X				X
Amyloid-related serum protein	2	1	1	1		2				X		
Angiogenin	2	1			1	1	X					X
Anti-HER-2 heavy chain	2	3	3	1	1	4				X		X
Anti-HER-2 light chain		1			2	1						X
Antibody 4D5 heavy chain	2	3	3	1	2	5	X					X
Antibody 4D5 light chain		1			2	1	X					X
Antibody 17-1A heavy chain	1	3	2	1	2	7		X				
Antibody 17-1A light chain	1	2	1		1	4	X					X
Antibody light chain kappa	1	3	1		1	4	X					X
Antibody OKT3 heavy chain	1	2	1			5	X					X
Antibody OKT3 light chain	1	3	1	1	2	9	X					X
Antibody OKT4 heavy chain	2	3	2	2	1	5	X					X
Antibody OKT4 light chain		1			2	1		stable				X
Atrial natriuretic peptide		1				1	X	X			X	X
Brain derived neurotrophic factor		1		1		3	X	X				X
Calbindin	1		1	1			X					X
Calmodulin	2		6			9	X		X			X
Carbonic anhydrase	3		3	2	1	1			X			X
CD4		2		1	4	4		X				
CD4-PE40	1	2	1	2	5	1					X	X

Protein												
Chloroperoxidase	1	2		1	1	1	3				X	X
Cholera toxin B subunit			3				3		X	X		X
Ciliary neurotrophic factor			1	1			4				X	
Crystallin-A			1				3	X		X		X
Cytochrome c			1				2	X				X
DNase			2				5	X			X	X
Epidermal GF (human)			2		2		1	X				X
Epidermal GF (murine)	1		2				1	X		X		X
Erythrocyte protein 4.1	1		2	2			6		X			X
Fibroblast GF acidic	2		3				2	X				
Fibroblast GF basic	1		4	2			2	X			X	X
Glucagon					1		1			X		
Granulocyte CSF			1			3	3	X				X
Growth hormone (bovine)	1		1				5	X			X	X
Growth hormone (human)	2						3	X			X	X
Growth hormone (porcine)	1		1				3	X				X
Growth hormone rel factor	1				1			X	X			X
Hemoglobin				1			2		X			
Hirudin			2		1		1		X	X		X
Histone					2				X			
HXGT			1				6					
Insulin							1	X			X	X
Insulin-like growth factor I								X			X	X
Insulinotropin											X	X
Interferon-α-2b	1						5		X			X
Interferon-β	1				1		3					X
Interferon-γ			1				4	X	X		X	X
Interleukin 1-RA						1	4	X			X	X

(continued)

Table II. (*Continued*)

Protein	# NG	# NS	# DG	# DP	# QG	# M	Hot-spot formul.	Other formul.	Hot-spot work-up	Other work-up	Oxidation	Pred reac
Interleukin 1α						3		X				X
Interleukin 1β (human)		1		1	2	6		X				X
Interleukin 1β (murine)	1		1	2	1	4	X					X
Interleukin 2	1					4	X	X		X		X
Interleukin 11			1	2		2		X			X	X
Lung surfactant						1					X	X
Lysozyme	1					2	X					X
Myelin basic protein		1	1		3	2			X			X
Neocarzinostatin		1	2	1	1			X				
Nerve growth factor		2	1	1		2	X				X	X
Parathyroid hormone		1				2				X		
Relaxin						2		X			X	X
RNAase A	1				1	4			X			X
RNAase U2	2		1		1				X			X
Secretin			1		1		X					X
SHMT	2		2	2	1	8	X					X
Tissue factor-243		1				1		stable				X
Tissue growth factor-β		4				1		stable				X
Tissue plasminogen activator	2		2		2	6	X					X
Trypsin		4			2	2	X					X
VEGF				1	1	6		X				X

[a]Note: Data for antibody E25 and TPO were not included in this analysis. It is not expected that the omission of these proteins changes the results significantly.

that may cause protein degradation does not mimic optimal formulation reaction conditions.

It has long been known that many proteins react at the traditional hot spots, but the predictive value of this general knowledge has not yet been tested. For example, what is the probability of primary reaction at Asn-Ser for a new, unstudied protein? The main objective of our analysis is to determine if the frequency of motifs of a particular type affects the propensity for proteins to degrade at a hot spot or at some other motif. In addition, the association between oxidation and the frequency of methionine residues was investigated.

In assessing hot-spot degradation, the following evaluations were conducted separately for proteins studied under formulation conditions and those studied under work-up reaction conditions. Note that the number of proteins used in the statistical analysis differs slightly from the total number of proteins in this compendium, largely because some proteins are structurally similar and so would unduly weight the analysis if all were used. For each hot-spot type, the frequency distribution was compared between proteins which exhibited degradation at a hot spot and those which did not. This comparison was carried out by formal contingency table analysis. A two-tailed Fisher's exact test was used to assess significance of the association between degradation at a hot spot and frequency of a particular motif for each of the five hydrolytic hot-spot types. An additional evaluation investigated this association with the frequency of hot spots of any type. The results are shown in Appendix A. For proteins studied under formulation conditions, results are summarized in Tables AIa–f and Figs. A1a–f, respectively. The corresponding Tables AIIa–f and Figs. AIIa–f present results for the proteins investigated under work-up conditions. The relationship between oxidation and frequency of Met residues is summarized in Table AIII; Fig. A3 provides a graphical summary.

By convention, p-values less than 0.05 are reported as representing a statistically significant association; however, all p-values should be interpreted with caution, since not all 73 of the proteins analyzed can be considered to provide independent information (e.g., results for the antibodies are unlikely to be independent because of sequence similarity outside of the CDR region). Since only 21 proteins were studied under work-up conditions, p-values were not reported for the association between degradation and hot-spot frequency; small sample sizes and discreteness of the distributions involved render formal hypothesis tests suspect in this case. For proteins studied under work-up conditions, graphs and tables are provided for descriptive purposes only.

The frequency distribution of Met residues was compared across proteins which did and did not undergo oxidation in similar fashion. This analysis was carried out for all 73 proteins combined, without distinguishing between those studied under formulation and work-up conditions. The analyses support the following conclusions:

- There is a pronounced shift in the frequency distribution of the -Asn-Gly-motif among proteins which degrade at a hot spot under formulation conditions. The majority (86%) of proteins not exhibiting hot-spot degradation lack an -Asn-Gly- motif, whereas a majority (59%) of those which do degrade at a hotspot have at least one -Asn-Gly- motif (Table AIa/Fig. AIa). The p-value of 0.004 suggests that this is not a random event.

- Similarly, the frequency of the -Asn-Ser- motif appears positively associated with hot-spot degradation under formulation conditions (Table AIb/Fig. AIb). The majority (71%) of proteins not exhibiting hot-spot degradation lack an -Asn-Ser- motif, whereas nearly half (40%) of those which do degrade at a hot spot have at least one -Asn-Ser- motif. The p-value for this analysis is 0.002 suggesting that this is not a random event.

- The tendency to degrade at a hot spot under work-up conditions does not appear to be associated with frequency of the other motifs: -Asp-Gly- ($p = 0.22$), -Asp-Pro- ($p = 1.00$), or -Gln-Gly- ($p = 0.27$. (Tables AIc–e/Figs. AIc–e). There may be several reasons for this. First, if these motives are unreactive on the time scale studied, then large values of p will be obtained. Second, if reaction goes undetected because of experimental difficulty (such as might be the case for iso-Asp formation from Asp), this will also result in an apparent lack of association.

- Not surprisingly, there is a significant association between degradation at a hydrolytic hot spot and the overall number of hot spots. The significance of this association, however, may be driven in part by the structural zero in Table AIf (proteins without any hot spot cannot degrade at a hot spot).

- In general, patterns for degradation under work-up conditions appear similar to those for the proteins studied under formulation conditions. An exception may be the pattern of -Asn-Ser- motifs (compare Tables AIIb and AIb), although the sample size (20) is too small to draw definitive conclusions.

- Since oxidation occurred for relatively few (11) of the 73 proteins, the ability to assess the relationship to the frequency of Met residues is limited. The p-value of 0.62 shows that there is no correlation between oxidation and the presence of Met (i.e., many proteins containing Met do not oxidize).

5. GENERAL CONCLUSIONS REGARDING PROTEIN DEGRADATION IN AQUEOUS SOLUTION

This literature compilation on the chemical reaction of proteins was assembled to establish boundaries to the reactivity of Asn, Asp, Gln, and possibly Met, in the context of neighboring amino acid sequence, regional hydrophobicity, and backbone flexibility. An extensive review of the literature, as well as several unpublished reports, afforded numerous proteins that selectively hydrolyze, deamidate, undergo iso-Asp formation, or oxidize in aqueous solution. Inspection of the primary amino acid sequence alone gives a modest indicator of the most reactive motifs; it was found that the general rules already established predict the majority of reactive sites observed (Asn-Gly, Asn-Ser, Asp-Gly, Gln-Gly, Asp-Pro, and Met). Of the proteins of which we have compiled reliable degradation data, only 5 (CD4, CNTF, acidic-FGF, GCSF, and neocarzinostatin) degraded primarily at "unusual" sites of degradation, and not at the available and predicted hot spots. We calculated the hydropathy/flexibility plots (termed "hydroflex" plots) to provide a way of further examining the degradation of peptides and proteins. By doing so we found that some residues predicted to react based on their amino acid sequence (but did not react experimentally) were calculated to be in hydrophobic regions of limited flexibility. Further, the hydrolytic protein degradation studies have been carried out under two types of conditions: those carefully controlled studies in aqueous solution at near-neutral pH where the integrity of the initial protein was well known (termed formulation studies) and those where degradation was observed after isolation from biological media or where the protein may have degraded upon work-up (herein termed, work-up studies). We present several examples of work-up degradation that do not adhere to the above rules (based on the predicted hot spots), possibly because of enzymatic catalysis or extreme reaction conditions used for protein isolation and purification. For these reasons, work-up degradation results should not be used to predict protein reactivity in aqueous formulations. Finally, the prediction of Met reactivity based on primary amino acid sequence was not successful, possibly because of the limited protein oxidation data available, because of the complex nature of protein oxidation by a variety of different oxidative catalysts (Knepp *et al.*, 1996), or because protein conformation prohibits reaction of Mets found in the protein core. Some general conclusions are emphasized.

1. Data used to predict protein reactivity in aqueous formulations should be carefully scrutinized before making general conclusions. Several of the exceptions to the rule for protein degradation in aqueous solution come from examples in the literature where the nature of the "unusual" degradation is unknown and may be caused by enzymatic degradation, heterogeneity of protein expression at the gene level, or hydrolytic or oxidative degradation upon work-up. These examples are not representative test cases for protein degradation in aqueous formulations.

2. Hydropathy seems to be a better predictor for protein degradation than does calculated flexibility. Inspection of more than 70 hydroflex plots shows that most of the reactive hot spots lie in regions predicted to be hydrophilic. In large part this is due to the nature of the calculation (for example, Asn, Asp, and Gln have large negative Kyte parameters, lowering the overall value of calculated hydrophobicity). For example, the literature average (over 500,000 protein entries included in this calculation) hydropathy for all residues is -0.32 (statistically corrected for the amount of each amino acid found in nature); similarly the hydropathy values for NG, NS, DG, QG, DP, and M (again statistically corrected and using a window of six amino acids in

the hydropathy calculation) are -0.81, -0.89, -0.84, -0.84, -1.06, and 0.04, respectively.

3. Met oxidation is not a major pathway for degradation for most proteins and is difficult, if not impossible, to predict based on primary sequence alone. Many of the proteins studied had several Met amino acids and yet did not show oxidative degradation; other proteins, however, showed oxidation as the primary degradation pathway. A few proteins also showed oxidation as a minor degradation pathway. For the handful of proteins that showed oxidation at Met, there was no observable correlation between Met reactivity and hydrophobicity. Again, the average Met hydrophobicity (statistically corrected) over the entire database was 0.04; the value, along with the standard deviation of the calculated hydropathy for reactive Mets was 0.2 ± 1.6.

4. There appears to be a fairly good correlation between degradation at hot spots and the number of available hot spots for reaction. Proteins with only a few hot spots (or the lesser reactive hot spots such as Gln-Gly) tended to react at non-hot-spot sites, whereas proteins with numerous hotspots, particularly if they included Asn-Gly, Asn-Ser, and Asp-Gly, tended to react primarily at these sites. There were exceptions to this conclusion, but they were few and did not represent the norm.

5. Based on the above, the design of protein stability experiments in aqueous formulations should focus initially on the identity of hot-spot degradation pathways, with emphasis on Asn-Gly and Asn-Ser (as applicable). Less attention should be focused on Gln-Gly, as this motif appears to be less reactive than Asp-Gly, Asp-Pro, or even Met.

APPENDIX A

There was a pronounced shift in the frequency distribution of the -Asn-Gly- motif among proteins which degraded at a hot spot under formulation conditions. The majority (86%) of proteins not exhibiting hot-spot degradation lacked an -Asn-Gly- motif, whereas a majority (59%) of those which degraded at a hot spot had at least one -Asn-Gly- motif. The p-value of 0.004 suggests that this is not a random event.

Table AIa. Hot-Spot Degradation under Formulation Conditions by Frequency of Asn-Gly motifs

Degrades	Frequency					
	0	1	2	3+	Total	
No	18 (86%)	2 (10%)	1 (5%)		21	
Yes	13 (41%)	12 (37%)	7 (22%)		32	
Total	31 (59%)	14 (26%)	8 (15%)		53	$p = 0.004$

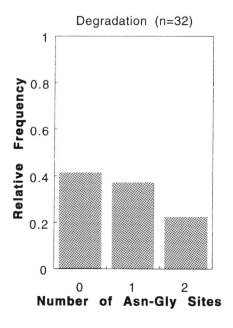

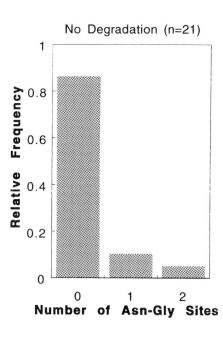

The frequency of the -Asn-Ser- motif appeared positively associated with hot-spot degradation under formulation conditions. The majority (71%) of proteins not exhibiting hot-spot degradation lacked an -Asn-Ser- motif, whereas nearly half (40%) of those which degraded at a hot spot had at least one -Asn-Ser- motif. The p-value for this analysis is 0.002, suggesting that this is not a random event.

Table AIb. Hot-Spot Degradation under Formulation Conditions
by Frequency of Asn-Ser motifs

Degrades	Frequency					
	0	1	2	3+	Total	
No	15 (71%)	3 (14%)	2 (10%)	1 (5%)	21	
Yes	6 (19%)	15 (47%)	4 (13%)	7 (22%)	32	
Total	21 (40%)	18 (34%)	6 (11%)	8 (15%)	53	$p = 0.002$

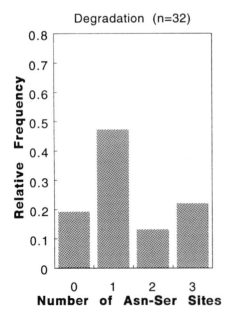

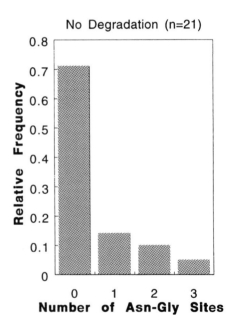

The tendency to degrade at the -Asp-Gly- hot spot under formulation conditions did not appear to be associated with frequency of the -Asp-Gly- motif. The p-value for this analysis was 0.22, suggesting that this was a random event. The reaction of Asp-Gly is often difficult to detect because of experimental difficulty (such as iso-Asp formation from Asp), and may account, at least in part, for the apparent lack of association.

Table AIc. Hot-Spot Degradation under Formulation Conditions by Frequency of Asn-Gly Motifs

Degrades	Frequency				Total	
	0	1	2	3+		
No	14 (67%)	3 (14%)	2 (9.5%)	2 (9.5%)	21	
Yes	11 (34%)	11 (34%)	5 (16%)	5 (16%)	32	
Total	25 (47%)	14 (26%)	7 (13%)	7 (13%)	53	$p = 0.22$

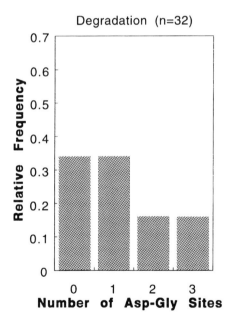

Degradation (n=32)

Relative Frequency

Number of Asp-Gly Sites

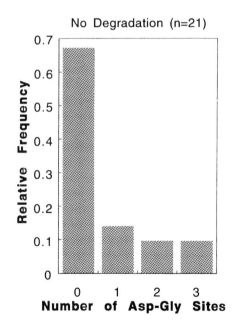

No Degradation (n=21)

Relative Frequency

Number of Asp-Gly Sites

The tendency to degrade at the -Asp-Pro- hot spot under formulation conditions did not appear to be associated with frequency of the -Asp-Pro- motif. The p-value for this analysis was 1.00, suggesting that this was a random event. The reaction of Asp-Pro is favored at low pH's and becomes less favorable as the pH is raised. Because many formulations are made at near-neutral pH, it is likely that this reaction is minimized and may account, at least in part, for the apparent lack of association.

Table AId. Hot-Spot Degradation under Formulation Conditions by Frequency of Asp-Pro Motifs

		Frequency				
Degrades	0	1	2	3+	Total	
No	15 (71%)	4 (19%)	2 (9.5%)		21	
Yes	21 (66%)	7 (22%)	4 (12%)		32	
Total	36 (68%)	11 (21%)	6 (11%)		53	$p = 1.00$

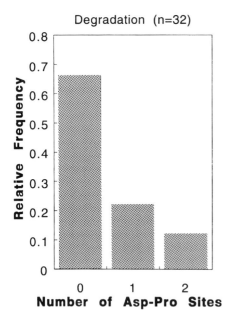

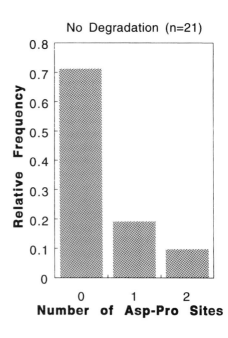

The tendency to degrade at the -Gln-Gly- hot spot under formulation conditions did not appear to be associated with frequency of the -Gln-Gly- motif. The p-value for this analysis was 0.27, suggesting that this was a random event. The reaction of Gln-Gly was observed only rarely in all of the proteins tabulated, even though this motif was found often. It is likely that the apparent lack of association of this motif with reactivity is caused by just that—lack of reactivity under formulation conditions.

Table AIe. Hot-Spot Degradation under Formulation Conditions by Frequency of Gln-Gly Motifs

	Frequency					
Degrades	0	1	2	3+	Total	
No	12 (57%)	3 (14%)	3 (14%)	3 (14%)	21	
Yes	17 (53%)	9 (28%)	6 (19%)	0	32	
Total	29 (55%)	12 (23%)	9 (17%)	3 (6%)	53	$p = 0.27$

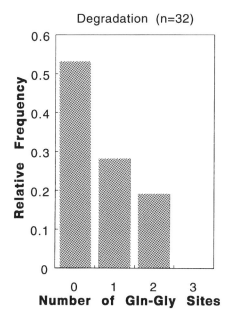

Degradation (n=32)

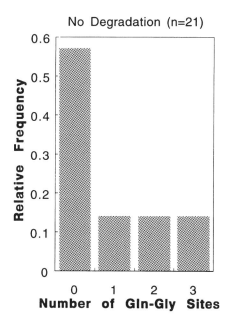

No Degradation (n=21)

The tendency to degrade at any hot spot under formulation conditions was tightly associated with the frequency of hot spots. The p-value for this analysis is 0.0004 suggesting that this was not a random event. The small p-value for this association may in part be driven by the structural zero in the degradation plot; no degradation at a hot spot is possible if the protein does not have a hot spot.

Table AIf. Hot-Spot Degradation under Formulation Conditions by Frequency of Any Motif

				Frequency						
Degrades	0	1	2	3	4	5	6	7+	Total	
No	9	2	0	3	2	2	0	3	21	
Yes	0	3	7	5	4	2	3	8	32	
Total	9	5	7	8	6	4	3	11	53	$p = .0004$

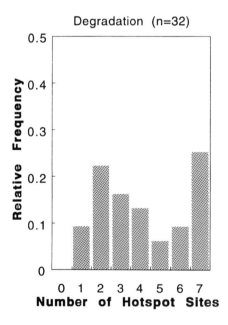

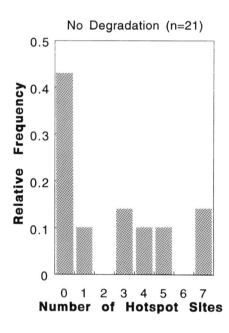

**Table AIIa. Hot-Spot Degradation
under Work-up Conditions
by Frequency of Asn-Gly Motifs**

| | Frequency | | | | | |
Degrades	0	1	2	3+	Total	
No	8	2	1	0	11	
Yes	2	4	2	1	9	
Total	10	6	3	1	20	$p = 0.103$

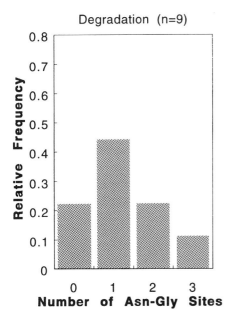

Degradation (n=9)

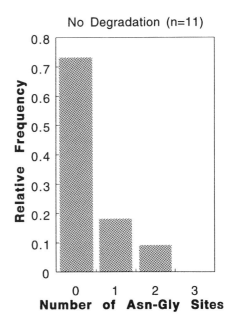

No Degradation (n=11)

**Table AIIb. Hot-Spot Degradation
under Work-up Conditions
by Frequency of Asn-Ser Motifs**

| Degrades | Frequency | | | | |
---	0	1	2	3+	Total
No	6	4	1		11
Yes	9	0	0		9
Total	15	4	1		20

$p = 0.056$

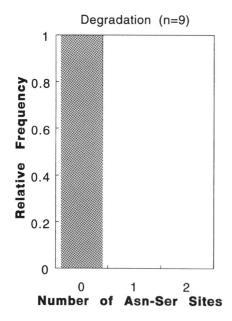

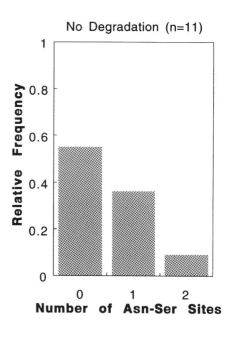

**Table AIIc. Hot-Spot Degradation
under Work-up Conditions
by Frequency of Asp-Gly Motifs**

		Frequency				
Degrades	0	1	2	3+	Total	
No	7	3	0	1	11	
Yes	2	3	2	2	9	
Total	9	6	2	3	20	$p = 0.098$

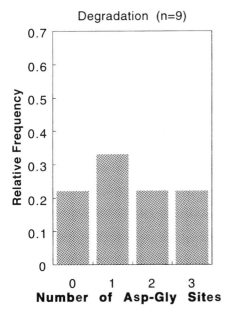

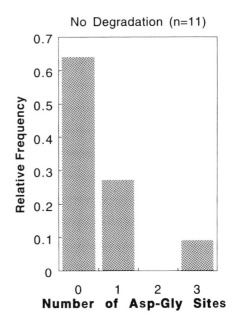

Table AIId. Hot-Spot Degradation under Work-up Conditions by Frequency of Asp-Gly Motifs

Degrades	Frequency					
	0	1	2	3+	Total	
No	7	4	0		11	
Yes	7	0	2		9	
Total	14	4	2		20	$p = 0.058$

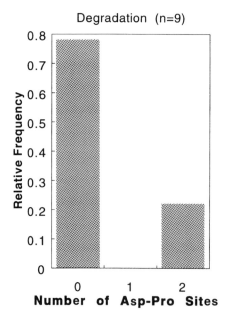

Degradation (n=9)

Relative Frequency

Number of Asp-Pro Sites

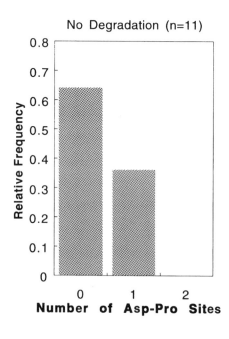

No Degradation (n=11)

Relative Frequency

Number of Asp-Pro Sites

**Table AIIe. Hot-Spot Degradation
under Work-up Conditions
by Frequency of Gln-Gly Motifs**

Degrades	Frequency					
	0	1	2	3+	Total	
No	7	2	2	0	11	
Yes	3	4	1	1	9	
Total	10	6	3	1	20	$p = 0.413$

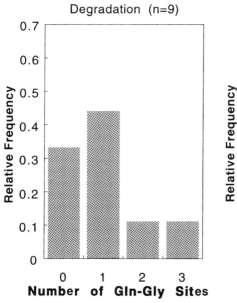

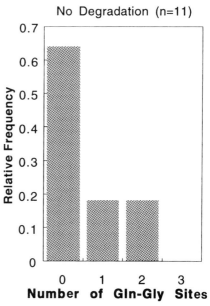

**Table AIIf. Hot-Spot Degradation under Work-up
Conditions by Frequency of Any Motif**

Degrades	0	1	2	3	4	5	6	7+	Total	
No	0	6	2	1	0	1	0	1	11	
Yes	0	2	0	1	3	0	1	2	9	
Total	0	8	2	2	3	1	1	3	20	$p = 0.133$

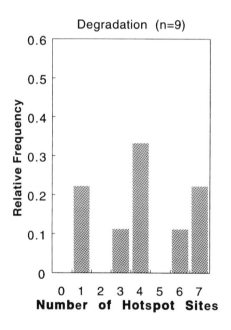

Degradation (n=9)

Number of Hotspot Sites

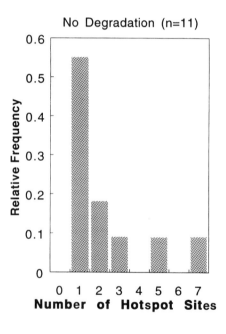

No Degradation (n=11)

Number of Hotspot Sites

These plots are intriguing and provocative, in that the did not find a correlation of oxidation with number of Met residues. This is perhaps somewhat surprising, in that one might have intuitively expected that proteins with many Met residues maight be more prone to oxidation that those with few. Indeed, there existed a single example where oxidation was the predominant pathway, and yet the protein is devoid of Met (oxidation occurred at Trp).

Table AIII. Oxidation by Frequency of Met Residues

Oxidation?	0	1	2	3	4	5	6	7+	Total	
No	8	11	10	10	8	5	4	4	60	
Yes	1	5	3	0	2	0	0	0	11	
Total	9	16	13	10	10	5	4	4	71	$p = 0.062$

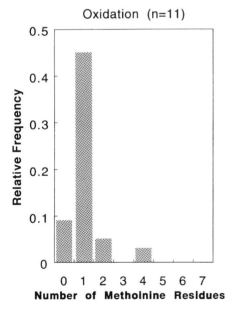

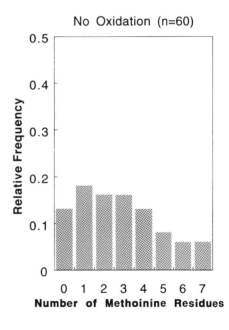

ACKNOWLEDGMENTS. This chapter would not have come together without the help of Jessica Burdman and Milianne Chin. Several others have contributed to this compendium: Sid Advant (*Protein Design Labs*), Dana Aswad (*UC Irvine*), Nancy Babour (*Bristol Myers*), John Battersby (*Genentech, Inc.*),Tom Bewley (*Genentech Inc.*), Ron Borchardt (*University of Kansas*), Bill Charman (*Monash University*), Diane Corbo (*R. W. Johnson*), Bim Dhingra (*Circa Pharmaceuticals Inc.*), Marcia Federici (*SKB*), John Frenz (*Genentech, Inc.*), Gerry Gitlin (*Biogen, Inc.*), Leo Gu (*Syntex Research*), Andy J. Jones (*Genentech, Inc.*), Victoria Knepp (*Alza, Corp.*), Leah Lipsich (*Boehringer Ingelheim*), Mike Mulkerrin (*Genentech, Inc.*), Rajiv Nayar (*Miles Laboratories*), John O'Connor (*Genentech, Inc.*), James "J.Q." Oeswein (*Genentech, Inc.*), Rodney Pearlman (*Megabios, Inc.*), Laurie Peltier (*Amylin*), Steve Prestrelski (*Alza Corp.*), Shelly Prince (*Univ. of Oklahoma*), Lynda Sanders (*Syntex Research*), Richard Senderoff (*Zymogenetics*), Paula Shadle (*SKB*), Mike Spellman (*Genentech, Inc.*), Robert Strickley (*Univ. of Utah*), Patricia Smialkowski (*SmithKline Beecham*), Glen Teshima (*Genentech, Inc.*), Jim Wells (*Genentech, Inc.*), and Tonie Wright (*Medical College of Virginia*).

REFERENCES

Abdel-Meguid, S. S., Shieh, H. S., Smith, N. W., Dayrenger, H. E., Violand, B. N., and Bentls, L. A., 1987, Three-dimensional structure of a genetically engineered variant of porcine growth hormone, *Proc. Natl. Acad. Sci. USA* **84(18):**6434–6437.

Artigues, A., Birkett, A., and Schirch, V., 1990, Evidence for the in vivo deamidation and isomerization of an asparaginyl residue in cytosolic serine hydroxymethyltransferase, *J. Biol. Chem.* **265:**4853–4858.

Aswad, D. W., 1984, Stoichiometric methylation of porcine adrenocorticotropin by protein carboxyl methyl transferase requires deamidation of asparagine-25, *J. Biol. Chem.* **259:**10714–10721.

Battersby, J. E., Hancock, W. S., Canova-Davis, E., Oeswein, J. Q., and O'Connor, B., 1994, Diketo-piperazine formation and N-terminal degradation in recombinant human growth hormone, *Int. J. Peptide Res.* **44:**215–222.

Bischoff, R., Lepage, P., Jaquinod, M., Cauet, G., Asker-Klein, M., Cleese, D., Laporte, M., Bayol, A., Dorsselaer, A. V., and Roitsch, C., 1993, Sequence specific deamidation: Isolation and biochemical characterization of succinimide intermediates or recombinant hirudin, *Biochemistry* **32:**725–734.

Blomback, B., 1967, Derivatives of glutamine in peptides, in: *Enzyme Structure*, Vol. 11 (C. H. W. Hirsh, ed.), Academic Press, New York, pp. 398–411.

Bodansky, M., Ondetti, M. A., Levine, S. D., and Williams, N., 1967, Synthesis of secretin. II. The stepwise approach, *J. Am. Chem. Soc.* **89:**6753–6757.

Bornstein, P., and Balian, G., 1970, The specific nonenzymatic cleavage of bovine ribonuclease with hydroxylamine, *J. Biol. Chem.* **245:**4854–4856.

Brange, J., Langkjaer, L., Havelund, S., and Vølund, A., 1992, Chemical stability of insulin. 1. Hydrolytic degradation during storage of pharmaceutical preparations, *Pharm. Res.* **9:**715–726.

Brophy, R. T., and Lambert, W. J., 1994, The adsorption of insulinotropin to polymeric sterilizing filters, *J. Pharm. Sci. Tech.* **48:**92–94.

Cacia, J., Keck, R., Presta, L. G., and Frenz, J., 1996, Isomerization of an aspartic acid residue in the complementarity region of a recombinant antibody (in preparation).

Campbell, R. M., Lee Y., Rivier, J., Heimer, E. P., Felix, A. M., and Mowles, T. F., 1991, GRF analogs and fragments: correlation between receptor binding, activity and structure, *Peptides* **12:**569–574.

Canfield, R. E., 1963, The amino acid sequence of egg white lysozyme, *J. Biol. Chem.* **238**:2698–2707.

Canova-Davis, E., Baldonado, I. P., and Teshima, G. M., 1990, Characterization of chemically synthesized human relaxin by high performance liquid chromatography, *J. Chromatogr.* **508**:81–96.

Canova-Davis, E., Kessler, T. J., Lee, P., Fei, D. T. W., Griffin, P., Stults, J. T., Wade, J. D., and Rinderknecht, E., 1991, Use of recombinant DNA derived human relaxin to probe the structure of the native protein, *Biochemistry* **30**:6006–6013.

Capasso, S., Mazzarella, L., and Zagari, A., 1991, Deamidation via cyclic imide of asparaginyl peptides: dependence on salts, buffers and organic solvents, *Pept. Res.* **4**:234–238.

Chaudhary, V. K., Mizukami, T., Fuerst, T. R., Fitzgerald, D. J., Moss, B., Pastan, I., and Berger, E. A., 1988, Selective killing of HIV-infected cells by recombinant human CD4-*Pseudomonas* exotoxin hybrid protein, *Nature* **335**:369–372.

Chazin, W. J., Kördel, J., Thulin, E., Hofmann, T., Drakenberg, T., and Forsén, 1989, Identification of an isoaspartyl linkage formed upon deamidation of bovine calbindin D9k and structural characterization by 2D ^{1}H NMR, *Biochemistry* **28**:8646–8653.

Chou, F. C., Chou, C., Shaperia, R., and Kibler, R. F., 1976, Basis of microheterogeneity of myelin basic protein, *J. Biol. Chem.* **251**:2671–2679.

Cipolla, D., Gonda, I., Meserve, K. C., Weck, S., and Shire, S. J., 1994, Formulation and aerosol delivery of recombinant DNA-derived human deoxyribonuclease (rhDNase), in: *Formulation and Delivery of Proteins and Peptides* (J. L. Cleland and R. Langer, eds.), ACS Press, pp. 322–342.

Cipolla, D. C., and Shire, S. J., 1991, Analysis of oxidized human relaxin by reverse phase HPLC, mass spectrometry and bioassays, in: *Techniques in Protein Chemistry II*, (J. J. Villafranca, ed.), Academic Press, New York, pp. 543–555.

Cleland, J. L., Powell, M. F., and Shire, S. J., 1993, The development of stable protein formulations: a close look at protein aggregation, deamidation, and oxidation, *Crit. Rev. Ther. Drug Carrier Syst.* **10**:307–377.

Darrington, R. T., and Anderson, B. D., 1994, The role of intramolecular nucleophilic catalysis and the effects of self-association on the deamidation of human insulin at low pH, *Pharm. Res.* **11**:784–793.

Darrington, R. T., and Anderson, B. D., 1995, Evidence for a common intermediate in insulin deamidation and covalent dimer formation: Effects of pH and aniline trapping in dilute acidic solutions, *J. Pharm. Sci.* **84**:275–282.

Darrington, T., 1995, personal communication.

Daumy, G. O., Wilder, C. L., Merenda, J. M., McColl, A. S., Geoghegan, K. F., and Otterness, I. G., 1991, Reduction of biological activity of murine recombinant interleukin-1b by selective deamidation at asparagine 149, *FEBS* **278**:98–102.

DiAugustine, R. P., Gibson, B. W., Aberth, W., Kelly, M., Ferrua, C. M., Tomooka, Y., Brown, C. F., and Walker, M., 1987, Evidence for isoaspartyl[1] (deamidated) forms of mouse epidermal growth factor, *Anal. Biochem.* **165**:420–429.

Eisenberg, D., 1984, Three dimensional structure of membrane and surface proteins, *Annu. Rev. Biochem.* **53**:595–623.

Engelman, D. M., Steitz, T. A., and Goldman, A., 1986, Identifying nonpolar transbilayer helices in amino acid sequences of membrane proteins, *Annu. Rev. Biophys. Chem.* **15**:321–353.

Everett, R., 1995, personal communication.

Everett, R. R., Felice, C. J., Adomaitis, M., Plucinsky, M. C., and Siegel, R. C., 1995, Glutamate to pyroglutamate: Identification of a novel protein degradation mechanism, Ninth Symp. Protein Society.

Flatmark, T., 1966, On the heterogeneity of beef heart cytochrome c. III. A kinetic study of the non-enzymatic deamidation of the main subfractions (Cy I–Cy III), *Acta. Chim. Scand.* **20**:1487–1496.

Foster, L., personal communication, 1996.

Frenz, J., Shire, S. J., and Sliwkowski, M. B., Purified forms of DNase. US Patent 5,279,823 (1994).

Friedman, A. R., Ichhpurani, A. K., Brown, D. M., Hillman, R. M., Krabill, L. F., Martin, R. A., Zurcher-Neeley, H. A., and Guido, D. M., 1991, Degradation of growth hormone releasing factor analogs in neutral aqueous solution is related to deamidation of asparagine residues, *Int. J. Pept. Protein Res.* **37**:14–20.

Fukawa, H., 1967, Changes of glutamine-peptides on heating in aqueous media, *J. Chem. Soc. Jpn.* **88:**459–463.

Galletti, P., Iardino, P., Ingrosso, D., Manna, C., and Zappia, V., 1989, Enzymatic methyl esterification of a deamidated form of mouse epidermal growth factor, *Int. J. Pept. Protein Res.* **33:**397–402.

Geigert, J., Panschar, M., Forng, S., Huston, H. N., Wong, D. E., Wong, D. Y., Taforo, C., and Pemberton, M., 1988, The long term stability of recombinant (Serine-17) human interferon-b, *J. Interf. Res.* **8:**539–547.

Gitlin, G., Tsarbopoulos, A., Patel, S. T., Sydor, W., Pramanik, B. N., Jacobs, S., Westreich, L., Mittelman, S., and Bausch, J. N., 1996, Isolation and characterization of a monomethioninesulfoxide variant of interferon α-2b, *Pharm. Res.*, in press.

Grossenbacher, H., Marki, W., Coulot, M., Muller, D., and Richter, W. J., 1993, Characterization of succinimide-type dehydration products of recombinant products of recombinant hirudin variant 1 by electrospray tandem mass spectrometry, *Rapid Commun. Mass Spectrom.* **7:**1082–1085.

Gu, L. C., Erdos, E. A., Chiang, H., Calderwood, T., Tsai, K., Visor, G. C., Duffy, J., Hsu, W., and Foster, L. C., 1991, Stability of interleukin-1b (IL-1b) in aqueous solution: Analytical methods, kinetics, products and solution formulation implications, *Pharm. Res.* **8:**485–490.

Hageman, M. J., 1995, personal communication.

Hallahan, T. W., Shapiro, R., Strydom, D. J., and Vallee, B. L., 1992, Importance of asparagine-61 and asparagine-109 to the angiogenic activity of human angiogenin, *Biochemistry* **31:**8022–8029.

Halliwell, B., and Gutteridge, M. C., 1990, Role of free radicals and catalytic metal ions in human disease: An overview, *Methods Enzymol.* **186:**1–85.

Hamburger, R., Azaz, E., and Donbrow, M., 1975, Autooxidation of polyoxyethylenic non-ionic surfactants and of polyethylene glycols, *Pharm. Acta Helv.* **50:**10–17.

Harris, R. J., 1995, personal communication.

Harris, R. J., Kwong, M. Y., Molony, M. S., and Ling, V. L., 1995, *Mass Spectrometry in the Biological Sciences*, Humana Press.

Harris, R. J., Wagner, K. O., and Spellman, M. W. 1990, Structural characterization of a recombinant CD4-IgG hybrid molecule, *Eur. J. Biochem.* **194:**611–620.

Hayashi, T., Ohe, Y., and Hayahi, H., 1982, Human spleen histone H4. Isolation and amino acid sequence, *J. Biochem.* **92:**1995–2000.

Heller, D. L., and Qi, H., 1994, Stabilization of a 31 amino acid peptide formulation in a viscous dextran vehicle. AAPS 9th Natl. Meeting, San Diego, CA.

Henderson, L. E., Henriksson, D., and Nyman, P. O., 1976, Primary structure of human carbonic anhydrase C, *J. Biol. Chem.* **251:**5457–5463.

Hendy, G. N., Kronenberg, H. M., Potts Jr., J. T., and Rich, A., 1981, Nucleotide sequence of cloned cDNAs encoding human preproparathyroid hormone, *Proc. Natl. Acad. Sci. USA* **78:**7365–7369.

Herman, A., Sahakian, N., Taniguchi, G., Rohde, M., and Stoney, K., 1995, unpublished results.

Hershenson, S., Thompson, S., Luedke, E., Callahan, W., and Garcia, A., 1995, unpublished results.

Hopp, T. P., 1985, Prediction of protein surfaces and interaction sites from amino acid sequences, in: *Synthetic Peptides in Biology and Medicine* (K. Alitalo, P. Partanen, and A. Vaheri, eds.), Elsevier, Amsterdam, pp. 3–12.

Hopp, T. P., 1986, Protein surface analysis. Methods for identifying antigenic determinants and other interaction sites, *J. Immunol. Methods* **88:**1–18.

Hopp, T. P., and Woods, K. R., 1981, Prediction of protein antigenic determinants from amino acid sequences, *Proc. Natl. Acad. Sci. USA* **78:**3824–3828.

Hopp, T. P., and Woods, K. R., 1983, A computer program for predicting protein antigenic determinants, *Mol. Immunol.* **20:**483–489.

Hora, M., 1995, personal communication.

Hühmer, A. F. R., Gerber, N. C., Ortiz de Montellano, P. R., and Schöneich, C., 1996, Peroxynitrile reduction of calmodulin stimulation of neuronal nitric oxide synthase, *Chem. Res. Toxicol.* **9:** 484–491.

Inaba, M., Gupta, K. C., Kuwabara, M., Takahashi, T., Benz Jr., E. J., and Maede, Y., 1992, Deamidation of human erythrocyte protein 4.1: Possible role of aging, *Blood* **79**:3355–3361.

Ingram, R., and Warne, N., 1994, The stability of rhIL-11 as a function of pH, time, and temperature, AAPS 9th Natl. Meeting, San Diego, CA.

Johnson, B. A., Shirokawa, J. M., and Aswad, D. W., 1989a, Deamidation of calmodulin at neutral and alkaline pH: Quantitative relationships between ammonia loss and the susceptibility of calmodulin to modification by protein carboxyl methyltransferase, *Arch. Biochem. Biophys.* **268**:276–286.

Johnson, B. A., Shirokawa, J. M., Hancock, W. S., Spellman, M. W., Basa, L. J., and Aswad, D. W., 1989b, Formation of isoaspartate at two distinct site during in vitro aging of human growth hormone, *J. Biol. Chem.* **264**:14262–14271.

Johnson, D. M., and Gu, L. C., 1988, Absorption of drugs to bioavailability and bioequivalence, in: *Encyclopedia of Pharmaceutical Technology*, 1 (J. Swarbrick and J. C. Boylan, eds.), Marcel Dekker, New York, pp. 415–449.

Kanaya, S., and Uchida, T., 1986, Comparison of the primary sequences of ribonuclease U2 isoforms, *Biochem. J.* **240**:163–170.

Keck, R. C., 1995, Structural characterization of deamidated species formed during in vitro aging of recombinant interferon gamma, in preparation.

Kenigsberg, P., Fang, G., and Hager, L. P., 1987, Post-translational modifications of chloroperoxidase from *Caldariomyces fumago*, *Arch. Biochem. Biophys.* **254**:409–415.

Keutmann, H. T., Sauer, M. M., Hendy, G. N., O'Riordan, J. L. H., and Potts Jr., J. T., 1978, Complete amino acid sequence of human parathyroid hormone, *Biochemistry* **17**:5723–5729.

Keyt, B., and Cleland, J., 1995, personal communication.

Knepp, V. M., Whatley, J. L., Muchnik, A., and Calderwood, T. S., 1996, Identification of antioxidants for prevention of peroxide-mediated oxidation of recombinant human ciliary neurotrophic factor and recombinant human nerve growth factor, *J. Pharm. Sci. Tech.* **50**:163–171.

Kossiakoff, A. A., 1988, Tertiary structure is a principal determinant to protein deamidation, *Science* **240**:191–194.

Kroon, D. J., 1994, personal communication.

Kroon, D. J., Baldwin-Ferro, A., and Lalan, P., 1992, Identification of sites of degradation in a therapeutic monoclonal antibody by peptide mapping, *Pharm. Res.* **9**:1386–1393.

Kwong, M. Y., and Harris, R. J., 1985, Identification of succinimide sites in proteins by N-terminal sequence analysis after alkaline hydroxylamine cleavage, *Protein Sci.* **3**:147–149.

Kyte, J., and Doolittle, R., 1982, A simple method of displaying the hydropathic character of a protein, *J. Mol. Biol.* **157**:105–132.

Lauren, S. L., Arakawa, T., Stoney, K., and Rohde, M. F., 1993, Covalent dimerization of recombinant human interferon-γ, *Arch. Biochem. Biophys.* **306**:350–353.

Lim, A., Canova-Davis, E., Ling, V., Eng, M., Truong, L., Henzel, B., Stults, J., Harris, R., Gorrell, J., Heinsohn, H., McHugh, C., Weissburg, R. P., and Powell, M. F., 1996, Stability of rhTPO: Aggregation, oxidation, deamidation, diketopiperazine formation, AAPS Meeting, South San Francisco, CA, March, 1996.

Lin, L., Kunitani, M., and Hora, M., 1996, Interferon-b-1b (Betaseron): A model for hydrophobic therapeutic proteins, in: *Formulation, Characterization, and Stability of Protein Drugs: Case Histories* (R. Pearlman and Y. John Wang, eds.), Plenum Press, New York, pp. 275–301.

Maeda, H., and Kuromizu, K., 1977, Spontaneous deamidation of a protein antibiotic, neocarzinostatin, at weakly acidic pH, *J. Biochem.* **81**:25–35.

Maneri, L., 1994, personal communication.

McCrossin, L. E., Charman, W. N., Currie, G. J., and Charman, S. A., 1994, Degradation rates of Asn-99 and Cys-181–Cys-189 residues in native porcine growth hormone or the respective isolated tryptic peptides, AAPS 9th Natl. Meeting, San Diego, CA.

McGinity, J. W., Hill, J. A., and La Via, A. L., 1975, Influence of peroxide impurities in polyethylene glycols on drug stability, *Pharm. Sci.* **64**:356–357.

McKerrow, J. H., and Robinson, A. B., 1974, Primary sequence dependence on the deamidation of rabbit muscle aldolase, *Science* **183**:85.

Midelfort, C. F., and Mehler, A. H., 1972, Deamidation in vivo of an asparagine residue of rabbit muscle aldolase, *Proc. Natl. Acad. Sci. USA* **69**:1816–1819.

Nabuchi, Y., Fujiwara, E., Ueno, K., Kuboniwa, H., Asoh, Y., and Ushio, H., 1995, Oxidation of recombinant human parathyroid hormone: effect of oxidized position on the biological activity. *Pharm. Res.* **12**:2049.

Nguyen, T. H., Burnier, J., and Meng, W., 1993a, The kinetics of relaxin oxidation by hydrogen peroxide, *Pharm. Res.* **10**:1563–1571.

Nguyen, T. H., and Ward, C., 1993b, Stability characterization and formulation development of Alteplase, a recombinant tissue plasminogen activator, in: *Stability and Characterization of Protein and Peptide Drugs: Case Histories*, 5 (Y. J. Wang and R. Pearlman, eds.), Plenum Press, New York, pp. 91–134.

Nyberg, F., Bergman, P., Wide, L., and Roos, P., 1985, Stability studies on human pituitary prolactin, *Upsala J. Med. Sci.* **90**:265–277.

O'Kelley, P., Thomsen, L., Tilles, J. G., and Cesario, T., 1985, Inactivation of interferon by serum and synovial fluids, *Proc. Soc. Exp. Biol. Med.* **178**:407–411.

Oliyai, C., and Borchardt, R. T., 1993, Chemical pathways of peptide degradation. IV. Pathways, kinetics, and mechanism of degradation of an aspartyl residue in a model hexapeptide, *Pharm. Res.* **10**:95–102.

Ota, I. M., and Clarke, S., 1989, Enzymatic methylation of L-isoaspartyl residues derived from aspartyl residues in affinity-purified calmodulin. The role of conformational flexibility in spontaneous isoaspartyl formation, *J. Biol. Chem.* **264**:54–60.

Ota, I. M., Ding, L., and Clarke, S., 1987, Methylation at specific altered aspartyl and asparaginyl residues in glucagon by the erythrocyte protein carboxyl methyltransferase, *J. Biol. Chem.* **262**:8522–8531.

Paranandi, M. V., Guzzetta, A. W., Hancock, W. S., and Aswad, D. W., 1994, Deamidation and isoaspartate formation during in vitro aging of recombinant tissue plasminogen activator, *J. Biol. Chem.* **269**: 243–253.

Patel, K., 1993, Stability of adrenocorticotropic hormone (ACTH) and pathways of deamidation of asparaginyl residue in hexapeptide segments, in: *Stability and Characterization of Protein and Peptide Drugs: Case Histories*, (Y. J. Wang and R. Pearlman, eds.), Plenum Press, New York, pp. 201–220.

Patel, K., and Borchardt, R. T., 1990, Chemical pathways of peptide degradation. II. Kinetics of deamidation of an asparaginyl residue in a model hexapeptide, *Pharm. Res.* **7**:703–711.

Patel, S. T., and Gitlin, G., 1995, personal communication.

Pearlman, R., and Nguyen, T., 1992, Pharmaceutics of protein drugs, *J. Pharm. Pharmacol.* **44** (Suppl 1):178–185.

Poulter, L., Green, B. N., Kaur, S., and Burlingame, A. L., 1990, The characterization of native and recombinant proteins by electrospray mass spectrometry, in: *Biological Mass Spectrometry* (A. L. Burlingame and J. A. McCloskey, eds.), Elsevier, Amsterdam, pp. 119–128.

Presta, L. G., Lahr, S. J., Shields, R. L., Porter, J. P., Gorman, C. M., Fendley, B. M., and Jardieu, P. M., 1993, Humanizatiion of an antibody directed against IgE, *J. Immunol.* **151**:2623–2632.

Ragone, R., Facchiano, F., Facchiano, A., Facchiano, A. M., and Colonna, G., 1989, Flexibility plot of proteins, *Protein Eng.* **2**:497–504.

Robinson, A. B., and Rudd, C. J., 1974, *Deamidation of Glutaminyl and Asparaginyl Residues in Peptides and Proteins*, Academic Press, New York.

Robinson, A. B., Scotchler, J. W., and McKerrow, J. H., 1973a, Rates of nonenzymatic deamidation of glutaminyl and asparaginyl residues in pentapeptides, *J. Am. Chem. Soc.* **95**:8156–8159.

Robinson, A. B., and Tedro, S., 1973b, Sequence dependent deamidation rates for model peptides of hen egg, *Int. J. Pept. Protein Res.* **5**:275–278.

Sasaoki, K., Hiroshima, T., Kusumoto, S., and Nishi, K., 1989, Oxidation of methionine residues of recombinant human interleukin 2 in aqueous solutions, *Chem. Pharm. Bull. (Tokyo)* **37**:2160–2164.

Sasaoki, K., Hiroshima, T., Kusumoto, S., and Nishi, K., 1992, Deamidation at asparagine-88 in recombinant human interleukin-2, *Chem. Pharm. Bull. (Tokyo)* **40**:976–980.

Schultz, J., 1967, Cleavage at aspartic acid, *Methods Enzymol.* **11**:255–263.

Seid-Akhavan, M., Winter, W. P., Abramson, R. K., and Rucknagel, D. L., 1976, Hemoglobin Wayne: A frameshift mutation detected in human hemoglobin alpha chains, *Proc. Natl. Acad. Sci. USA* **73**: 882–886.

Senderoff, R. I., Wootton, S. C., Boctor, A. M., Chen, T. M., Giordani, A. B., Julian, T. N., and Radebaugh, G. W., 1994, Aqueous stability of human epidermal growth factor 1-48, *Pharm. Res.* **11**:1712–1720.

Sepetov, N. F., Krymsky, M. A., Ovchinnikov, M. V., Bespalava, Z. D., Isakova, O. L., Soucek, M., and Lebl, M., 1991, Rearrangement, racemization and decomposition of peptides in aqueous solution, *Pept. Res.* **4**:308–313.

Shahrokh, Z., Eberlein, G., Buckley, D., Paranandi, M. V., Aswad, D. W., Stratton, P., Mischak, R., and Wang, Y. J., 1994, Major degradation products of basic fibroblast growth factor: Detection of succinamide and iso-aspartate in place of aspartate-15, *Pharm. Res.* **11**:936–944.

Shen, F. J., Kwong, M., Keck, R. G., and Harris, R. J., 1996, Application of t-butylhydroperoxide to study sites of potential methionine oxidation in recombinant antibodies, in: *Techniques in Protein Chemistry*, Vol. 7 (D. Mershak, ed.), Academic Press, San Diego.

Shire, S. J., 1995, personal communication.

Sletten, K., Marhaug, G., and Husby, G., 1983, The covalent structure of amyloid-related serum protein SAA from two patients with inflammatory disease, *Z. Physiol. Chem.* **364**:1039–1046.

Son, K., and Kwon, C., 1995, Stabilization of human epidermal growth factor (hEGF) in aqueous solution, *Pharm. Res.* **12**:451–454.

Stadtman, E. R., 1990, Metal ion catalyzed oxidation of proteins: biochemical mechanism and biological consequences, *Free Radical Biol. Med.* **9**:315–325.

Steinberg, S. M., and Bada, J. L., 1983, Peptide decomposition in the neutral pH region via the formation of diketopiperazines, *J. Org. Chem.* **48**:2295–2298.

Stephenson, R. C., and Clarke, S., 1989, Succinimide formation from aspartyl and asparaginyl peptides as a model for the spontaneous degradation of proteins, *J. Biol. Chem.* **264**:6164– 6170.

Stevenson, C. L., Donlan, M. E., Freedman, A. R., Kubiak, T. M., and Borchardt, R. T., 1993, The effect of secondary structure on the rate of deamidation of several growth hormone releasing factor analogs, *Int. J. Pept. Protein Res.* **42**:497–503.

Sunahara, N., Kawata, S., Kaibe, K., Furuta, R., Yamayoshi, M., Yamada, M., and Kurooka, S., 1989, Differential determination of recombinant human interleukin-1α and its deamidated derivative by two sandwich enzyme immunoassays using monoclonal antibodies, *J. Immunol. Methods* **119**:75–82.

Svanti, J., and Milstein, C., 1972, The complete amino acid sequence of a mouse kappa light chain, *J. Biochem.* **128**:427–444.

Takao, T., Watanabe, H., and Shimonishi, Y., 1985, Facile identification of protein sequences by mass spectrometry, *Eur. J. Biochem.* **146**:503–508.

Teh, L., Murphy, L. J., Huq, N. L., Surus, A. S., Friesen, H. G., Lazarus, L., and Chapman, G. E., 1987, Methionine oxidation in human growth hormone and human chorionic somatomammotropin, *J. Biol. Chem.* **262**:6472–6477.

Teshima, G., and Canova-Davis, E., 1992, Separation of oxidized human growth hormone variants by reversed-phase high-performance chromatography, *J. Chromatogr.* **625**:207–215.

Teshima, G., Hancock, W. S., and Canova-Davis, E., 1995a, Effect of deamidation and isoaspartate formation on the activity of proteins, in: *Deamidation and Isoaspartate Formation in Peptides and Proteins* (D. Aswad, ed.), CRC Press, Boca Raton, FL, pp. 167–191.

Teshima, G., Porter, J., Yim, K., Ling, V., and Guzzetta, A., 1991a, Deamidation of soluble CD4 at asparagine-52 results in reduced binding capacity for the HIV-1 envelope glycoprotein gp120, *Biochemistry* **30**:3916–3922.

Teshima, G., Stults, J. T., Ling, V., and Canova-Davis, E., 1991b, Isolation and characterization of a succinimide variant of methionyl human growth hormone, *J. Biol. Chem.* **266**:13544–13547.

Teshima, G., and Wu, S., 1996, Capillary electrophoresis analysis of proteins, in: *Methods in Enzymology* (B. C. Kange and W. S. Hancock, eds.) in press.

Teshima, G., and Yim, K., 1995b, personal communication.

Tomizawa, H., Yamada, H., Ueda, T., and Imoto, T., 1994, Isolation and characterization of 101-succinimide lysozyme that possesses the cyclic imide at Asp-101-Gly102, *Biochemistry* **33**:8770–8778.

Tsuda, T., Uchiyama, M., Satao, T., Yoshino, H., Tsuchiya, Y., Ishikawa, S., Ohmae, S., Watanabe, S., and Miyake, Y. J., 1990, Mechanism and kinetics of secretion degradation in aqueous solutions, *J. Pharm. Sci.* **79**:223–227.

Tyler-Cross, R., and Schirch, V., 1991, Effects of amino acid sequence, buffers, and ionic strength on the rate and mechanism of deamidation of asparagine residues in small peptides, *J. Biol. Chem.* **266**: 22549–22556.

Venkatesh, Y. P., and Vithayathil, P. J., 1984, Isolation and characterization of monodeamidated derivatives of bovine pancreatic Ribonuclease A, *Int. J. Peptide Protein Res.* **23**:494–505.

Violand, B. N., Schlittler, M. R., Toren, P. C., and Siegel, N. R., 1990, Formation of isoaspartate 99 in bovine and porcine somatotropins, *J. Protein Chem.* **9**:109–117.

Violand, B. N., Siegel, M. R., Kolodziej, E. W., Toren, P. C., Cabonce, M. A., Siegel, N. R., Duffin, K. L., Zobel, J. F., Smith, C. E., and Tou, J. S., 1992, Isolation and characterization of porcine somatotropin containing a succinimide residue in place of aspartate 129, *Protein Sci.* **1**:1634–1641.

Volkin, D. B., and Middaugh, C. R., 1996, The characterization, stabilization, and formulation of acidic fibroblast growth factor, in *Formulation, Characterization, and Stability of Protein Drugs: Case Histories* (R. Pearlman and Y. John Wang, eds.), Plenum Press, New York, pp. 181–217.

Voorter, C. E. M., Roersma, E. S., Bloemendal, H., and de Jong, W. W., 1987, Age-dependent deamidation of chicken αA-crystallin, *FEBS Lett.* **221**:249–252.

Wang, J., 1995, personal communication.

Wang, J. H., Yan, Y. W., Garett, T. P., Liu, J. H., Rodgers, D. W., Garlick, R. L., Tarr, G. E., Husain, Y., Reinherz, E. L., and Harrison, S. C., 1990, Atomic structure of a fragment of human CD4 containing two immunoglobulin-like domains, *Nature* **348**:411–418.

Watanabe, C., 1991, Genentech Sequence Analysis Programs, Genentech, Inc., San Francisco.

Wearne, S. J., and Creighton, T. E., 1989, Effect of protein conformation on rate of deamidation: Ribonuclease and its ligands, *Proteins Struct. Funct. Genet.* **5**:8–12.

Wilson, J. M., Landa, L. E., Kobayashi, R., and Kelley, W. N., 1982, Human hypoxanthine-guanine ribosyltransferase, *J. Biol. Chem.* **257**:14830–14834.

Wingfield, P. T., Mattaliano, R. J., McDonald, H. R., Craig, S., Clore, G. M., Gronenborn, A. M., and Schmeissner, U., 1987, Recombinant-derived interleukin-1α stabilized against specific deamidation, *Protein Eng.* **1**:413–417.

Wood, D. C., Salsgiver, W. J., Kasser, T. R., Lange, G. W., Rowold, E., Violand, B. N., Johnson, A., Leimgruber, R. M., Parr, G. R., Siegel, N. R., Kimack, N. M., Smith, C. E., Zobel, J. F., Ganguli, S. M., Garbow, J. R., Bild, G., and Krivi, G. G., 1989, Purification and characterization of pituitary bovine somatotropin, *J. Biol. Chem.* **264**:14741–14747.

Wright, C. S., and Raikhel, N., 1989, Sequence variability in three wheat germ agglutinin isolectins: products of multiple genes in polyploid wheat, *J. Mol. Evol.* **28**:327–336.

Wright, H. T., 1991a, Sequence and structure determinants of the nonenzymatic deamidation of asparagine and glutamine residues in proteins, *Protein Eng.* **4**:283–291.

Wright, H. T., 1991b, Nonenzymatic deamidation of asparaginyl and glutaminyl residues in proteins, *CRC Crit. Rev. Biochem. Mol. Biol.* **26**:1–52.

Yao, Y., Yin, D., Jas, G. S., and Kuczera, K., Williams, T. D., Schöneich, C., and Squier, T. C., 1996, Oxidative modification of carboxyl-terminal vicinal methionine in calmodulin by hydrogen peroxide inhibits calmodulin-dependent activation of the plasma membrane Ca-ATPase, *Biochemistry* **35**:2767–2787.

2

Characterization, Stability, and Formulations of Basic Fibroblast Growth Factor

Y. John Wang, Zahra Shahrokh, Sriram Vemuri, Gert Eberlein, Irina Beylin, and Mark Busch

1. INTRODUCTION

Basic fibroblast growth factor (bFGF) as described in this chapter is a recombinant, human, single-chain, nonglycosylated polypeptide that contains 154 amino acids (Fig. 1), with a molecular mass of about 18 kDa (17,123 Dalton, as determined by mass spectrometry). It is a primary inducer of mesoderm formation in embryogenesis, and can modulate both cell proliferation and cell differentiation *in vitro* and *in vivo*. As a mitogen and chemoattractant, bFGF is a potent mediator of wound healing, angiogenesis, and neural outgrowth. Its clinical utility for wound healing, collateral blood vessel formation in myocardial infarct, and osteogenesis in bone fractures is being evaluated.

bFGF is one of at least nine structurally homologous fibroblast growth factors, several of which are characterized by heparin binding and by potent mitogenic activity on a variety of mesoderm- and neuroectoderm-derived cells such as fibroblasts, endothelial cells, smooth muscle cells, chondrocytes, osteoblasts, and melano

Y. John Wang, Sriram Vemuri, and Mark Busch • Pharmaceutical Research and Development and Quality Control, Scios Inc., Mountain View, California 94043. *Zahra Shahrokh* • Department of Research and Development, Genentech Inc., South San Francisco, California 94080. *Gert Eberlein* • Research and Development, Matrix Pharmaceutical Inc., Menlo Park, California 94025. *Irina Beylin* • Development, Alza Corporation, Palo Alto, California 94303.

Formulation, Characterization, and Stability of Protein Drugs, Rodney Pearlman and Y. John Wang, eds., Plenum Press, New York, 1996.

```
   1                              10
(Met) Ala Ala Gly Ser Ile Thr Thr Leu Pro Ala Leu Pro Glu │Asp Gly│ Gly

        20                                      30
Ser Gly Ala Phe Pro Pro Gly His Phe Lys │Asp Pro│ Lys Arg Leu Tyr Cys

               40                                        50
Lys │Asn Gly│ Gly Phe Phe Leu Arg Ile His Pro │Asp Gly│ Arg Val │Asp Gly│

                              60
Val Arg Glu Lys Ser │Asp Pro│ His Ile Lys Leu Gln Leu Gln Ala Glu Glu

    70                                      80
Arg Gly Val Val Ser Ile Lys Gly Val Cys Ala Asn Arg Tyr Leu Ala (Met)

            90                                      100
Lys Glu │Asp Gly│ Arg Leu Leu Ala Ser Lys Cys Val Thr Asp Glu Cys Phe

                         110
Phe Phe Glu Arg Leu Glu Ser Asn Asn Tyr Asn Thr Tyr Arg Ser Arg Lys

120                                     130
Tyr Thr Ser Trp Tyr Val Ala Leu Lys Arg Thr Gly Gln Tyr Lys Leu Gly

        140                                     150
Ser Lys Thr Gly Pro Gly Gln Lys Ala Ile Leu Phe Leu Pro (Met) Ser Ala

    155
Lys Ser
```

Figure 1. Primary sequence of bFGF. The final bFGF product does not contain methionine at position 1. The positions of asp-pro, asp-gly, and asn-gly, potential degradation sites (Section 6), are highlighted.

cytes (Burgess and Maciag, 1989). The two most prominent FGFs are distinguished by their isoelectric points: acidic FGF (aFGF) having a pI of 5–6 and bFGF having a pI of 9.8. These two FGFs share 55% sequence identity and are referred to in some literature as FGF-1 and FGF-2, respectively. Other members of this family include keratinocyte growth factor (FGF-7), androgen-induced growth factor (FGF-8), int-2 protein (FGF-3), and K (for Karposi sarcoma)-FGF (FGF-4), etc. All nine members of the FGF family share 35–55% sequence homology and two conserved cysteines.

There are various lengths of human bFGF reported in the literature. The predominant form in initial isolations from tissue was 146 residues (Pro[1]-Ala-Leu ... Ser[146]), the N-terminus can be extended at least to 11 amino acids: Gly-Thr-Met-Ala[1]-Ala[2]-Gly[3]-Ser[4]-Ile[5]-Thr[6]-Thr[7]-Leu[8]. Intermediate lengths begin with Ala[1] or Ala[2]. These different lengths may result from translation initiation occurring at different codons or from protease action during isolation and purification of bFGF from different sources of cells. Different forms of bFGF having the following N-terminal sequences have been developed by various pharmaceutical companies worldwide: Gly-Thr-Met ... 157 residues by Synergen (Squires *et al.* 1988; Florkiewicz and Sommer, 1989); Ala-Ala-Gly ... 154 residues by Scios Inc. (Abraham *et al.*, 1986; Thompson *et al.*, 1991; Thompson, 1989) and Farmitalia Carlo Erba (Adami *et al.*,

1992); and Pro-Ala-Leu ... 146 residues by Takeda (Koichi *et al.*, 1989), Chiron (Eriksson *et al.*, 1991), and Amgen (Fox *et al.*, 1988). Bovine bFGF (146 residues), which can be sourced conveniently, differs only in position 112 (in the 146-residue numbering scheme) where threonine is substituted with serine and in position 128 where serine is substituted with proline.

Both bFGF and aFGF display a strong interaction with the glycosaminoglycans (GAG) such as heparin and heparan sulfate, and it has been demonstrated that heparin protects bFGF and aFGF against trypsin, heat, and acid inactivation (Gospodarowicz and Cheng, 1986). GAGs, also known as mucopolysaccharides, are long unbranched polysaccharide chains composed of repeating disaccharide units. They are called glycosaminoglycans because one of the two sugar residues in the repeating disaccharides is always an amino sugar (*N*-acetylglucosamine or *N*-acetylgalactosamine). GAGs are highly negatively charged due to the presence of sulfate or carboxyl groups, or both, on many of the sugar residues. The major GAGs are heparin (6–25 kDa), keratin sulfate (1–1.8 kDa), heparan sulfate (5–12 kDa), chondroitin (5–50 kDa), and hyaluronic acid ($4-10^3$ kDa), where the sulfates per disaccharide units decreased from 2–3 to 0 in that order. Except hyaluronic acid, GAGs are covalently linked to proteins, through serine, to form proteoglycan (mucoproteins). The hydrophilicity of GAGs attracts a large amount of water and effectively fills the extracellular space.

For some time it was generally believed that, unlike aFGF, bFGF is not potentiated by heparin in a mitogenic assay (Sommer and Rifkin, 1989). However, recent data demonstrated the need for heparin or heparan sulfate in bFGFs binding to soluble FGF receptor in a cell-free environment (Ornitz *et al.*, 1992). In Sommer's experiment (1989), the residual amount of heparan sulfate on the cell surface obscured the effect of added heparin; thus potentiation would not be observed in the cell proliferation assay. Although the physiological significance of the interaction of FGF with GAG is not clear, it is possible that, *in vivo*, FGF molecules are protected by binding to GAG and stored in the extracellular matrix as an FGF–GAG complex. During injury or the process of wound healing, FGF could be released to bind high-affinity receptors, through the action of heparinase or protease, thus triggering a cascade events of chemoattraction, angiogenesis, etc. The reserved amount of FGF in tissue is important, as FGF's lack classical secretory signal peptides and do not appear to be secreted by cultured cells.

In production of recombinant bFGF at Scios Inc. (Shadle *et al.*, 1993; Scheuermann *et al.*, 1992), cDNA encoding for 155 residue bFGF (Met + 154 residues) is performed in a plasmid vector in *E. coli* B cells. After fermentation, the bacterial cells are lysed by a homogenizer to release bFGF. The first step of purification is ion-exchange chromatography carried out on SP-Sephadex. The subsequent purification can be any one of the following: heparin–Sepharose, copper chelating, or hydrophobic-interaction chromatography. The final step is ion-exchange or size-exclusion chromatography to collect the monomer of FGF in pH 5 citrate buffer containing EDTA as a stabilizer. The purified protein, with Met^1 truncated, has >98% purity by SDS-PAGE.

2. PHYSICOCHEMICAL CHARACTERIZATION AND ANALYSIS

2.1. Structure and the Conformation

Eriksson *et al.* (1991, 1993), Zhu *et al.* (1991), Zhang *et al.* (1991), and Ago *et al.* (1991) reported detailed structure and conformation data on bFGF based on X-ray crystallographic analysis. Basic FGF (146 residues) crystals were prepared by the hanging drop vapor diffusion technique from a solution of ammonium sulfate, citrate (or Tris), and dithiothreitol. The structure was determined by X-ray diffraction at 1.6-Å or 2.5-Å resolution. bFGF is a globular protein of ~4 nm diameter with hydrophobic residues lining the core and a large number of charged residues on the surface. The backbone structure is that of a β barrel consisting of 12 antiparallel β strands connected by β turns and arranged in a pattern of approximate threefold axis of symmetry. The ribbon structure is shown in Fig. 2. The three-dimensional structure of basic FGF is also similar to that of interleukin-1 β, which has minimal sequence homology to FGF.

A single tryptophan exists near the surface of the protein, the position of which is conserved in the structure of all the related proteins. The fluorescence from this tryptophan is quenched in the native protein and increases upon unfolding (Shahrokh *et al.*, 1994b; Copeland *et al.*, 1991); hence fluorescence spectroscopy is a useful method to follow structural perturbations of the protein (more discussion in Section 2.3).

An unusual cluster of positively charged residues (Lys-138, Lys-134, Lys-128, Arg-129, Lys-144) is found on one side of the protein which is considered to be the heparin binding region of the protein. The receptor binding domain is in this vicinity and is made of peptide segment 115–124 (including Tyr-123 and Trp-124). The segments of the first 25 (through His-Phe from the N-terminus) and last 3 (from C-terminus) residues are disordered because the structures were too flexible to be resolved by crystallographic analysis.

There are two exposed cysteines (Cys-78 and -96) and two conserved, buried cysteines (Cys-34 and -101). The protein is capable of formation of disulfide-linked multimers via the two exposed SH groups (Thompson and Fiddes, 1992) and, as a result, multimerization is a major formulation problem, particularly at high pHs where disulfide bond formation is promoted. Interestingly, the protein has been crystallized at both pH 5.3 (Zhang *et al.*, 1991) and 8.1 (Eriksson *et al.*, 1991) and the structures are nearly superimposable. Based on crystallographic data, the distances between any pair of cysteines are too far to form disulfide linkages. Thus native bFGF is expected to have all four cysteines in reduced form. Although Fox *et al.* (1988) had found only two free SH groups based on DTNB titration and therefore suggested a disulfide bond between the two conserved 34 and 101 cysteines, this result was probably caused by an artifact in analysis.

Close packing of positive charges in the heparin binding region generates a significant amount of structural energy that causes latent instability. Polyanions such as heparin interact with this region, resulting in a large stabilization effect. Such

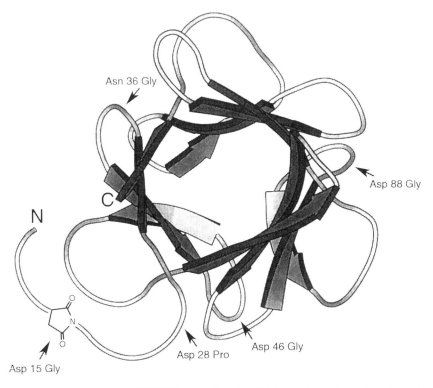

Figure 2. The folded structure of bFGF. There are 12 antiparallel β-strands that form a β-barrel structure with a hydrophobic core (modified drawing from Eriksson *et al.*, 1993). The locations of degradation sites (succinimide, asp-pro, asp-gly, asn-gly) are shown.

stabilization protects aFGF and bFGF against thermal and pH-induced denaturation, as well as protease cleavage. It is the degree of sulfation of heparin which seems to be critical to its protective activity. Interestingly, sulfate ions (which were included in the buffers during crystallization) can be found within the crystal structure (Eriksson *et al.*, 1993), bound to those lysine residues that are also involved in heparin binding. These observations all suggest that sulfates and heparins are structural stabilizers for bFGF in solution; however, they do not protect the cysteines in bFGF against formation of either intra- or inter-molecular disulfide bonds.

2.2. UV Spectroscopy

UV spectroscopy can be a convenient assay for protein concentration during manufacturing. The uncertainty associated with the UV method, however, derives from the fact that the extinction coefficient is calculated from protein concentration determined by methods such as nitrogen content (Kjeldahl), quantitative amino acid analysis, or colorimetric assay of protein (Bradford or bicinchoninic acid assay), and each of these methods may have artifacts affecting its accuracy and precision. Nevertheless, the UV method can still be valuable in determining content uniformity of the product, protein concentration after aggregates are removed by filter, and, qualitatively, in assessing trends of protein aggregation. The absorbance maximum of bFGF at 277 nm arises from one tryptophan and seven tyrosines; the absorptivity is nearly equal to the sum of absorptivities of these amino acids. We have demonstrated that UV absorbance of bFGF is not affected by pH, citrate concentration, etc. (Eberlein *et al.*, 1994).

2.3. Fluorescence Spectroscopy

In the bFGF molecule, a single tryptophan located near the receptor binding site enables us to examine the state of the protein (native versus unfolded) through fluorescence spectroscopy. This method is one of the limited number of approaches for evaluating a protein's folded structure within aggregates and precipitates (Shahrokh *et al.*, 1994b).

The fluorescence excitation spectrum of bFGF shows one asymmetric component that peaks at 277 nm (Fig. 3A). Excitation at this wavelength gives a broad asymmetric emission spectrum which peaks at 306–308 nm (Fig. 3B). bFGF has seven tyrosines (Fox *et al.*, 1988; Sluzky *et al.*, 1994) which give rise to the emission spectrum of native bFGF, whereas the emission of the single tryptophan near the surface is quenched. Tryptophan-specific excitation at 290 nm gives rise to a broad spectrum slightly above the background (Fig. 3B), confirming the quenched state of tryptophan in native bFGF. The quenched state of tryptophan in native bFGF might be due to a charge interaction with neighboring lysine and arginine residues.

Denaturation of bFGF with guanidine (Gn)HCl (5.6 M, 5 hr, 22°C) results in a dramatic rise in emission at 350 nm (Fig. 3B) and excitation at 280 nm (Fig. 3A), concomitant with a marked decrease in tyrosine emission. Apparently tryptophan emission is unquenched upon protein unfolding, whereas the decrease in tyrosine emission might have been due to an interaction with GnHCl, as noted for other proteins (Copeland *et al.*, 1991). Thermal and acid denaturation also result in quenching of the tyrosines and unquenching of tryptophan, although a blue-shift of the emission peak is observed. The fluorescence behaviors of both bFGF and aFGF are similar and unlike textbook proteins such as albumin, where tryptophan emission is quenched upon protein unfolding (Copeland *et al.*, 1991).

The ratio of peak emissions at 350 nm and 308 nm appears to be a sensitive index of bFGF denaturation. Thus, a fluorescence index (F_{350}/F_{308}) of 0.21 and 1.9 identifies full native and fully denatured bFGF, respectively (Sluzky *et al.*, 1994). The

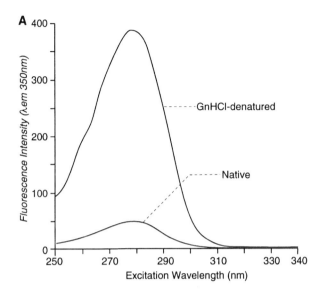

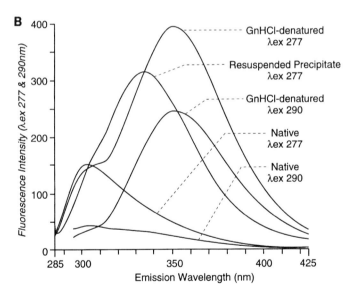

Figure 3.   Fluorescence spectra of soluble bFGF. (A) The excitation spectra of native (in pH 6.5 phosphate buffer and 1 mM EDTA) and denatured (+5.6 M GnHCl) bFGF. (B) The emission spectra of native and denatured soluble bFGF, as well as 3× washed precipitates found after storage (35°C, 2.5 days).

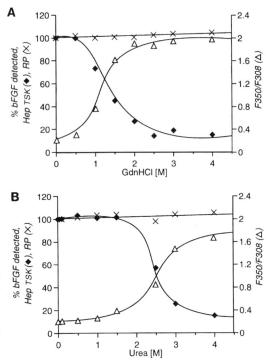

Figure 4. Chaotrope-dependent bFGF denaturation. Degree of unfolding is expressed as the ratio of fluorescence intensities at 350 to 380 nm (△). The recovery of bFGF from HepTSK (◆) and RP (×) columns following denaturation in (A) GnHCl and (B) urea is shown.

equilibrium denaturation profile using this ratio is consistent with a two-state model with midpoints at 1.2 M GnHCl and 2.7 M urea (Fig. 4).

bFGF is highly susceptible to precipitation. The folded structure of bFGF within the precipitates can be evaluated by fluorescence spectroscopy, which confirms its denatured state (Shahrokh *et al.*, 1994b). The emission spectra of bFGF suspensions containing precipitates or aggregates are very reproducible so long as a uniform suspension is maintained. The sum of the emission spectra of native soluble bFGF and denatured/precipitated bFGF is superimposable on the spectrum of unfractionated suspension, demonstrating the utility of fluorescence in quantitative analysis of denatured aggregates in turbid protein formulations.

2.4. Circular Dichroism (CD) and Fourier-Transform Infrared Spectroscopy (FTIR)

The far-UV CD spectra of a 153-residue, double serine mutein (Wu *et al.*, 1991) and the 146-residue bFGF (Fox *et al.*, 1988) are comparable, with a minimum at 202 nm, resembling that of an unordered protein or a protein rich in distorted antiparallel β-sheet. Further analysis suggested that the molecule consisted of 50% in β-sheet and no α-helix present. Heat-induced aggregates showed a CD spectrum indicative of helix-like structures. The helicity was also enhanced in trifluoroethanol and sodium dodecyl sulfate.

The secondary structure of bFGF was also examined by Prestrelski *et al.* (1991) using Fourier-transform infrared spectroscopy (FTIR). Their results confirmed that bFGF contains predominantly β-structure (~42%) and β-turns (~20%). About 17% of the protein backbone assumes irregular or disordered conformations. The CD and FTIR observations of the native protein are consistent with the X-ray crystallographic analyses.

2.5. Reverse-Phase HPLC (RP-HPLC)

Reverse-phase HPLC is a well-established technique for the analysis and purification of peptides and proteins and offers high-resolution separations of closely related molecules. From the mobile phase, bFGF adsorbs onto the hydrophobic surface of the column and remains there until the organic solvent, acetonitrile in this case, reaches a sufficient concentration (about 28–39%), and displaces bFGF from the hydrophobic surface. With a C-4 coated silica column (5-micron particle size, 300-Å pore size) bFGF is eluted at 35% acetonitrile when 0.1% TFA is used as a modifier. Disulfide-linked dimers and an unidentified bFGF-like protein (possibly monomer with internal disulfide) can be readily separated by this method (Shahrokh *et al.*, 1994d). Also dimers of different linkages (i.e., 78-78, 78-96, 96-96) can be resolved into three distinct peaks only by RP-HPLC (Shahrokh *et al.* 1994d; Asta-fieva *et al.*, 1996).

Cysteines in bFGF are readily oxidized to cysteic acid during manufacturing processes which utilize copper chelate chromatography (Scheuermann *et al.*, 1992). bFGF with buried cysteic acid is detectable when the protein is unfolded by the RP-HPLC eluant, i.e., TFA and a high content of organic solvent. Under these conditions, the oxidized species is resolved from the native protein. Although these chemical changes in bFGF are detectable by RP-HPLC, they do not affect biological activity, since the oxidation sites are remote from the receptor and heparin binding regions.

2.6. Ion-Exchange HPLC (HPIEC)

In order to complement the utility of the RP-HPLC technique, analytical methods for bFGF using ion-exchange HPLC were developed. The interaction of a protein with an ion exchange column is not exclusively dependent on the total charges exhibited by the molecule under the solvent conditions (usually aqueous buffer systems). Rather, it can be attributed to the asymmetric spatial distribution of charges on the protein and their electrostatic interactions with the surface of the chromatographic material. Thus, the interaction of the protein is strongly dependent on the maintenance of the three-dimensional structure of the protein during the chromatographic process. Disruption of that structure is likely to result in significant changes in the elution behavior of the protein molecule. Therefore, this method is most suitable as a stability-indicating method. The column used for this method is a PolyCAT A (PolyLC, Inc., Columbia, MD). The column is run at ambient temperature, using a 6.8-mM/min ammonium sulfate gradient at pH 6. This method is capable of separating most known degradation products (cyclic imide, deamidated species, dimers, etc.). Details are discussed in Section 6.

2.7. Affinity HPLC Methods

FGF's strong affinity for heparin, which can only be disrupted at >1.7 M NaCl, serves as a basis for the analysis of bFGF. Heparin affinity chromatography can be performed on Sepharose-based heparin-TSK HPLC. This method is capable of distinguishing monomeric and multimeric forms of bFGF, but has little utility or selectivity for the other chemical or minor conformational modifications of bFGF that must be addressed in the development of a stability-indicating assay for a protein pharmaceutical. Interaction with heparin-bound column-packing material relies on maintenance of bFGF's tertiary structure (or at least that of its heparin-binding domain), because the interaction involves bringing into proximity basic residues distant from each other in the sequence (10, 11). Figure 4 shows the correlation of the degree of unfolding as determined by the ratio of fluorescence intensity at 350 to 308 nm and bFGF recovery from heparin TSK HPLC. The mirror images of the two curves substantiate the fact that hep-TSK can discriminate denatured bFGF from the native form, whereas RP-HPLC is unable to discern the difference.

Though FGFs can be easily purified by heparin affinity chromatography, those interested in the clinical use of FGF purified in this fashion should be concerned about residual amounts of heparin which may leach from the column, and, because of strong binding to the growth factors, can not be completely removed.

2.8. Size-Exclusion HPLC (HP-SEC)

Like many proteins, bFGF and its multimers can be separated on size-exclusion chromatography using, for example, TSK-Gel (2000SW). Because bFGF is rich in positively charged amino acids, elution from the silica-based TSK gel requires at least 0.5 M NaCl in the mobile phase. Even then, native bFGF monomer elutes at an apparent molecular weight (MW) of 14.0 ± 0.6 kD (~80% of actual MW). Similar nonideal elution from SEC columns has been observed for many proteins due to nonspecific interactions.

3. BIOLOGICAL METHODS OF EVALUATION

3.1. Cell Proliferation Assays

The mitogenic activity of bFGF can be assessed using target cells such as a baby hamster kidney fibroblast cell line (BHK-21) or adrenal cortex capillary endothelial (ACE) cells. After incubation of these cells with bFGF at various concentrations, the increase in the number of cells, as a measure of cell proliferation, can be determined by either Coulter particle counter or protein analysis by the bicinchoninic acid method at 595 nm. Mitogenicity can also be measured by incorporation of ^{3}H-thymidine into DNA of 3T3 fibroblast cells in tissue culture plates.

Angiogenic activity of bFGF and three Cys-to-Ser muteins was tested on the chick embryo chorioallantoic membrane (Seno *et al.*, 1988). A polypropylene disk carrying certain concentrations of bFGF was grafted onto the membrane. The potency was determined by the percentage of the number of embryos which demonstrated angiogenesis toward the disk.

3.2. *In Vivo* Animal Models

Unlike many biotechnology derived products which are administered by parenteral route, growth factors can be administered topically (locally) for treatment of dermal wounds, nonunion fractures, etc. Efficacy of a growth factor product can be significantly influenced by the product strength, dosing regimen, and excipients. It is essential that formulation aspects be optimized prior to the initiation of expensive clinical trials. Once a formulation is chosen, if there are any major subsequent changes such as significant modification in purification process, addition of anti-microbial preservative, or revision of formulation aids, etc., it will be prudent that, in addition to physicochemical characterization, the efficacy be tested by *in vivo* animal models.

In general, animal models (an excellent review of this topic can be found in Abraham and Klagsbrun, 1995) can be divided into two categories: models of unimpaired healing and models of impaired healing. The latter has the advantage of an expanded magnitude of disparity between active and placebo; however, the disadvantage is the concern whether the underlying impairment mechanism truly reflects the clinical situation.

Among models of unimpaired healing, Davidson *et al.* (1985, 1988) was the first to carry out wound-healing studies with highly purified bFGF injected into polyvinyl alcohol sponge disks which had been implanted under the skin of rats. Efficacy was measured by increased granulation tissue and accumulation of DNA. Recombinant bFGF was tested by Fiddes *et al.* (1991) utilizing a similar approach. A rabbit ear dermal ulcer model (Mustoe *et al.*, 1991) was used to test mutant forms of bFGF (Seno *et al.*, 1988). In this test, circular wounds were made by excision of punch biopsies down to the cartilage. Efficacy was measured by migration of new granulation tissue and epithelium from the wound periphery.

Healing of surgical wounds can be measured by tensile strength of the wound area. To test the effect of bFGF in this type of model, McGee *et al.* (1988) made dorsal incisions in normal rats, closed the wounds with sutures, and injected bFGF 3 days afterward. There was about a 40% increase in tissue strength of the bFGF-treated incisions relative to controls.

Of all the unimpaired models, the partial thickness dermal wound model has been tested the most. The ability of bFGF to stimulate growth of keratinocytes in culture suggested that bFGF, in addition to its effects on granulation tissue formation, might also serve to accelerate epidermal wound healing. The rate of epithelialization could be accelerated by a single application of 1 μg bFGF/cm^2 on pig skin (Hebda *et al.*, 1990). Effects of the treatment protocol, vehicle types, dressing material, etc., can be carefully assessed by this model.

Diabetics or patients with circulatory illnesses are known to have impaired wound healing. Conceivably, the exogenous application of growth factors may facilitate healing. A number of laboratories have tested the ability of bFGF to modulate wound repair in animal models of impaired healing. Diabetes induced by streptozotocin (Broadley *et al.*, 1988), prednisolone treatment (Klingbeil *et al.*, 1991), protein malnourishment (Albertson *et al.*, 1993), ischemia made by cutting and cauterizing arteries (Ahn and Mustoe, 1990), and bacterial contamination (Stenberg *et al.*, 1991) are examples of methods which induce healing impairment. To illustrate the utility of a healing-impaired wound model, Fig. 5 shows the effect of bFGF on the closure

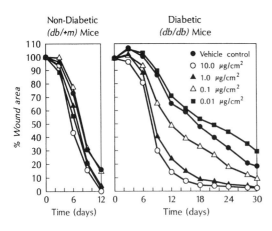

Figure 5. Effect of varying doses of bFGF on the closure of full-thickness excisional wounds in diabetic (db/db) and heterozygous control (db/+m) mice. Single bFGF doses of 10, 1.0, 0.1, and 0.01 μg/cm^2 were applied on the day of wounding. The number of animals in each treatment group ranged from 7 to 10.

of full-thickness excisional wounds in diabetic (db/db) mice. Similar results were observed in genetically obese (ob/ob) mice (Klingbeil *et al.*, 1991; Fiddes *et al.*, 1991).

4. THERMAL STABILITY

4.1. Use of a Differential Scanning Calorimeter

Protein denaturation upon thermal stress can be conveniently studied with a differential scanning calorimeter (DSC) where T_m, the midpoint of the endothermic peak profile in the thermogram, reflects the denaturation point of the protein. This technique can be used to identify optimal pH, buffer species, stabilizer, etc., where protein conformation is most stable. Typically, for bFGF, temperature-dependent changes in heat capacity are generated from a 1-mg/ml solution, heated at 1°C/min to 95°C (Vemuri *et al.*, 1994).

At pH 5 and 7, the T_m's observed for bFGF were 52°C and 63°C, respectively. In comparison, aFGF is considerably less stable, showing a T_m of 42°C in phosphate buffer pH 6.5 (Copeland, 1991).

4.2. Thermal Stability as a Function of pH

The pH dependence of thermal denaturation of bFGF was studied in a phosphate–citrate–borate buffer system (Vemuri *et al.*, 1994). An endothermic change in the thermogram is apparent above pH 4. An upward shift in T_m from 50 to 64°C was observed as the pH was changed from 4 to 9 (Fig. 6). As is evident in Fig. 6, the T_m reached a plateau between pH 7 and 9. The data suggest that the bFGF conformation is thermally most stable between pH 7 and 9. Thermograms in the pH range of 2 to 4 have nondiscernible peaks, possibly due to multiple pathways of thermal denaturation.

Protein denaturation in the acidic pH range can be corroborated by fluorescence spectroscopy. The fluorescence emission spectra of bFGF (pH 5) at room temperature showed a single peak at 308 nm (Fig. 3). When the temperature of the sample was raised to 65°C for 30 min beyond its T_m value (i.e., 61°C) the emission peak shifted to 342 nm. Similarly, when the pH of the bFGF solution was adjusted to 3, the fluorescence spectrum was affected and showed increased fluorescence intensity with a maximum at 342 nm (Vemuri *et al.*, 1994). These observations suggest that protein denaturation induced by heat and acidic pH causes shifts in fluorescence emission. A ratio of fluorescence intensity 342/308 can be used as an index to follow the stability of bFGF under stress conditions (Shahrokh *et al.*, 1994b).

As is evident from Fig. 7, the fluorescence intensity ratio increased as the pH was reduced from 5 to 2, but did not change when the pH was raised from 5 into

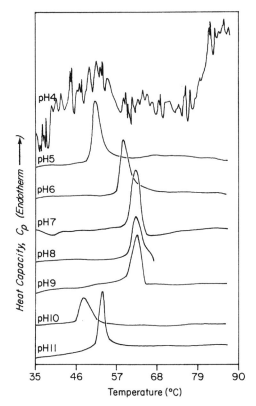

Figure 6. pH-dependent change in DSC endothermic peak of bFGF. Experiments were performed at 1 mg ml^{-1} bFGF in phosphate–citrate–borate buffer.

the alkaline region up to pH 8. A slight increase in the fluorescence intensity ratio was noted at pH 9, probably due to formation of tyrosinate. The increased fluorescence intensity ratio in the acidic region is attributed to the unfolding of protein. Although sulfated ligands protect bFGF against thermal denaturation (see the following section) these ligands cannot offer any protection against acid-induced denaturation (Vemuri *et al.*, 1994).

4.3. Effect of Sulfated Ligand

Since bFGF is a heparin binding protein, under certain conditions heparin and other sulfated ligands will influence the thermal stability of the growth factor. The

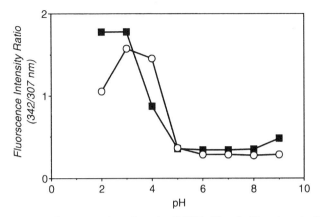

Figure 7. pH-dependent fluorescence intensity ratio of bFGF with and without heparin. (■) bFGF alone, (○) bFGF: heparin at 1:0.3 weight ratio.

effect of heparin on the thermal denaturation of bFGF is dramatic. A weight ratio as low as 0.3:1 of heparin to bFGF shifted the endothermic peak from 61 to 90°C. Copeland *et al.* (1991) showed a T_m shift from 42 to 67°C by the addition of heparin to a formulation of aFGF. Similar results were reported using low-molecular-weight heparin, sucrose octasulfate, and inositol hexasulfate for both bFGF (Vemuri *et al.*, 1994) and aFGF (Tsai *et al.*, 1993). The common ion in all these compounds is sulfate; however, the greatest increase in T_m that can be derived from sodium sulfate is only 9°C, suggesting that the multivalent interaction of the ligands with bFGF is important to structural stabilization through relief of tension that is caused by charge repulsion in the lysine/arginine-rich region.

Physical protection of bFGF against thermal denaturation is probably responsible for the preservation of biological activity described by Koichi *et al.* (1989), where 100% biological activity was detected by Balb/c 3T3 cell proliferation assay, after incubation of 100 μg/ml bFGF with 4.6 μg/ml dextran sulfate salt at 56°C for 30 min, whereas unprotected bFGF, under the same conditions, showed only 11% activity remaining.

4.4. Thermal Stability Determined by Circular Dichroism

The far-UV CD spectrum of bFGF (pH 7, 20 mM phosphate buffer) at 0°C was indistinguishable from that at 25°C. However, as the temperature of the sample solution was raised from 25 to 75°C, dramatic changes occurred. The ellipticity at 187 nm decreased as the temperature was raised to 41°C, disappeared completely at 50°C, and became positive at 55°C. The 187-nm band was attributed to tyrosine side chains; ellipticity of this band decreased and eventually disappeared when the pH was increased from 7 to 10.7 and then to 11.7 (Wu *et al.*, 1991). The fact that CD changes at 187 nm occurred at lower temperatures (50–55°C) than the T_m (62°C) measured by DSC at the same pH suggests that the tyrosine-rich region (four out of seven tyrosine residues are located between positions 112 and 124) is more sensitive to thermal stress than the whole molecule is. Perhaps the perturbation of structure in this region precedes the complete conformational change as observed in the DSC experiment.

5. OXIDATION OF CYSTEINES

There are four cysteines in bFGF, and all of them are very reactive in solution. Mechanistic study of the singular cysteine in captopril showed that disulfide formation can be effectively retarded by the addition of a metal chelating agent, EDTA, and maintenance of pH below 6 and that sulfite-type antioxidants were ineffective as stabilizers (Timmins *et al.*, 1982). A change in the reaction rate from first order to zero order occurs as the captopril concentration decreases. The apparent zero-order rate constant shows a first order dependency on oxygen tension and second-order dependency on cupric ion concentration (Lee and Notari, 1987).

5.1. Disulfide Formation

Basic FGF purified from *E. coli* expression system (Shadle *et al.*, 1993; Scheuermann *et al.*, 1992) is in the fully reduced form and when chromatographed on heparin-TSK elutes as a single peak at 1–2 M of NaCl (Thompson and Fiddes, 1992). When bFGF is air oxidized, it elutes as a heterogeneous mixture, with up to six peaks on heparin-TSK chromatography (Fig. 8B). Treatment of the oxidized bFGF with reducing agents reverts the mixture to the homogeneous form (Fig. 8A), indicating that the heterogeneity is due to the formation of disulfide bonds. Interestingly, when analyzed by SDS-PAGE, these six fractions from heparin-TSK chromatography all migrated as a single monomer band with minor bands of higher-molecular-weight forms. This observation can be explained by rapid thiol-disulfide exchange occurring when the multimeric bFGF is mixed with the denaturing sample buffer prior to electrophoresis. In order to properly assess the molecular weight of these six fractions, bFGF should be treated with a thiol-alkylating agent, iodoacetamide (500 mM). Following such treatment, species migrating on SDS-PAGE as monomer, dimer, trimer, and higher multimers were distinctively observed from each corresponding heparin-TSK fractions (Thompson and Fiddes, 1992).

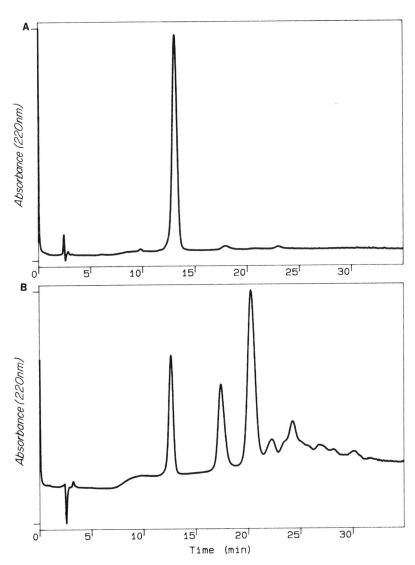

Figure 8. Heparin-TSK HPLC analysis of bFGF that has undergone a significant degree of multimerization. Chromatography was carried out on a 7.5 cm × 7.5 mm column either after (A) or before (B) reduction with dithiothreitol. The native bFGF also elutes as the 13-min peak.

5.2. Prevention of Cysteine Oxidation

When bFGF (at pH 7.4 or 5.0, 25°C) was analyzed by RP-HPLC and heparin affinity HPLC, Foster *et al.* (1991) observed substantial loss of the bFGF main peak in 24 hr. A similar extent of loss was also observed on the BHK bioassay indicating that such chemical change also resulted in losses in biological potency. To preserve the reduced form of bFGF, 1 mM EDTA (disodium or calcium disodium salt) was incorporated into the formulation. Similar to the experience with captopril, which has a single sulfhydril group, spiked cupric ion accelerated the loss of bFGF (Foster *et al.*, 1991). In addition, pH 5 is slightly better than pH 7 with respect to bFGF recovery. When formulated as such, bFGF showed greater than 90% recovery by RP-HPLC for several months at 5°C (Table I). Based on this observation a liquid formulation was evaluated in toxicology studies and early clinical trials.

5.3. Sites of Cysteine Oxidation

Any of the four cysteines residue positions (34, 78, 96, and 101) in bFGF can potentially form intra- or intermolecular disulfides. Using site directed mutagenesis,

**Table I. Stability Data by Heparin Affinity HPLC
and Reversed-Phase HPLC for bFGF[a] in
Polypropylene Containers at 4°C[b]**

Storage time (days)	% bFGF remaining[c]	
	Heparin-TSK HPLC	Reversed-phase HPLC
0	100.0	100.0
4	95.2	99.6
9	97.8	
14	98.7	102.0
16	97.4	109.9
17	103.7	104.9
19	96.9	102.3
33	102.6	102.3
41	104.4	102.0
61	105.2	101.6
93	97.1	99.8
125	88.4	95.8
156	96.0	95.2
190	90.4	

[a]Solution contains 50 mM sodium acetate, pH 5.0, with 1 mM calcium
disodium EDTA with isotonicity adjusted by addition of sodium chloride.
[b]Data from Foster *et al.* (1991).
[c]Percent initial based on main peak area.

one can substitute serines for cysteines and produce a total of 15 muteins (1, 4, 6, and 4 muteins for 4, 3, 2, and 1 serine replacements, respectively). From the behavior of these muteins on heparin affinity HPLC, where only the 78,96 double serine mutein remained as a single peak, one can deduce that cysteines at 78 and 96 positions were the most reactive (Seno *et al.*, 1988; Thompson and Fiddes, 1992). The other two cysteines, 34 and 101, are less reactive and this may be attributed to conformational restraint (Eriksson *et al.*, 1991) or formation of an intramolecular disulfide (Thompson and Fiddes, 1992). Since heparin affinity HPLC can detect bFGF and its multimers in the native conformation, it is possible that oxidative changes of inner cysteines (34 and 101) would not have been detected, so long as tertiary structure is maintained.

Muteins of improved stability are valuable for pharmaceutical purposes. The most stable one is Ser^{78}, Ser^{96}-bFGF, and its angiogenic activity by chick embryo chorioallantoic membrane assay is comparable to that of native bFGF (Seno *et al.*, 1988).

6. COVALENT BOND MODIFICATION DETECTED BY HPIEC

In bFGF, there are two solvent-exposed methionines, seven aspartates, and five asparagines, all of which are potential sites of degradation by oxidation, chain cleavage, and deamidation, respectively. These sites (except Met) are highlighted in Fig. 1. Three of the aspartates (15, 46, 88) and one of the asparagines (36) are adjacent to a by glycine and are located in regions of the protein that are predicted to have high flexibility; both of these conditions are thought to favor succinimide formation.

By HP-IEC, fresh bFGF was ~98% main peak. Incubation in citrate buffer, pH 5 at 25°C (for a few weeks), resulted in the appearance of a significant component which eluted ~1.4 min later than the main peak. Moreover, there was an increase in a number of minor components that eluted at ~16 min and ~17–19 min later relative to the main peak (Fig. 9).

6.1. Monomer–Multimer Distribution

In order to identify bFGF degradation products, aged bFGF was fractionated by HP-IEC. From HP-SEC (Fig. 10), the apparent molecular weights of fresh monomeric and dimeric bFGF were calculated to be 13.5 ± 0.4 kDa (which is less than the theoretical value of 17.1 kDa) and 29.6 ± 0.5 kDa, respectively. Fractions 2 through 8 all eluted at a position with an apparent molecular weight of 13.7 kDa, suggesting that they were monomeric bFGF (F5 is shown in Fig. 10B). F10–14 (~1.4 min post-main peak) also eluted as a monomer (see F12 in Fig. 10B). F22–24 (~6.5 min post-main peak) eluted as a truncated monomer missing ~3700 Da (F23 in Fig. 10B). F27–33

A

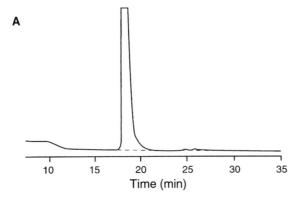

B

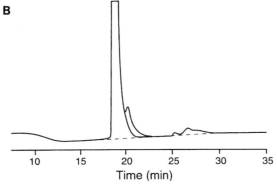

Figure 9. HP-IEC profiles of bFGF: (A) fresh sample; (B) sample aged at pH 5 (25°C, 13 weeks). A 6.8 mM/ min ammonium sulfate gradient at pH 6 was used.

eluted where the dimers should elute (F27 in Fig. 10B) (Shahrokh *et al.*, 1994c). The disulfide linkage of the dimers was previously confirmed by (a) their dissociation to monomers in the presence of 20–30 mM DTT, (b) their increased concentration at higher pH's, and (c) their absence in the cysteine-to-serine mutant (Thompson and Fiddes, 1992). F34–39 contained trimer and truncated dimer forms.

6.2. Identification of Asp^{28}-Pro Cleaved and Asp^{15}-Gly Cleaved bFGF

By LC/MS, F5 consisted of bFGF(2–155) with a corrected mass of 17,127 ± 3 amu, and a minor des-ala bFGF component (designated as bFGF(3–155). The exact mass difference between F5 [using bFGF(2–155)] and the major component in F23 was 2596 amu (Fig. 11). A minor component missing 1334 amu was also detected in F23 by LC/MS (not shown). N-terminal sequencing revealed the presence of two components in nearly equal proportions; one beginning with pro-lys-arg and the other

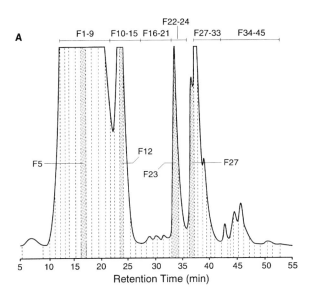

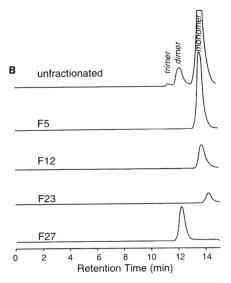

Figure 10. Fractionation of degraded bFGF by HP-IEC (A) and characterization by HP-SEC (B). 12 mg bFGF in citrate-EDTA, pH 5 was aged at 25°C for 13 weeks, filtered and fractionated by HP-IEC.

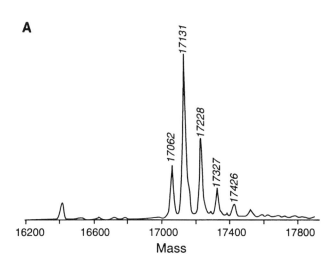

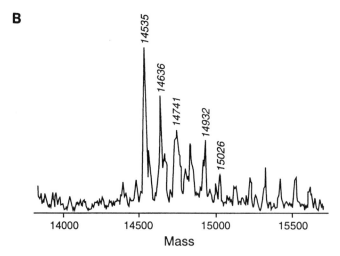

Figure 11. LC/mass spectrometry of bFGF degradation products. Mass spectra of a fraction within the main HP-IEC peak (F5, A), and the two post-main-peak components (F23, B and F12, C). The des-ala component (missing 79 ± 3 amu) and the phosphate and/or sulfate adducts (multiples of 100 ± 5 amu) are seen. B and C show the degradation products of bFGF at Asp[28] and Asp[15], respectively.

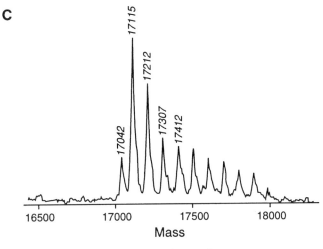

Figure 11. (*Continued*)

with gly-gly-ser. These data are consistent with co-elution of two cleavage products in F23: bFGF(29–155), which was cleaved at the asp[28]-pro site (missing 2596 Da), and bFGF(16–155), which was cleaved at the asp[15]-gly site (missing 1334 Da). The positions of these degradation sites are illustrated in Figs. 1 and 2.

6.3. Identification of Succinimide at Aspartate[15]

N-terminal sequencing of F12 stopped at aspartate[15], which could have been due to the formation of either an iso-asp or a succinimide at this position. By LC/MS, a mass which was 18 ± 2 amu smaller than F5 was obtained (Fig. 11). The loss of mass of one water equivalent and the elution at a more basic position on the HP-IEC are consistent with the presence of a succinimide rather than iso-asp at aspartate[15].

Supporting evidence for the presence of succinimide at aspartate[15] in F12 came from the observation that treatment of F12 at pH 8 (37°C, 2 hr) converted this species to the main peak on HP-IEC. Addition of a reducing agent to prevent disulfide-linked multimerization at high pH had no effect. This conversion was accompanied by minimal deblocking of sequencing through aspartate[15], suggesting that the vast majority of the conversion products were the iso-asp derivative and/or D-isomers. Direct determination of the iso-asp content of the pH 8-treated F12 using the isoaspartyl methyltransferase (PIMT) assay showed 38% iso-asp. By using PIMT, isoaspartate was found in the N-terminal cluster of tryptic fragments that spans residues 2 through 50 and contains the asp[15]-gly sequence. Other asparagine containing segments, such as fragment 107–116, did not show the transformation to isoaspartate (Shahrokh *et al.*, 1994a).

Based on the X-ray diffractogram of bFGF crystals, the first 25 amino acids from the N-terminus are in disorder (Fig. 2) and most likely are not participating in receptor or heparin binding activities. Therefore, modification at asp[15] would not likely affect the biological properties of bFGF.

7. AGGREGATION DETERMINED BY UV SPECTROMETRY

UV spectrometry is unsurpassed for precision and sensitivity for quantifying aggregates. Typically with bFGF solutions, a loss of 2% due to aggregation can cause an absorbance increase of 20% due to turbidity. This small amount of protein loss, 2%, which is hardly discernible by HPLC assays, may be verified by the difference in UV absorbance between filtered control and aged samples. Concomitantly, the magnitude of the UV absorbance increase (i.e., 20%) allows formulators to screen a variety of excipients and to determine the optimal pH (Fig. 12). In spite of these advantages, one should recognize the limitations; i.e., this method does not provide information on the shelf life of the product. In addition, because many experiments were carried out at elevated temperatures, such as 30°C for the results reported herein, the exact stability trend at storage temperature, namely 5°C, needs to be assessed by products stored in vials and analyzed periodically by more specific stability indicating assays (Eberlein *et al.*, 1994). These stability differences are due to non-Arrhenius behavior arising from competing reactions that can have vastly different temperature dependencies.

7.1. Effect of pH and Buffer Type

In a 30°C thermostated cuvette, a plot of bFGF absorbance versus time shows a sigmoidal curve. The maximal rate of absorbance change at 277 nm is used for comparing stability of the formulations. The lag time, which represents the nucleation phase, and eventually leads to aggregation, is ignored in these analyses. Examples of these UV analyses are shown in Fig. 13.

The effects of pH on protein aggregation were examined in a pH range of 2.8 to 8.0 using citrate as a buffer. Precipitation of bFGF was fast at pH 2–5 and negligible at pH values above 6. At pH 5, the formation of light-scattering particles increased in proportion to increases in citrate buffer concentrations. When the effect of buffer species was compared, citrate buffer at pH 3.7 caused aggregation, whereas acetate buffer at pH 3.8 did not. The relative instability between citrate and acetate buffers was confirmed by a study at 5°C, 25°C, and 37°C where the amount of soluble bFGF, as determined by RP-HPLC, was indeed higher in the acetate-buffered sample than

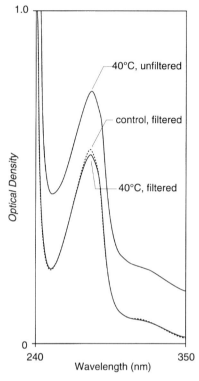

Figure 12. Filtered 1 mg/ml bFGF solutions before and after 12 hr incubation at 30°C in 100 mM citrate pH 5. After incubation there was a ~10 times increase in absorbance due to turbidity compared to the protein loss after filtration.

in the citrate-buffered sample. On the other hand, at pH 5.5–5.7, phosphate, acetate, and citrate buffers all showed similar aggregation rates (Eberlein *et al.*, 1994).

7.2. Effect of Excipients

In surveys of stabilizers for protein and peptide formulations (Wang, 1992; Wang and Hanson, 1988) surfactants have been used in many protein formulations as stabilizers against aggregation. Unlike those proteins, bFGF does not benefit from surfactants such as polysorbate 80 and sodium dodecylsulfate to reduce rate of aggregation, suggesting that aggregation may not be initiated by hydrophobic inter-actions. Agents that increase viscosity of the product also do not mitigate the formation of aggregates.

In contrast, salts or carbohydrates which can modify the solvation characteristics of the protein demonstrate some advantages. At a concentration above 2.6 M,

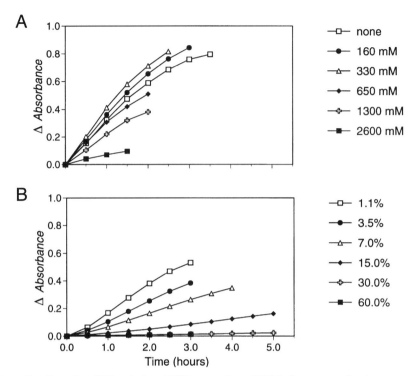

Figure 13.   Examples of UV analysis on bFGF aggregation at 30°C, in the presence of various concentrations of (A) NaCl in citrate buffer pH 4.7, (B) sucrose in citrate buffer pH 5.0.

NaCl inhibits the formation of aggregates. Sucrose blocks aggregation at concentrations of 30% and above.

Preservatives, such as benzyl alcohol and methyl paraben, are detrimental to the stability with regards to aggregate formation. Benzalkonium chloride, a cationic preservative, works at very low concentration and causes minimal adverse effects, but still there is a concentration-dependent increase in aggregation (Eberlein *et al.*, 1994).

Timasheff (1989) theorized that solutes or cosolvents either penetrate the hydration layer of the protein and interact with it or are excluded from the hydration layer and thus stabilize the protein structure. Sodium chloride and sucrose may be preferentially excluded from the protein domain, thus stabilizing it, whereas surfactants decrease the surface tension of water and destabilize the hydration layer. Positively charged benzalkonium chloride may be repulsive to the positively charged bFGF and minimally affect it at low concentrations; at high concentrations, however, benzalkonium ion may ion-pair with one or more of the 16 negatively charged groups on the surface of bFGF, penetrate the water layer around the protein, and disrupt the hydrophobic interaction in the core with its long hydrophobic side chains. Benzalkonium chloride interaction with the hydrophobic core of bFGF may lead to unfolding and aggregation of the denatured protein. Further work would be necessary to confirm these speculations.

7.3. Effect of Sulfated Ligands

In the presence of heparin or low-molecular-weight heparin, the aggregation reaction is extremely slow such that only a lag phase can be observed. To minimize aggregation, a 1:5 heparin/bFGF ratio (w/w) at pH 6.5 is optimal. A high degree of sulfation seems to be necessary to stabilize bFGF. If dextran is sulfated with more than 3 sulfates per disaccharide unit, it will stabilize bFGF as well. Thus, it was not surprising to see that low-sulfated ligands such as chondroitin A, B, or C, actually increased the aggregation rate. Ethylene glycol chitin has no effect (Eberlein *et al.*, 1994).

The aforementioned results for bFGF in comparison to aFGF are strikingly similar. Tsai *et al.* (1993) found that a surprisingly wide variety of polyanions, including small sulfated and phosphorylated compounds, stabilized acidic FGF. These polyanionic ligands were capable of delaying the heat-induced (40°C) aggregation by 10–1000-fold when the samples contained 0.5× or 10× ligand by weight and were monitored at 350 nm.

8. CHARACTERIZATION OF bFGF AGGREGATES AND PRECIPITATES

Aging of a pH 5 bFGF solution at 25°C resulted in the appearance of a few white or translucent particles within several days, and eventually the formation of white fluffy precipitates which coated the bottom surface of the container. These changes were caused by denaturation, aggregation, and precipitation as confirmed by fluorescence spectroscopy (see Section 2.3). Denaturation, the unfolding of bFGF monomer, is followed by aggregation, i.e., the multimerization of denatured bFGF primarily through hydrophobic interactions. When the aggregates are sufficiently large that they can be removed by a 0.2-μm filter, they are, in a pharmaceutical sense, precipitates. In addition to the use of filters, the precipitates can be collected from the pellet after samples are centrifuged (2500 g, 5 min) and the supernatant carefully removed.

8.1. Absence of Soluble Aggregates

The presence of any soluble aggregates following 0.2-μm filtration was assessed by HP-SEC. GnHCl (2 M) was placed in the mobile phase to ensure recovery of any denatured species without unfolding of the native bFGF (Sluzky *et al.*, 1994). In aged samples, small amounts of dimer, trimer, and tetramer could be observed. However, these species did not contribute to the UV scattering, as the ratio of peak-to-trough optical density was not affected (Section 8.2). Despite a significant portion of precipitate that could be removed by filtration, no species larger than tetramer or pentamer were detected (Fig. 14). This observation is quite different from experiences reported with other proteins such as α1-antitrypsin, γ-interferon, interleukin-2, growth hormone, etc., where distinct peaks of large soluble aggregate can be identified on HP-SEC (Watson and Kenney, 1988; Vemuri *et al.*, 1993).

8.2. Quantitation of Insoluble Aggregates/Precipitates

RP-HPLC determines the combined quantity of all forms of bFGF, both native and denatured, in a denatured state. Between the filtered and the control samples, the difference in the total area under HPLC peaks gives an estimate of the amount of insoluble aggregates. UV spectroscopy of the unfiltered aged sample provides a sensitive method for early detection of aggregation. When the A277/A245 ratio falls below 2, visible precipitates will soon follow. With only a minimal amount (<2%) of aggregated bFGF (as determined by the difference between filtered aged sample and control sample) a >20% increase in optical density at 277 nm was observed (Eberlein

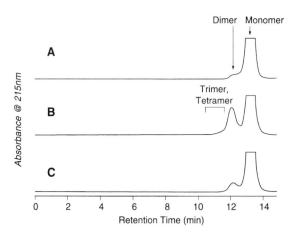

Figure 14.   Size-exclusion HPLC analysis of soluble bFGF aggregates. bFGF samples (2 mg/ml) were aged at 4°C for ~1 yr. Filtered aged samples (B and C) and controls (−70°C, A) were analyzed by HP-SEC. The mobile phase consisted of 100 mM phosphate–EDTA buffer, pH 6, plus 2 M GnHCl and 1 M NaCl to ensure recovery of potentially denatured aggregated species. Species up to tetramers were detected which were disulfide linked and DTT dissociable. More multimeric species were detected at higher pH (B and versus C), as expected for disulfide reactions. B, pH 6.5, 1 yr, 4°C; C, pH 5, 1 yr, 4°C.

et al., 1994). Fluorescence spectroscopy also quantitates the insoluble aggregates since the signal of denatured species is distinct from the signal representing the native form (Shahrokh *et al.*, 1994b).

8.3. Mass Balance

Whereas analysis of the filtered sample provides an indirect estimate of the insoluble aggregates, for direct quantitative analysis and proof of mass balance in bFGF formulations, the precipitates had to be solubilized and analyzed. GnHCl (4 M) is effective in the complete recovery of protein from a sample that had >60% of precipitable bFGF (Sluzky *et al.*, 1994). Using any one of the three methods, UV spectroscopy, RP-HPLC, or HP-SEC (with 2 M GnHCl in the mobile phase), one could show total mass of unfractionated samples equal to the sum of protein amounts from supernatant, wash, and precipitates (Shahrokh *et al.*, 1994c).

8.4. Characterization of Precipitates

Fluorescent spectroscopy of an aged bFGF sample shows that precipitated bFGF resembles bFGF denatured by a chaotrope. To investigate whether these precipitates are associated by hydrophobic interaction or disulfide bonds, the precipitates must be solubilized by GnHCl and characterized by RP-HPLC and HP-SEC. Unfortunately, GnHCl treatment dissociates disulfide linkages in bFGF, similar to the results obtained with SDS-PAGE (discussed in Section 5.1); consequently, direct analysis of precipitates is not possible (Fig. 15).

The dimer fraction collected from HP-IEC developed into three distinct peaks on RP-HPLC. When these three dimers (Cys-78–Cys-78, 78–96, and 96–96) were treated with GnHCl, they quantitatively formed equal amounts of monomeric bFGF with four free thiols and another kind of monomer which was reducible by DTT to native monomeric bFGF (Fig. 15). This reducible monomer (peak A) is bFGF with an intramolecular disulfide linkage (96–101). The content of multimers prior to addition of the chaotrope, GnHCl, could be back-calculated as at most twice the amount of peak A because of quantitative conversion of multimer to two equally distributed species, one of which is peak A.

Figure 16 shows the HPLC profiles of GnHCl solubilized precipitates and the corresponding supernatant. By HP-SEC, the majority of the species were monomeric, except for 5% of nondissociable dimer which was present in the precipitates (Fig. 16, top). By RP-HPLC, about 30% of the non-main-peak species were present in the precipitates, which were threefold more than that observed in the supernatant. In particular, peak A represents 22% and 10% of the total peak area in the precipitates and supernatant, respectively, suggesting twice the amount of those quantities could

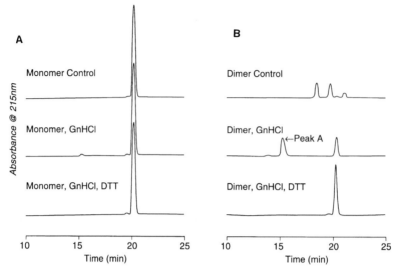

Figure 15. Dimer dissociation by GnHCl. Whereas 4 M GnHCl minimally affected the RP-HPLC profile of a purified monomer (A), the three purified dimer forms (B, top) collapsed to two monomeric forms (B, middle), one eluting at the position of the original native main peak (~20 min) and the other eluting at 14 min (peak A). Peak A converted to the main peak with 20 mM DTT treatment (B, bottom). The monomer and dimeric forms were purified by HP-IEC.

have been multimeric prior to GnHCl treatment. The identities of other minor species remain to be determined.

From these deductions, the major component in bFGF precipitation seems to be disulfide scrambled bFGF. In the example illustrated in Fig. 16, up to 44% of the precipitates might have originated from dimers as evidenced by an increase in the amount of intradisulfide monomer. The GnHCl-solubilized precipitates also showed a small fraction of undissociated dimer by HP-SEC. Since disulfide-linked species are dissociated by GnHCL treatment through thiol-disulfide exchange, this dimer could be formed through transamidation or β-elimination.

8.5. Aggregation in the Presence of Glycosaminoglycan

Since GAGs increase the thermal stability of bFGF, their utility in improving shelf life of a solution formulation of bFGF was investigated. Solutions of bFGF with or without heparin at 35°C showed visual aggregation in about 10 days. When monomer concentration as a function of time was monitored by heparin affinity HPLC, in the presence of heparin, an initial lag phase was observed (similar to UV

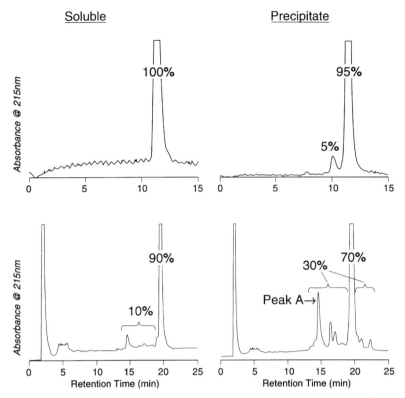

Figure 16. HPLC profiles of purified, solubilized bFGF precipitates. An aged sample (35°C, 2.5 days, pH 5) was centrifuged. The supernatant and the triply washed precipitates were solubilized with 4 M GnHCl and analyzed by HP-SEC (top) and RP-HPLC (bottom). The precipitates were enriched in nonreducible dimers (~11 min peak, top right) and other degradation peaks (compare bottom right and left chromatograms). Peak A co-eluted with the intramolecular disulfide-linked monomers.

analysis in Section 5.3). This was followed by a rapid decrease in monomer concentration which is greater than that seen in the absence of heparin. The accelerated loss of monomer correlated with increased dimer concentration. Thus although GAGs were considered conformation stabilizers, they accelerated the loss of monomer (Shahrokh *et al.*, 1994c).

Heparin with a molecular weight of 14–16 kDa has 10–14 potential binding sites for bFGF. Conceivably these binding sites, all positioned in linear order adjacent to each other, would bring several FGFs into close contact, which could in turn promote multimerization, and lead to the accelerated loss of monomer, as observed. Although multimerization of bFGFs and their complexation with heparin eventually leads to

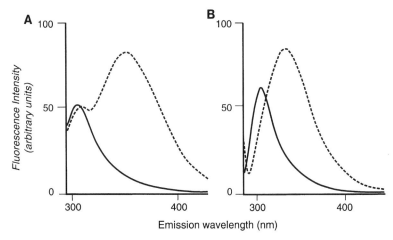

Figure 17. Fluorescence emission spectra of bFGF precipitates. (A) Emission spectra of native soluble bFGF (——) and denatured bFGF (----) in 5.5 M GnHCl (λ_{ex} 277 nm) after dilution to 0.1 mg/ml. (B) Emission spectra of resuspended precipitates with (——) or without heparin (----) (at −0.1 mg/ml). Note the narrower spectral width of precipitates in the presence of heparin compared to that of soluble monomer without heparin. Emission spectra were obtained on a Shimadzu model RF540 fluorimeter scanned at 400 nm/min. The experiment used 5 nm excitation and emission slits and 4 mm × 10 mm excitation and emission pathlengths.

aggregation and precipitation, the protein's native structure is maintained in these aggregates. As illustrated in Fig. 17, fluorescence spectroscopy for resuspended precipitates formed in the presence of heparin was comparable to that of native protein. Moreover, these precipitates could be resolubilized with 1 M NaCl, unlike precipitates formed in the absence of heparin where chaotropes are required to resolubilize such precipitates.

Supporting evidence of this scheme comes from the observation that the Cys-78/96 double mutein of bFGF (which remained monomeric) showed no precipitation with heparin and was an order of magnitude more stable than the wild-type bFGF. Interestingly, aFGF, which has ~55% sequence homology to bFGF and is structurally similar, did not show increased multimerization by heparins. In fact, other investigators have shown that heparin prevented Cu-oxidation of the cysteines of aFGF. These differences in behavior could be explained solely on a structural basis: aFGF has three cysteines: two at positions 16 and 83, which are buried, and one at position 117, which is exposed. This exposed cysteine of aFGF is in a region near the heparin binding domain which sterically protects the cysteine from oxidation. In contrast, the two exposed cysteines of bFGF are far away from the heparin binding domain and therefore are not protected against oxidation.

9. FORMULATIONS

Because of bFGF's wide range of potented clinical indications coupled with its affinity to glycosaminoglycan, there are many types of dosage forms and formulation options that can be developed for bFGF.

9.1. Aqueous Solution

An aqueous solution of bFGF requires a metal chelant (Foster *et al.*, 1991) or an antioxidant (Adami *et al.*, 1992; Farmitalia WO 92/01442, p. 4) to preserve the thiol groups.

As expected, numerous patents (Ungheri *et al.*, 1992) and articles (Kajio *et al.*, 1992) have described the use of heparin and glycosaminoglycan as stabilizers. Koichi *et al.* (1989) listed β-1,3-glycansulfate, dextran sulfate, and cyclodextrin sulfate, all having an average molecular weight 7500 and about 16–20% sulfur content. In an aqueous medium, when bFGF is brought into contact with an equimolar amount of glycan sulfate, a di- or tri- basic carboxylic acid (50 mM–0.4 M) is required as a stabilizer. The stabilized formulation of Koichi *et al.* (1989) is resistant to stress (37°C, 24 hr), trypsin, and pepsin digestion.

A solution product can be applied topically by a mechanical pump spray or dropper. If adsorbed to a calcium sulfate carrier, it can be used to enhance bone growth (Rosenblum, 1991). When adsorbed to Gelfoam (a freeze-dried gelatin sponge produced by the Upjohn Co.), it can be used to promote angiogenesis on skin flaps. Marks *et al.* (1991) described the use of a collagen sponge soaked with a solution of growth factor that faciliated early dermal and epidermal wound healing.

9.2. Freeze-Dried Formulation

The conformation of protein can be qualitatively assessed by infrared spectroscopy. By comparison of second-derivative FTIR spectra of protein in solution, in dehydrated (freeze-dried formulation) and rehydrated states (postreconstitution), one can assess the possible protein damage due to freeze-drying.

Prestrelski *et al.* (1993) reported that bFGF when freeze-dried in Tris buffer, exhibited a moderate conformational change (e.g., band broadening) and a slight shift in certain bands. When excipients such as sucrose, lactose, and glucose were each added to the formulation, the dehydrated state exhibited spectra which resembled the solution prior to lyophilization, suggesting these excipients preserved the conformation of native bFGF and can be considered as a suitable formulation aids for bFGF.

Upon reconstitution, the rehydrated bFGF again exhibited a moderate conformational change when it was freeze-dried in buffer, but exhibits almost the native conformation when sucrose (4-to-1 weight ratio) was included prior to freeze-drying. In general, bFGF is less susceptible to conformation change as compared with two other proteins, γ-IFN and casein. bFGF also seems to be insensitive to the selection of additives because it exhibited a comparable conformation change when freeze-dried with any of the eight polyols (carbohydrates, alcohols) tested.

In a patent (Adami *et al.*, 1992), polysorbate (polyoxyethylene sorbitan fatty acid ester) and cysteine were found to act synergistically to provide increased stability to a freeze-dried formulation containing mannitol and dithiothreitol. Also discussed was the use of an antimicrobial preservative agent. Benzalkonium chloride at a concentration of about 0.005% by weight is particularly suitable because its efficacy is well documented and it is commonly used in ophthalmic preparations, presumably having the minimal irritation propensity.

9.3. Powder Formulation

The affinity between bFGF and glycosaminoglycan can be utilized to prepare solid dosage forms of bFGF (Fukunaga *et al.*, 1992, 1994), potentially useful for oral administration to treat peptic ulcer. The aluminum salt of β-cyclodextrin sulfate (ACDS) was prepared from β-cyclodextrin by first reacting with trimethylammonium sulfate, then crystallizing, and finally redissolving in water prior to addition of aluminum chloride. To the ACDS suspension, bFGF solution was added, and the resultant mixture was freeze-dried to prepare a powdery composition of bFGF and ACDS. This preparation was shown to be resistant to simulated gastric juice (pH 1.2 and pepsin).

As described in another patent, a stabilizer, sodium dextran sulfate (MW 7500) was added to a citrate solution (pH 8.0) of bFGF mutein CS23 (equivalent to Ser[78], Ser[96]-bFGF); then 1 ml of this solution was added to 5 g of water-insoluble polymer such as hydroxypropyl cellulose. The mixture was stirred and dried at room temperature under reduced pressure. This powder formulation can be incorporated into a traditional oral tablet or oleaginous topical formulations. (Akiyama *et al.*, 1993)

9.4. Microspheres

To deliver bFGF for burn or wound healing, bFGF can be loaded into water-insoluble, water-swellable microspheres. The powder of these spheres has gel-forming capabilities. As an example, bFGF and dithiothreitol (as an antioxidant) are dissolved in water, pH 6.0, into which starch microspheres having an average diameter of 20 microns had been added. The suspension is allowed to stand at room temperature for 30 min, and is then lyophilized into white flowing powder. In order to enhance stability, the microspheres may be composed of an anionic polymer such as heparin, chondroitin sulfate, cellulose sulfate, alginate, or hyaluronate. Although numerous examples were cited in the patent as stabilizers, it is understood that bFGF requires specific spatial orientation of the anions for stabilization (DePonti *et al.*, 1992).

Another approach, which is not too different from the previous example, utilizes heparin-Sepharose beads to adsorb and stabilize bFGF. These beads are then encapsulated in a microspherical controlled-release device using a natural polymer, alginate. Release kinetics can be enhanced by enzymatic bond cleavage with heparinase (Edelman *et al.*, 1991).

9.5. Gel Formulation

Gel formulations for use in wound healing and containing a growth factor have been reported for many growth factors. specifically EGF and PDGF (Finkenauer *et al.*, 1989), aFGF (Matuszewska *et al.*, 1994), and TGF-α (Tan *et al.*, 1993). The aqueous gel formulations typically comprise a thickening agent, which can be a cellulose derivative (methylcellulose, hydroxyethylcellulose, carboxymethylcellulose), a hydroxyethyl polymer (poloxamers), a polyacrylamide (carbopol), hyaluronic acid, or natural gums (Zatz *et al.*, 1989). These gel formulations can be used for dermal wounds or for the induction of bone formation when bFGF in a carboxymethylcellulose gel is impregnated in a demineralized bone matrix (Aspenberg *et al.*, 1991).

Fibrin gel is a unique vehicle. It is formed by the addition of thrombin to a fibrinogen solution. As a naturally occurring and partially human-derived product, the material appears to have no tissue toxicity, promotes a firm seal in seconds to minutes, is reabsorbed in days to weeks following application and appears to promote local tissue growth. Fibrin gel containing bFGF was found to stimulate bone fracture repair (Kawaguchi *et al.*, 1994). Experiments using radiolabeled bFGF revealed that 64% of the dose injected to the fracture site remained after 6 hr, 33% remained after 24 hr, and 9% was present 3 days after injection.

Due to the high content of water in the gels, stability of the growth factor is a concern. It has been mentioned in patents (Akiyama *et al.*, 1993; DePonti *et al.*, 1992) that the gels can be lyophilized to provide a stable dosage form which can be reconstituted at the time of use. One needs to follow this suggestion with caution, as this type of lyophilized cake often forms a hard gummy substance upon reconstitution. This is because a gel forms on the outer surface and prevents further penetration of water. As a result, content uniformity within this dosage form is questionable. Also during a routine stability study, we were surprised to note that bFGF reduced the viscosity of the hydroxyethyl cellulose gel (Shahrokh *et al.*, 1995). Viscosity loss was identified as arising from cleavage of cellulose polymer chains by a cellulase-like substance which was a host-cell-derived impurity. Even though *E. coli*, the host bacteria for bFGF expression, is not known to produce cellulase-like enzymes, nevertheless, a minute quantity of endogluconase was not removed by an elaborate purification process via copper chelating HPLC (Scheurermann *et al.*, 1992). Replacing the copper column with a hydrophobic interaction column step completely avoided such problems (Shadle *et al.*, 1993).

9.6. Target to FGF Receptor

bFGF can be used as a guide for targeted delivery of toxins to specific cells. Saporin, a ribosome-inactivating protein, is itself not toxic to the cell; however, if saporin is conjugated to bFGF, it is taken up by cells that express bFGF receptor and is a potent toxin that causes cell death. The potency of this conjugate is proportional to the number of receptors expressed on the surface of the treated cells (Lindner *et al.*, 1991).

10. CONCLUSION

This chapter presents the current knowledge regarding the pharmaceutical aspects of bFGF. Detailed analyses by crystallography, UV, fluorescence spectrometry, CD, FTIR, and DSC illustrate the conformation and the physicochemical properties of this protein molecule. Quantitation of bFGF and assessment of covalent modifications and conformation states can be accomplished by RP-HPLC, Hep-TSK HPLC, HPIEC, and/or HP-SEC; all four methods are complementary. Moreover, *in vivo* and *in vitro* testing methods were reviewed. These biological methods are valuable in confirming biological potency of bFGF preparations.

Degradation of bFGF was studied in great length. First, the most labile moieties, cysteine residues, were found to cause dimer and multimer formation through disulfide linkages. During long-term storage of the products, succinimide formation at Asp^{15}, a minute change in a large molecule, can be detected by HPIEC; the pathway of this degradation was confirmed by LC-MS, alkaline conversion, and PIMT. Cleavage sites, (i.e., Asp^{28}-Pro and Asp^{15}-Gly) were also identified by HPIEC, HP-SEC, and LC-MS. Like many other proteins, bFGF is prone to aggregation and precipitation. Aggregation rates were studied by UV analyses at 30°C to screen formulation parameters. The aggregates were further isolated and characterized by RP-HPLC, HP-SEC, and fluorescence spectrometry. Scrambled disulfide linkages, rather than hydrophobic interactions, were the primary binding force for the aggregate formation. Interestingly, aggregates formed in the presence of GAGs preserved the native conformation, whereas in aggregates formed in the absence of

GAGs, the conformation resembled that of bFGF denatured by a chaotrope or by high temperature.

Finally, many examples of formulating bFGF for treatment of dermal wounds, bone fractures, and other potential indications were reviewed and discussed.

It is anticipated that additional data and knowledge related to better understanding of the bFGF molecule will continue to surface. Recent studies on conformation and structure of bFGF receptor, and on the ternary interaction among bFGF, FGF receptors, and GAG, certainly will shed light on the biological roles of bFGF and GAG. This knowledge will benefit bFGF scientists in improving clinical formulations and treatment regimens.

ACKNOWLEDGMENTS. The authors acknowledge the following people who have at one time contributed to the bFGF project in the Pharmaceutical R & D Department of Scios Inc.: Linda Foster, Vanitha Sampath, William Lee, Michelle Chow, Rich Ennis, Victoria Sluzky, David Battaglia, Pam Stratton, Robert King, and Amy Wong. We also want to acknowledge the helpful suggestions from our colleagues: Douglas Buckley, Judy Abraham, Jeff Higaki, and Diane Blumenthal. The encouragement from Armin Ramel is greatly appreciated.

REFERENCES

Abraham, J. A., and Klagsbrun, M., 1996, Modulation of wound repair by members of the fibroblast growth factor family, in: *The Molecule and Cellular Biology of Wound Repair*, 2nd ed. (R. A. F. Clark, ed.), Plenum Press, New York.

Abraham, J. A., Mergia, A., Whang, J. L., Tumolo, A., Friedman, J., Hjerrid, K. A., Gospodarowicz, D., and Fiddes, J. C., 1986b, Nucleotide sequence of a bovine clone encoding the angiogenic protein, bFGF, *Science* **233**:545–548.

Abraham, J. A., Whang, J. L., Tumolo, A., Friedman, J., Gospodarowicz, S., and Fiddes, J. C., 1986a, Human bFGF: nucleotide sequence and genomic organization, *EMBO J.* **5**:2523–2528.

Adami, M., Dalla Casa, R., Gambini, L., Magrini, R., Mariani, R., and Perrone, G., 1992, Stable pharmaceutical compositions containing a fibroblast growth factor, International Patent Appl. WO 92/01 442.

Ahn, S. T., and Mustoe, T. A., 1990, Effects of ischemia on ulcer wound healing: a new model in the rabbit ear, *Ann. Plast. Surg.* **24**:17–23.

Ago, H., Kitagawa, Y., Fujishima, A., Matsuura, Y., and Katsube, Y., 1991, Crystal structure of basic fibroblast growth factor at 1.6 Å resolution, *J. Biochem.* **110**:360–363.

Akiyama, Y., Yoshioka, M., and Kitamori, N., 1993, Stabilized FGF composition and production thereof, U.S. Patent 5189148.

Aspenberg, P., Thorngren, K.-G., and Lohmander, L. S., 1991, Fibroblast growth factor increases or inhibits induced bone formation, depending on dose, Transactions 1st Annual Meeting of the European Orthopedic Research Society.

Astafieva, I. V., Eberlein, G. A., and Wang, Y. J., 1996, Absolute on-line molecular mass analysis of basic fibroblast growth factor and its multimers by reversed-phase liquid chromatography with multi-angle laser scattering detection, *J. Chromatog. A*, in press.

Broadley, K. N., Aquino, A. M., Hicks, B., Ditesheim, J. A., McGee, G. S., Demetriou, A. A., Woodward,

S. C., and Davidson, J. M., 1988, Growth factors bFGF and TGFβ accelerate the rate of wound repair in normal and in diabetic rats, *Int. J. Tiss. Reac.* **10:**345–353.

Burgess, W. H., and Maciag, T., 1989, The heparin-binding (fibroblast) growth factor family of proteins, *Annu. Rev. Biochem.* **58:**575–606.

Copeland, R. A., Ji, H., Halfpenny, A. J., Williams, R. W., Thompson, K. C., Herber, W. K., Thomas, K. A., Bruner, M. W., Ryan, J. A., Marquis-Omer, D., Sanyal, G., Sitrin, R. D., Yamazaki, S., and Middaugh, C. R., 1991, The structure of human acidic fibroblast growth factor and its interaction with heparin, *Arch. Biochem. Biophys.* **239:**53–61.

Davidson, J., Buckley, A., Woodward, S., Nichols, W., McGee, G., and Demetriou, A., 1988, Mechanisms of accelerated wound repair using epidermal growth factor and basic fibroblast growth factor, in: *Growth Factors and Other Aspects of Wound Healing: Biological and Clinical Implications*, Alan R. Liss, New York, pp. 63–75.

Davidson, J. M., Klagsbrun, M., Hill, K. E., Buckley, A., Sullivan, R., Brewer, P. S., and Woodward, S. C., 1985, Accelerated wound repair, cell proliferation, and collagen accumulation are produced by a cartilage-derived growth factor, *J. Cell Biol.* **100:**1219–1227.

DePonti, R., Torricelli, C., Confalonieri, C., Adami, M., Martini, A., and Lardini, E., 1992, Delivery system for growth factors, U.K. Patent Appl. 2 245 831 A.

Eberlein, G. A., Stratton, P. A., and Wang, Y. J., 1994, Stability of rhbFGF as determined by UV spectroscopy, *PDA J. Pharm. Sci. Tech.* **48:**224–230.

Edelman, E. R., Langer, R. S., Klagsburn, M., and Mathiowitz, E., 1989, Controlled release systems containing heparin and growth factors, International Patent Appl. WO/12464.

Eriksson, A. E., Cousens, L. S., and Matthews, B. W., 1993, Refinement of the structure of human basic fibroblast growth factor at 1.6 Å resolution and analysis of presumed heparin binding sites by selenate substitution, *Protein Sci.* **2:**1274–1284.

Eriksson, A. E., Cousens, L. S., Weaver, L. H., and Matthews, B. W., 1991, Three dimensional structure of human basic fibroblast growth factor, *Proc. Natl. Acad. Sci. USA* **88:**3441–3445.

Fiddes, J. C., Hebda, P. A., Hayward, P., Robson, M. C., Abraham, J. A., and Klingbeil, C. K., 1991, Preclinical wound-healing studies with recombinant human basic fibroblast growth factor, *Ann. N.Y. Acad. Sci.* **638:**316–328.

Finkenaur, A. L., Cohen, J. M., Shalaby, S. W., Sandoval, E. A., Bezwada, R. S., and Kronenthal, R. L., 1989, Gel formulations containing growth factors, European Patent Appl. 0 312 208.

Florkiewicz, R. Z., and Sommer, A., 1989, High molecular weight human angiogenic factors, International Patent Appl. WO/91 06568.

Foster, L. C., Thompson, S. A., and Tarnowski, S. J., 1991, Methods and formulations for stabilizing fibroblast growth factor, International Patent Appl. W0/91 15509.

Fox, G. M., Schiffer, S. G., Rohde, M. F., Tsai, L. B., Banks, A. R., and Arakawa, T., 1988, Production, biological activity, and structure of recombinant basic fibroblast growth factor and an analog with cysteine replaced by serine, *J. Biol. Chem.* **263:**18452–18458.

Fukunaga, K., Hijikata, S., Ishimura, K., Sonoda, R., Irie, T., and Uekama, K., 1994, Aluminium β-cyclodextrin sulphate as a stabilizer and sustained-release carrier for basic fibroblast growth factor, *J. Pharm. Pharmacol.* **46:**168–171.

Fukunaga, K., Shigeki, H., Ishimura, K., Ohtani, Y., Kimura, K., Fujii, M., and Hata, Y., 1992, Composition of stabilized fibroblast growth factor, European Patent 0550 035 A2.

Gospodarowicz, D., and Cheng, J., 1986, Heparin protects basic and acidic FGF from inactivation, *J. Cell Physiol.* **128:**475–484.

Hebda, P. A., Klingbeil, C. K., Abraham, J. A., and Fiddes, J. C., 1990, Basic fibroblast growth factor stimulation of epidermal wound healing in pigs, *J. Invest. Dermatol.* **95:**626–631.

Kajio, T., Kawahara, K., and Kato, K., 1992, Stabilization of basic fibroblast growth factor with dextran sulfate, *Fed. Europ. Biochem. Soc.* **306:**243–246.

Kawaguchi, H., Kurokawa, T., Hanada, K., Hiyama, Y., Tamura, M., Ogata, E., and Matsumoto, T., 1994, Stimulation of fracture repair by recombinant human basic fibroblast growth factor in normal and streptozotocin-diabetic rats, *Endocrinology* **135:**774–781.

Klingbeil, C. K., Cesar, L. B., and Fiddes, J. C., 1991, Basic fibroblast growth factor accelerates tissue repair in models of impaired wound healing, in: *Clinical and Experimental Approaches to Dermal and Epidermal Repair: Normal and Chronic Wounds*, Alan R. Liss, New York, pp. 443–458.

Koichi, K., Kawahara, K., and Tomoko, K., 19889, Stabilized FGF composition and production thereof, European Patent Appl. 345660 A1.

Lee, T.-Y., and Notari, R. E., 1987, Kinetics and mechanism of captopril oxidation in aqueous solution under controlled oxygen partial pressure, *Pharm. Res.* **4:**98–103.

Lindner, V., Lappi, D. A., Baird, A., Majack, R. A., and Reidy, M. A., 1991, Role of bFGF in vascular lesion formation, *Circ. Res.* **68:**106–113.

Marks, M. G., Doillon, C., and Silver, F. H., 1991, Effects of fibroblasts and basic fibroblast growth factor or facilitation of dermal wound healing by type 1 collagen matrices, *J. Biomed. Mater. Res.* **25:** 683–696.

Matuszewska, B., Keogan, M., Fisher, D. M., Soper, K. A., Hoe, C., Huber, A. C., and Bondi, J. V., 1994, Acidic fibroblast growth factor: evaluation of topical formulations in diabetic mouse wound healing model, *Pharm. Res.* **11:**65–71.

McGee, G. S., Davidson, J. M., Buckley, A., Sommer, A., Woodward, S. C., Aquino, A. M., Barbour, R., and Demetriou, A. A., 1988, Recombinant basic fibroblast growth factor accelerates wound healing, *J. Surg. Res.* **45:**145–153.

Mustoe, T. A., Pierce, G. F., Morishima, C., and Deuel, T. F, 1991, Growth factor-induced acceleration of tissue repair through direct and inductive activities in a rabbit dermal ulcer model, *J. Clin. Invest.* **87:**694–703.

Ornitz, D. M., Yayon, A., Flanagan, G., Svahn, N., Levi, E., and Leder, P., 1992, Heparin is required for cell-free binding of basic fibroblast growth factor to a soluble receptor and for mitogenesis in whole cells, *Mol. Cell. Biol.* **12:**240–247.

Prestrelski, S. J., Arakawa, T., Kenney, W. C., and Byler, D. M., 1991, The secondary structure of two recombinant human growth factors, platelet-derived growth factor and basic fibroblast growth factor, as determined by Fourier-transform infrared spectroscopy, *Arch. Biochem. Biophys.* **285:**111–115.

Prestrelski, S. J., Fox, G. M., and Arakawa, T., 1992, Binding of heparin to basic fibroblast growth factor induces a conformational change, *Arch. Biochem. Biophys.* **293:**314–319.

Prestrelski, S. J., Tedischi, N., Arakawa, T., and Carpenter, J. F., 1993, Dehydration-induced conformational transitions in proteins and their inhibition by stabilizers, *Biophys. J.* **65:**661–671.

Rosenblum, S., Ricci, S. L., Frenkel, S. R., and Aleander, H., 1991, Diffusion of fibroblast growth factor from a calcium sulfate carrier, Proc. Combined Meeting of the Orthopedic Research Societies of USA, Japan, and Canada at Banff, Canada, p. 230.

Scheuermann, T. A., Tarnowski, J., and Silverness, K. B., 1992, Method to purify basic fibroblast growth factor, U.S. Patent 5136025.

Seno, M., Sasada, R., Iwane, M., Sudo, K., Kurokawa, T., Ito, K., and Igarashi, K., 1988, Stabilizing basic fibroblast growth factor using protein engineering, *Biochem. Biophys. Res. Com.* **151:**701–708.

Shadle, P. J., Silverness, K. B., and King, R. S., 1993, Process for purification of basic fibroblast growth factor, U.S. Patent 5331095.

Shahrokh, Z., Beylin, I., Eberlein, G., Busch, M., Kang, L., Wong, A., Anderson, C., Blumenthal, D., and Wang, Y. J., 1995, Cellulose cleaving activity from *E. coli* detected in topical formulations of recombinant proteins, *BioPharm.* **8:**32–38.

Shahrokh, Z., Eberlein, G. A., Buckley, D., Paranandi, M., Aswad, D., Stratton, P. A., Mischak, R., and Wang, Y. J., 1994a, Detection of succinimide in place of aspartate[15] as a major degradant of basic fibroblast growth factor, *Pharm. Res.* **11:**936–944.

Shahrokh, Z., Eberlein, G. A., and Wang, Y. J., 1994b, Probing the conformation state of protein precipitates by fluorescence spectroscopy, *J. Pharm. Biomed. Anal.* **12:**1035–1041.

Shahrokh, Z., Sluzky, V., Stratton, P. R., Eberlein, G. A., and Wang, Y. J., 1994c, Disulfide-Linked Oligomerization of Basic Fibroblast Growth Factor, in *ACS Symposium Series 567 on Protein Formulation and Delivery*, 1994, American Chemical Society, Washington, DC, Chap. 6.

Shahrokh, Z., Stratton, P. A., Eberlein, G. A., and Wang, Y. J., 1994d, Approaches to analysis of aggregates and demonstrating mass balance in pharmaceutical protein (bFGF) formulations, *J. Pharm. Sci.* **83:** 1645–1650.

Sluzky, V., Shahrokh, Z., Stratton, P. A., Eberlein, G. A., and Wang, Y. J., 1994, Chromatographic methods for quantitation of native, denatured and aggregated bFGF in solution formulations, *Pharm. Res.* **11:** 485–490.

Sommer, A., and Rifkin, D. B., 1989, Interaction of heparin with human basic fibroblast growth factor: protection of angiogenic protein from proteolytic degradation by a glycosaminoglycan, *J. Cell. Physiol.* **138:**215–220.

Squires, C. H., Childs, J., Eisenberg, S. P., Polverini, P. J., and Sommer, A., 1988, Production and characterization of human basic fibroblast growth factor from *Escherichia coli, J. Biol. Chem.* **263:** 16297–16302.

Stenberg, B. D., Phillips, L. G., Hokanson, J. A., Heggers, J. P., and Robson, M. C., 1991, Effect of bFGF on the inhibition of contraction caused by bacteria, *J. Surg. Res.* **50:**47–50.

Tan, E. L., Shah, H. S., Leister, K. J., Kozick, L. M., Pasciak, P., Vanderlaan, R. K., Yu, C.-D., and Patel, B., 1993, Transforming growth factor-α in a semisolid dosage form: Preservative and vehicle selection, *Pharm. Res.* **10:**1238–1242.

Thompson, S. A., 1989, Methods to stabilize basic fibroblast growth factor, U.S. Patent 5130418.

Thompson, S. A., and Fiddes, J. C., 1992, Chemical characterization of the cysteines of basic fibroblast growth factor, *Ann. N.Y. Acad. Sci.* **638:**78–88.

Thompson, S. A., Protter, A. A., BItting, L., Fiddes, J. C., and Abraham, J. A., 1991, Cloning, recombinant expression, and characterization of basic fibroblast growth factor, *Meth. Enzymol.* **198:**96–116.

Timasheff, S. N., and Arakawa, T., 1989, in: *Stabilization of Protein Structure by Solvents in Protein Structure—A Practical Approach* (T. F. Creighton, Ed.), IRL Press, London.

Timmins, P., Jackson, I. M., and Wang, Y. J., 1982, Factors affecting captopril stability in aqueous solution, *Intl. J. Pharm.* **11:**329–326.

Tsai, P. K., Volkin, D. B., Dabora, J. M., THompson, K. C., Bruner, M. W., Gress, J. O., Matuszewska, B., Keogan, M., Bondi, J. V., and Middaugh, C. R., 1993, Formulation design of acidic fibroblast growth factor, *Pharm. Res.* **10:**649–659.

Ungheri, D., Garofano, L., Battistini, C., Caminati, P., and Mazue, G., 1992, Synergistic composition comprising a fibroblast growth factor and a sulfated polysaccharide, for use as antiviral agent, European Patent Appl. 497 341 A2.

Vemuri, S., Beylin, I., Sluzky, V., Stratton, P. A., Eberlein, G. A., and Wang, Y. J., 1994, The stability of bFGF against thermal denaturation, *J. Pharm. Pharmacol.* **46:**481–486.

Vemuri, S., Yu, C. T., and Roosdrop, N., 1993, Formulation and stability of recombinant α₁-antitrypsin, in: *Stability and Characterization of Protein and Peptide Drugs* (Y. J. Wang and R. Pearlman, eds.), Plenum Press, New York, pp. 263–285.

Wang, Y. J., 1992, Parental products of proteins and peptides, in: *Pharmaceutical Dosage Forms: Parenteral Medications* (K. Avis, H. A. Lieberman, and L. Lachman, eds.), Marcel Dekker, New York.

Wang, Y. J., and Hanson, M., 1988, Parenteral formulations of proteins and peptides: stability and stabilizer, *J. Parenteral Sci. Tech.* **42:**S1–S26.

Watson, E., and Kenney, W. C., 1988, High-performance size-exclusion chromatograph of recombinant derived proteins and aggregated species, *J. Chromatogr.* **436:**289–298.

Wu, C.-S. C., Thompson, S. A., and Yang, J. T., 1991, Basic fibroblast growth factor is a β-rich protein, *J. Protein Chem.* **10:**427–436.

Yamazaki, S., and De Phillips, P. A., 1990, Method for the purification of therapeutically active recombinant acidic fibroblast growth factor, European Patent Appl. 0408 146A2.

Zatz, J., Berry, J., and Alderman, D., 1989, Viscosity imparting agents in disperse systems, in: *Pharmaceutical Dosage Forms: Disperse Systems* (H. Lieberman *et al.*, eds.), Marcel Dekker, New York, pp. 171–204.

Zhang, J., Cousens, L. S., Barr, P. J., and Sprang, S. R. 1991, Three-dimensional structure of human basic fibroblast growth factor, a structural homolog of interleukin 1β, *Proc. Natl. Acad. Sci. USA* **88:**3446–3450.

Zhu, X., Komiya, H., Chiroin, A., Faham, S., Fox, G. M., Arakawa, T., Hsu, B. T., and Rees, D. C., 1991, Three-dimensional structures of acidic and basic fibroblast growth factors, *Science Proc. Natl. Acad. Sci. USA* **251:**90–93.

3

The Characterization, Stabilization, and Formulation of Acidic Fibroblast Growth Factor

David B. Volkin and C. Russell Middaugh

1. INTRODUCTION

Acidic fibroblast growth factor (aFGF or FGF-1) is a 16-kDa protein present in a wide variety of tissues. It possesses a broad spectrum of biological activities and belongs to a group of at least nine structurally related proteins generally designated fibroblast growth factors (FGFs). These proteins are characterized by their affinity for sulfated polysaccharides such as heparin and the related heparan proteoglycans which are found on many cell surfaces and essentially all basement membranes. The two best-characterized members of the FGF family of proteins are acidic (aFGF or FGF-1) and basic (bFGF or FGF-2) fibroblast growth factor. These two proteins are potent mitogens for cells of mesodermal origin as well as for many of the cells derived from embryonic ectoderm. In addition, aFGF and bFGF are chemotactic for cells in culture. *In vivo*, aFGF and bFGF display angiogenic activity promoting vascular endothelial cell mitogenesis as well as chemotaxis and induction of proteases involved in tissue regeneration. Due to this wide range of biological activities, many potential therapeutic uses for aFGF and bFGF have been explored, including acceleration of wound healing, prevention of restenosis after angioplasty, regeneration of nerves, cartilage, and bone tissue, and the healing of gastric ulcers as well as retinal and tympanic membranes. Several reviews have been prepared on the structure and

David B. Volkin and C. Russell Middaugh • Department of Vaccine Pharmaceutical Research, Merck Research Laboratories, West Point, Pennsylvania 19486.

Formulation, Characterization, and Stability of Protein Drugs, Rodney Pearlman and Y. John Wang, eds., Plenum Press, New York, 1996.

biological activities of FGFs (Middaugh *et al.*, 1993; Burgess, 1991; Burgess and Maciag, 1989).

The biological activity of the FGFs is at least partially mediated through binding to cell surface receptors. Two distinct types of FGF receptors are found on the surface of cells: specific, high-affinity protein transmembrane receptors of the protein kinase family (K_d, 10–200 pM) and less-specific, lower-affinity cell surface heparan proteoglycans (K_d, 2–100 nM). FGFs are primarily found *in vivo* bound to cell surface proteoglycans, which results in a stabilized, sequestered form of these growth factors. In response to stress, it is believed that proteases and heparanases are either activated or secreted from injured cells, thereby releasing heparan-bound FGFs in an active form from the cell surface. FGFs can then bind to their high-affinity receptors, possibly inducing receptor dimerization, which in turn leads to tyrosine kinase activation and subsequent signal transduction and cell activation (mitogenesis, chemotaxis, angiogenesis, etc.). It appears that both natural and artificial heparin-like molecules also facilitate and perhaps potentiate the ability of FGFs to bind to their high-affinity receptors (Aviezer *et al.*, 1994; Li *et al.*, 1994; Pantoliano *et al.*, 1994; Walker *et al.*, 1994). While it has been shown that only four to eight monosaccharide units are required to stabilize FGFs against a variety of environmental insults, larger structures (greater than eight monosaccharide units) are generally required for biological activity (see review, Middaugh *et al.*, 1993). One hypothesis suggests that polyanion binding may bring two or more FGF molecules close together, leading to dimerization and ultimately activation of the high-affinity receptors (Ornitz *et al.*, 1992). Polyanions may also bind both FGF and FGF receptors simultaneously, thereby forming a ternary complex (Kan *et al.*, 1993). Another idea argues that an FGF molecule can bind to two receptors through different regions of the growth factor, in a manner analogous to human growth hormone and its receptor, with heparan sulfate stabilizing the resulting complex (Thompson *et al.*, 1994). The FGF high-affinity receptor contains an extracellular region (containing two or three immunoglobulin-like domains), a transmembrane region, and an intracellular tyrosine kinase domain. Numerous FGF receptors and spliced variants have been discovered so far, and characterization of their distribution and binding affinities has only recently been initiated (e.g., McKeehan and Kan, 1994). This is further complicated by recent evidence suggesting temporal nuclear location and possible activity for the FGFs (Jans, 1994). It is clear, however, that the extensive array of FGFs and receptors represents an extremely complex system of major biological importance.

Comparison of amino acid sequences reveal a 55% homology between acidic and basic FGF. X-ray crystallography and NMR have been used to reveal the three-dimensional structure of acidic and basic FGF from several species, including humans (see Section 3.3). As expected the overall tertiary structure is very similar for the two proteins. Both proteins are comprised of a series of tightly coupled anti-parallel beta-sheets designated a "beta-trefoil" (12 antiparallel beta-strands organized into a symmetrical threefold repeat of a four-stranded structure; Zhu *et al.*, 1991). The ribbon structure of bFGF is shown in Fig. 2 of Chapter 2. Both proteins contain a cluster of basic amino acid residues on the surface; a combination of site-directed mutagenesis, chemical modification, and photoaffinity labeling experiments has implicated Lys-112, Lys-118, and Arg-122 in human aFGF as part of the polyanion binding site (see Chavan *et al.*, 1994, and references therein). Although both proteins contain several cysteine residues, no disulfide bonds appear to be formed in the native structure. Despite these similarities, human bFGF and aFGF differ in molecular weight, isoelectric point, number of cysteine residues, and conformational stability. Most dramatically, heparin has the ability to potentiate the mitogenic activity of aFGF by about 20-fold. These differences are important in differentiating the formulation strategies required to stabilize and deliver acidic and basic FGFs for clinical use.

In this chapter, we discuss preformulation studies performed with recombinant human aFGF (an amino terminal truncated form containing 141 amino acid residues) which have emphasized a thorough examination of the protein's interaction with a variety of stabilizing polyanions as well as the determination of the causes and mechanisms of aFGF inactivation during storage. In particular, the physical instability of the growth factor due to unfolding and aggregation and chemical instability due to degradative covalent reactions such oxidation and deamidation are described. By combining this understanding of the physicochemical properties of aFGF in solution with the clinical and pharmaceutical needs for delivering and manufacturing a protein drug, stabilized topical formulations of human aFGF for the treatment of wounds have been successfully prepared and utilized for *in vivo* studies.

2. NATURE OF THE INTERACTION OF aFGF WITH HEPARIN

Fibroblast growth factors are only one of many groups of proteins that bind heparin. In fact, FGFs are typically purified in the laboratory by heparin affinity chromatography and were originally called heparin binding growth factors. Despite its widespread use clinically as an anticoagulant, heparin remains an incompletely characterized, chemically ill-defined, heterogeneous mixture of sulfated polysaccharides (Nachtmann *et al.*, 1983; Linhardt, 1991), although efforts to prepare smaller, better-defined analogues is an active area of research. Heparin is commonly synthesized *in vivo* as a proteoglycan containing long, extended polysaccharide chains attached to a small protein core. The polysaccharide chains consist of a repeating copolymer of 1,4-linked glucuronic and *N*-acetyl-glucosamine which are subsequently partially deacylated and sequentially *N*- and *O*-sulfated. Heparin is found in the body tissues of many animals, with an especially rich source being tissue containing large numbers of mast cells. Commercially, heparin is prepared from either porcine intestinal mucosa or bovine lung tissue. Purification involves proteolytic treatment of the tissue, extraction and complexation of the polysaccharides, followed by fractional precipitation (it is then treated with base and oxidizing agents

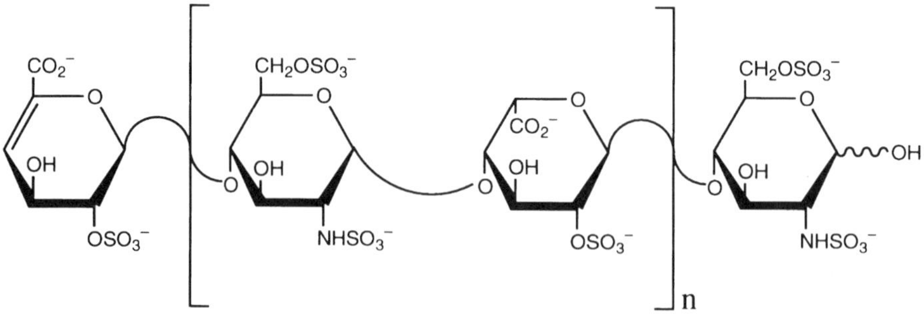

Figure 1. Predominant disaccharide sequence found in heparin consisting of trisulfated 1,4-linked L-iduronic acid and D-glucosamine. This sequence is estimated to account for 60–90% of the total sequence of commercially available heparins (Linhardt, 1991).

during processing to remove residual protein). Whether found attached to proteoglycan on the cell surface or in its highly purified state, heparin has at least three levels of structural complexity (see Fig. 1). First, the polysaccharide chains are a mixture of molecular weights ranging from 5000 to 40,000 ($n \sim 10$–50). Second, incomplete postpolymerization modifications during biosynthesis result in sequence heterogeneity. Approximately 60–90% of the primary sequence is trisulfated 1,4-linked L-iduronic acid and D-glucosamine as shown in Fig. 1. Third, these large heparin chains have an extended helical conformation in solution. These three structural characteristics play a key role in dictating the diverse biological activities of heparin, including its interaction with growth factors.

2.1. Conformational Stability: Thermal- and Denaturant-Induced Unfolding of aFGF in the Presence and Absence of Heparin

The effect of the interaction of aFGF with heparin on the protein's structural stability was initially examined by employing a spectrophotometric turbidity method. This technique monitors the kinetics of the temperature-induced aggregation of unfolded protein by measuring the amount of light scattering (turbidity) at 350 nm over time. As shown in Fig. 2, aFGF rapidly aggregates at 40°C in the absence of polyanions. The presence of increasing amounts of heparin (16 kDa) inhibits the rate and extent of the aFGF aggregation. No detectable aggregation was observed until the ratio of heparin to aFGF was reduced below 1:10 (on a weight and molar basis which are similar since both molecules have an average molecular weight of approximately 16 kDa). This result suggests that multiple binding sites are available on the heparin molecule for aFGF binding.

To more directly ascertain the stabilizing effect of heparin on the structure of

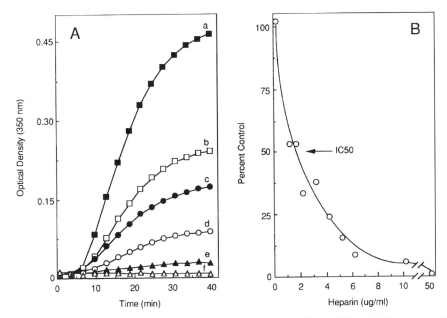

Figure 2. Effect of heparin on the heat-induced aggregation of aFGF at 40°C. (A) Time course of turbidity formation. Samples contained 0.1 mg/ml aFGF in a PBS buffer with (a) no heparin, (b) 0.015X, (c) 0.03X, (d) 0.05X, (e) 0.1X, and (f) 0.5X heparin by weight (B) Effect of heparin concentration on aFGF turbidity formation at 40°C. The Y-axis in B represents the maximum rate of turbidity formation (ΔOD 350 nm/min) normalized to sample (a) containing no heparin. The IC_{50} value is the concentration of heparin at which the rate of aFGF aggregation is 50% of the unliganded protein. Experimental details in Volkin *et al.* (1993) courtesy of Academic Press.

aFGF, the temperature-induced unfolding of the protein was examined by a combination of fluorescence and circular dichroism (CD) spectroscopies. The spectroscopic properties of aFGF in solution have been described in detail elsewhere (Copeland *et al.*, 1991). As shown in Fig. 3A, the far-UV circular dichroism spectrum displays a positive ellipticity peak at 228 nm and a negative band near 205 nm, characteristic of proteins rich in β-II type secondary structure (Wu *et al.*, 1992). In agreement with X-ray crystallography and NMR, CD analysis suggests native, human aFGF consists of approximately 55% beta-sheet, 20% turns, 10% alpha-helix, and 15% disordered structure. The effect of temperature on the secondary structure of aFGF can be conveniently monitored by changes in the CD ellipticity maximum at 228 nm. The fluorescence emission spectrum of aFGF displays characteristic tyrosine emission near 305 nm upon excitation at 280 nm (see Fig. 3B). Fluorescence-quenching studies indicate that seven of the protein's eight tyrosine residues are solvent exposed while the single tryptophan residue is partially inaccessible to solvent. Upon thermal unfolding, the single tryptophan residue of aFGF is unquenched, resulting in a

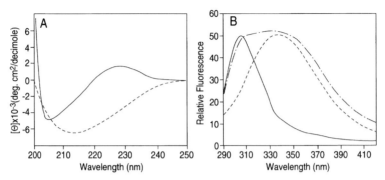

Figure 3. Optical spectroscopic properties of aFGF. (A) Far-UV circular dichroism spectra. The solid line is native while the dashed line is thermally unfolded protein. (B) Fluorescence emission spectrum with 280-nm excitation. The solid line is native, dash/dot line is partially unfolded, and dashed line is mostly unfolded protein. Experimental details in Copeland *et al.* (1991) courtesy of Academic Press.

tryptophan-dominated spectrum with an emission maximum found near 350 nm. Neither the fluorescence nor CD spectrum of aFGF changes upon the addition of heparin (or any other polyanion described in this chapter), implying that no major conformational changes occur in the vicinity of the single Trp residue or the overall secondary structure upon ligand binding (Copeland *et al.*, 1991).

The effect of heparin concentration on the thermal-induced unfolding of aFGF as measured by fluorescence spectroscopy is shown in Fig. 4. In the absence of a polyanions, aFGF unfolds at the surprisingly low temperature of about 30°C at neutral pH. Upon the addition of increasing amounts of heparin, the thermal unfolding temperature (T_m) increases to approximately 60°C. The ratio of heparin to protein required to induce one-half the maximum stabilization as measured by T_m values is 0.1× (by weight). Thus, heparin dramatically enhances the thermal stability of aFGF in solution with increases in the protein's thermal unfolding temperature of about 30°C as measured by fluorescence spectroscopy. A similar stabilization is detected by both CD and differential scanning calorimetric measurements, although temperature transitions are observed at approximately 10°C higher temperatures (Volkin *et al.*, 1993; Tsai *et al.*, 1993). This difference is thought to reflect the formation of a "molten globule" state by the growth factor in the physiological temperature region (Mach *et al.*, 1993b), a phenomenon that may be important for membrane transport of the protein (Wiedlocha *et al.*, 1992; Mach and Middaugh, 1995).

The thermodynamic parameters of the unfolding process of native aFGF were difficult to obtain from thermal denaturation experiments due to irreversible aggregation that occurs at high temperatures after partial unfolding. Urea-induced unfolding was therefore employed to monitor the reversible unfolding of aFGF, since this denaturant should help maintain the solubility of unfolded forms as well as not interfere with the presumed electrostatic interactions involved in the binding of

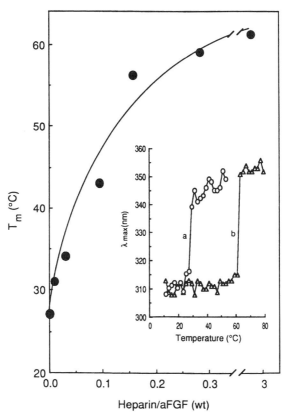

Figure 4. Effect of heparin concentration on the thermal unfolding temperature (T_m) of aFGF as measured by fluorescence spectroscopy. The inset is a representative experiment in which the aFGF fluorescence wavelength emission maximum (excitation at 280 nm) is measured as a function of temperature in the absence (a) and presence (b) of 3X heparin by weight. Experimental details in Volkin *et al.* (1993) courtesy of Academic Press.

polyanions to aFGF. As shown in Fig. 5, unliganded aFGF unfolds at a [urea]$_{1/2}$ of 2.3 M (the concentration of urea at the midpoint of the denaturant-induced transition from native to unfolded protein). As increasing amounts of heparin are added, the [urea]$_{1/2}$ increases to 3.6 M. By assuming simple two-state behavior, the equilibrium denaturation profiles were analyzed by linear extrapolation method to obtain the free energy change due to unfolding (Burke *et al.*, 1993). This analysis finds a ΔG_{app} value of 6.5 kcal/mol for the unliganded protein, a value not unexpected based on the molecular weight and thermal unfolding temperature of aFGF. In the presence of excess heparin the ΔG_{app} increases to 9.2 kcal/mol, implying about 2.5 kcal/mol of stabilization of the native form of aFGF upon binding to heparin (Burke *et al.*, 1993).

Another approach used to quantitatively characterize the interaction of aFGF

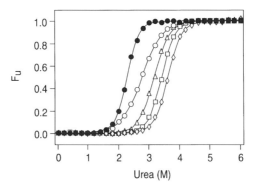

Figure 5. Effect of heparin concentration on the urea-induced unfolding of aFGF as measured by fluorescence spectroscopy. Samples contained 0.1 mg/ml protein in a PBS buffer containing 1 mM EDTA and the indicated amounts of urea. Heparin concentration by weight are from left to right are 0X, 0.1X, 0.33X, 1X, and 10X. Experimental details in Burke *et al.* (1993) courtesy of American Chemical Society.

with heparin is to examine the rate of denaturant induced unfolding and refolding of the protein in the presence and absence of heparin (Burke *et al.*, 1993; Mach and Middaugh, 1994). The rate of aFGF unfolding and refolding can be monitored by fluorescence spectroscopy as described above for thermal unfolding experiments, except that one measures the time course of the appearance of the fluorescence maxima at 350 nm (unfolding of aFGF in a denaturant-containing solution) or 305 nm (refolding of aFGF to native state upon dilution from a denaturant-containing solution), respectively. Unliganded aFGF unfolds in a solution of 4.4 M urea with a rate constant of 0.2 s^{-1}. The presence of 0.3× heparin inhibits the unfolding rate by 300-fold while the addition of 1–10× heparin slows the rate of aFGF unfolding by over 2000-fold compared to unliganded protein (Burke *et al.*, 1993). When aFGF is refolded by dilution from a denaturant containing solution (e.g., 0.1 M guanidine hydrochloride), polyanions have little or no effect on the kinetics of refolding at temperatures below 30°C. At temperatures above 30°C, however, aFGF absolutely requires a polyanion such as heparin to refold and the energetics of this process are strongly dependent on the nature of the stabilizing polyanion (Dabora *et al.*, 1991).

2.2. Size and Charge Requirements of Heparin Required to Stabilize aFGF

It is difficult to determine the precise molar ratios of aFGF to heparin used in these heparin stabilization experiments due to the inherent heterogeneity of commercial preparations of this polysaccharide. Therefore, to better understand the size requirements of heparin's interaction with aFGF, a series of well-defined heparin fragments (enzymatically prepared and purified oligosaccharides ranging in size from disaccharide to decasaccharide) were examined for their ability to stabilize aFGF against thermal unfolding as measured by both fluorescence and CD. Although the disaccharide did not alter the T_m of aFGF compared to the unliganded protein, higher-molecular-weight fragments (tetramer, hexamer, octamer, and decamer) all stabilized aFGF approximately to the same extent as heparin itself (T_m values from 53–61°C; Volkin et al., 1993a). In addition, the size requirement of oligosaccharide binding to aFGF was examined by incubating aFGF–heparin complexes with heparin lyases I and II and the size of protected oligosaccharides determined by gradient PAGE analysis. Results of these experiments show that a tetrasaccharide is the smallest oligosaccharide protected from enzymatic digestion. Furthermore, when partially enzymatically digested heparin was passed over an aFGF affinity column and then eluted with a salt gradient, the tetrasaccharide was found to be enriched in the high-affinity fraction. In addition, when aFGF was noncovalently bound to a heparin affinity column, purified tetrasaccharide was able to displace aFGF from the heparinized resin. Taken together, these experiments strongly suggest that the small-est fragment of heparin able to interact and stabilize aFGF is the hexasulfated tetrasaccharide fragment (see Fig. 1). These data are also in agreement with physical considerations based upon examination of the crystal structure of aFGF as described below.

To better understand the charge requirements of heparin stabilization of aFGF, a series of chemically modified heparin molecules of varying sulfation levels were examined for their ability to stabilize aFGF against both thermal- and urea-induced unfolding as measured by fluorescence spectroscopy. As the sulfur content of the derivatized heparin was increased (1.5% to 4.5–8% to 13.5% S), the T_m of aFGF rose from 28 to 49 to 61°C, respectively (Volkin et al., 1992, 1993). Similarly, urea unfolding experiments found that the midpoint of the unfolding transition and the value of ΔG_{app} dramatically increases as a function of the sulfur content of heparin ($[\text{urea}]_{1/2}$ values of 2.3, 2.5, and 3.5 M, respectively; Burke et al., 1993). In both sets of experiments, the completely desulfated heparin (1.5% S) appears to bind only very weakly if at all to aFGF as evidenced by T_m, $[\text{urea}]_{1/2}$, and ΔG_{app} values equal to those of unliganded protein. These findings support previous work establishing the primary role for the sulfate groups of heparin in its interaction with aFGF (for reviews, see Middaugh et al., 1993; Burgess, 1991; Burgess and Maciag, 1989).

2.3. Stoichiometry and Affinity of the aFGF–Heparin Interaction

To determine the number of aFGF molecules capable of binding to a heparin molecule, the size of aFGF–heparin complexes (at various molar ratios of protein to polysaccharide) was measured by static and dynamic light scattering (Mach et al., 1993a). As shown in Fig. 6A, the addition of small amounts of heparin (16 kDa) to a solution of aFGF (a molar ratio of aFGF/heparin of 500 to about 20) results in a sharp

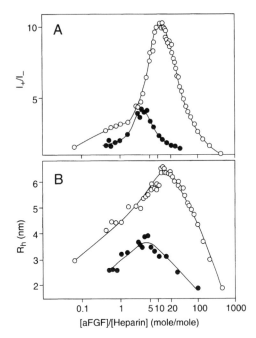

Figure 6. Size of aFGF-heparin complexes as a function of the protein/polysaccharide molar ratio as measured by static and dynamic light scattering. (A) Scattered light intensity of the mixtures of aFGF and heparin (I_+) normalized to the sum of the expected intensities from noninteracting aFGF and heparin (I_-). (B) Mean hydrodynamic radii of aFGF–heparin complexes. Open symbols are for 16-kDa heparin and solid symbols are for 4.8-kDa heparin. Experimental details in Mach *et al.* (1993) courtesy of American Chemical Society.

increase in the observed scattering intensity I_+ compared to the calculated intensity of noninteracting protein and polysaccharide mixtures I_-. At a molar ratio of about 15:1 aFGF/heparin, all of the aFGF molecules appear to be bound to a single heparin molecule producing a maximum in the light-scattering intensity. Further increases in the concentration of heparin produce excess binding sites and partial occupancy of a single heparin molecule with a consequent decrease in the average complex size and scattered light intensity. This trend continues until in the presence of excess amounts of heparin (molar ratios of aFGF/heparin of less than 1) there is on the average only one aFGF molecule bound per heparin molecule. In the presence of low-molecular-weight heparin (4.8 kDa), a similar titration pattern is observed with maximal occupancy at about 4:1 molar ratio of aFGF/heparin. When dynamic light scattering was utilized to monitor the hydrodynamic radius of aFGF–heparin complexes at various molar ratios of aFGF/heparin (Fig. 6B), a nearly equivalent titration pattern was observed for aFGF in the presence of high- and low-molecular-weight heparin. Modeling of the light-scattering experiments predicts that about 10 aFGF molecules bind 16-kDa heparin at high- affinity sites while 4–5 bind with weaker affinity. This corresponds to a maximal loading of one aFGF molecule bound per every 4.4 monosaccharide units of heparin (Mach *et al.*, 1992, 1993). The size of aFGF–heparin complexes was also examined by analytical ultracentrifugation. These experiments demonstrate a molecular mass of 30–35 kDa for aFGF–heparin complexes in the presence of a threefold weight excess of heparin. For ratios of heparin–aFGF of less than 1, the system is no longer homogeneous with a distribution of molecular weights observed. For example, a 10-fold excess of aFGF produces a range of molecular-weight complexes from 50 to 160 kDa corresponding to aFGF-heparin ratios of 2:1 up to 9:1 (Mach *et al.*, 1993a), in good agreement with the light-scattering results.

The high affinity of aFGF for heparin has been recognized since the initial affinity purification of the growth factor. For example, it requires 1.4 M NaCl to elute purified aFGF from a heparin affinity column. Surface plasmon resonance (SPR) measurements were utilized to quantitatively measure the association and dissociation of aFGF from a heparinized surface (Mach *et al.*, 1993a). In these experiments, biotinylated heparin was immobilized to the biosensor surface via streptavidin which was covalently linked to the carboxylated dextran matrix on the biosensor surface. Varying amounts of aFGF were then passed over the heparinized biosensor surface and the rate and extent of aFGF binding was monitored. It was shown that aFGF binds biotinylated heparin with an association rate constant of $2-11 \times 10^{-5}$ M^{-1} s^{-1}, a dissociation rate constant of 0.06–0.03 s^{-1} and an overall dissociation constant (K_d) of 50–140 nM. The K_d value for aFGF–heparin measured by surface plasmon resonance is in good agreement with affinity values estimated by other techniques (reviewed in Middaugh *et al.*, 1993). SPR measurements also indicated multiple aFGF molecules are bound to a single heparin chain with stoichiometric values of 8–10, similar to aFGF– heparin ratios determined by light scattering and analytical ultracentrifugation.

Based on these physical measurements, the nature of the interaction of aFGF with heparin has been quantitatively characterized. The growth factor binds heparin with high affinity (K_d of 50–140 nM) with the stoichiometry of this interaction depending on the molar ratio of protein to ligand in solution. An aFGF molecule can bind every 4–5 monosaccharide units on heparin with the smallest, high-affinity site consisting of a highly sulfated tetrasaccharide. The binding of aFGF to heparin does not cause any detectable conformational change in the protein. Nevertheless, the protein is dramatically stabilized against thermal- and denaturant-induced unfolding. This stabilization of aFGF occurs presumably by shifting the equilibrium between folded and unfolded protein by the preferential binding of heparin to native forms. As described in the introduction, the binding of heparin to aFGF also greatly enhances the growth factor's mitogenic activity as measured by a variety of *in vitro* and *in vivo* assays. Based on these biophysical experiments, some part of this enhancement is probably due to physical stabilization of the protein (although a direct role for heparin stabilization of the binding of aFGF to its high-affinity receptor appears likely as well). As will be discussed, the binding of heparin to aFGF not only confers physical stabilization, but also protects labile cysteine residues from oxidation, a chemical reaction leading to inactivation of the growth factor. The combination of physical and chemical stabilization data has provided insight into the location and nature of the aFGF polyanion binding site as will be considered next.

3. NATURE OF THE aFGF POLYANION BINDING SITE

3.1. Specificity of the aFGF Polyanion Binding Site

A question arises as to the specificity of the interaction of aFGF with heparin. Comparisons of the binding specificity of the many serum proteins that form complexes with heparin are of interest in this regard. Perhaps the best-known heparin binding protein is the protease inhibitor antithrombin III, a key protein involved in the regulation of the blood coagulation cascade. Antithrombin III binds to a particular pentasaccharide sequence within heparin and then undergoes a functional conformational change. This interaction is highly specific: removal of the 3-O-sulfate group in the third residue of the pentasaccharide dramatically decreases the polyanion's ability to bind to antithrombin III as well as diminishing the complex's antifactor Xa activity (Castellot *et al.*, 1986).

To explore the structural specificity of polyanion's interaction with aFGF, the turbidity method was again initially employed (Volkin *et al.*, 1993a; Tsai *et al.*, 1993). A large variety of polyanions, including non-heparin-sulfated polysaccharides, diverse low-molecular-weight sulfated and phosphorylated compounds as well as numerous other highly charged compounds were incubated with aFGF and the rate and extent of aFGF aggregation was monitored. A summary of many of these experiments are shown in Fig. 7 in which the ability of these ligands to inhibit the extent of aFGF aggregation after 30 min at 40°C is illustrated. The sulfated polymers varied greatly in their ability to stabilize aFGF. For example, under these conditions, heparin, dextran sulfate and pentosan polysulfate completely inhibited aFGF aggregate formation, chondrotin sulfates provided 10–100-fold stabilization while polyvinyl and keratan sulfate stabilized aFGF only 1–10 fold (compared to the unliganded protein). Many of the low-molecular-weight sulfated and phosphorylated compounds such as ATP, inorganic phosphates, and various polyanionic inositol compounds such as inositol hexasulfate and phytic acid (inositol hexaphosphate) also dramatically stabilized aFGF. Furthermore, quite different highly charged polymers such as poly A,G and poly Asp also provided some protection against heat-induced aggregation. In fact, many other diverse agents not shown in Fig. 7 such as double- and single-stranded DNA, the highly phosphorylated protein phosvitin, the sulfated sugar lactobionic acid as well as high concentrations of salts such as sulfates and phosphates all significantly inhibited aFGF aggregation. As might be expected, related but positively charged or uncharged derivative compounds such as poly Arg and unsulfated inositol did not provide any protection. The concentration dependence of the

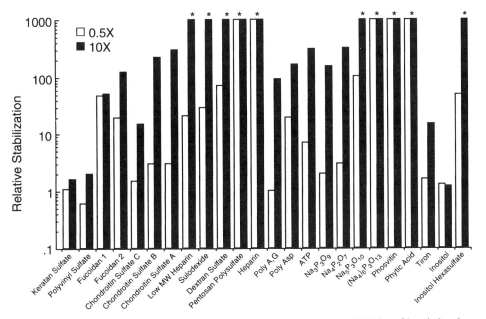

Figure 7.   Stabilization of aFGF by various polyanions as measured by the inhibition of heat induced aggregation at 40°C. The relative stabilization is the extent of aggregation (ΔOD 350 after 15 min) in the presence of 0.5X (open bars) and 10X (solid bars) ligands (by weight) normalized to unliganded protein. Asterisk indicates no aggregation was observed during the time course of the experiment. Experimental details in Tsai *et al.* (1993) courtesy of Plenum Publishing.

inhibition of heat induced aggregation by these substances fell into three general categories: sulfated polymers require molar ratios substantially below one (0.03–0.1) implying multiple aFGFs can bind to a single polymer molecule; lower-molecular-weight negatively charged compounds like tetrapolyphosphate or inositol hexasulfate appear to interact with high affinity at low to unitary stochiometries (0.6–2); and finally, small singly charged molecules like ammonium sulfate and phosphate salts appear to bind only weakly (ligand:to:aFGF molar ratio of >80).

To further quantify the ability of this diverse set of polyanions to interact with aFGF, two other protein stability-related parameters were investigated, namely, the effect polyanions on aFGF's thermal melting temperature (T_m) and the ability of polyanions to protect aFGF's three reduced cysteine residues from oxidation. A combination of fluorescence spectroscopy and circular dichroism was utilized to demonstrate that many of the compounds which inhibited thermally induced aggregation of aFGF also raise proportionally the protein's thermal unfolding temperature (Volkin *et al.*, 1992, 1993a). The charge requirements of the stabilizing ligands were probed with differentially phosphorylated inositol compounds. It was seen as the number of phosphate groups increased from 1 to 6 (P1, P2, P3, P4, P6), the thermal unfolding temperature of aFGF increased from 28 to 31 to 42 to 51 to 61°C respectively as measured by fluorescence spectroscopy. Similar effects of increasing stability with increasing ligand charge density were observed with differentially sulfated β-cyclodextrins both by thermal- and urea-induced unfolding of aFGF (Volkin *et al.*, 1993a; Burke *et al.*, 1993).

The ability of a wide variety of polyanions to protect aFGF from autooxidation was analyzed by measuring the percentage of thiol groups remaining in solution after incubation of aFGF–polyanion complexes with copper ions for 10 min. In the absence of a stabilizing polyanion only 40% of the protein's available thiol groups were titratable with Ellman's reagent, while the addition of heparin preserved greater than 97% of aFGF's cysteine residues under the same conditions. Other polyanions such as those listed in Fig. 7 varied in their ability to protect the cysteine residues against oxidation (75–97% protection). In general, compounds which were most effective at stabilizing aFGF were most effective at protecting the protein's sulfhydryl groups (Volkin *et al.*, 1993a). A summary of the stabilizing effects of representative polyanions on the conformational and chemical integrity of aFGF is shown in Table I. Based on these experiments it is clear that the specificity of the interaction of aFGF with polyanions is surprisingly weak with a wide variety of polyanions, including sulfated, phosphorylated, and highly charged polymers as well as polyanionic low-molecular-weight compounds, able to induce physical stabilization against both thermal unfolding and chemical oxidation. This lack of specificity provides numerous potential options for developing stable drug formulations of this unstable growth factor.

3.2. Interaction of aFGF with Other Selected Polyanions: Suramin, Sucrose Octasulfate, Nucleotides, and Chromatography Resins

A number of highly polyanionic compounds which have already been approved for human use were also examined for their effects on aFGF. Suramin, a symmetrical polysulfonated naphthylurea, has been used extensively to treat human parasitic diseases such as trypanosomiasis and onchocerciasis, and is currently being evaluated as an antitumor agent (Middaugh *et al.*, 1992; see references within). In this regard, suramin is believed to inhibit the binding of various growth factors to their receptors by direct interaction with the protein ligand. Until recently, the nature of this interaction was unclear. The interaction of suramin with aFGF provides an ideal model with which to elucidate the mechanism of this interaction (Middaugh *et al.*, 1992). To this end, initial observations showed that the weak fluorescence of a suramin solution is significantly enhanced by the addition of aFGF. Titration experiments reveal a maximum effect at a molar ratio of suramin to aFGF of 2:1. Both CD and Amide I' FTIR analysis of the secondary structure of aFGF in the presence of suramin suggest a small conformational change in the growth factor upon binding.

**Table I. Physical Stabilization of aFGF by Various
Polyanionic Ligands[a,b]**

Additive	T_m (°C)	Cu²⁺ Oxidation (% SH lost in 10 min)
Buffer alone	45	60%
Sodium sulfate MW 142	57	25%
Tetrapolyphosphate MW 440	66	<3%
Inositol hexaphosphate MW 660	70	<3%
Inositol hexasulfate MW 890	66	22%
Sulfated lactobionic acid amide MW 2,600	62	N.P.
Sulfated β-cyclodextrin MW ~2,500	65	<3%
Sulfated γ-cyclodextrin MW ~3,000	70	5%
Pentosan polyphosphate MW ~5,000	60	6%
Low MW heparin MW ~5,000	66	<3%
Dextran sulfate MW ~8,000	62	7%
Heparin MW ~16,000	64	<3%

[a]Thermal melting temperatures (T_m) were measured by circular dichroism. Samples contained 100 μg/ml aFGF (6 μM) in a phosphate-buffered saline solution, pH 7.2, with excess ligand (typically 3X by weight except when 120 mM sodium sulfate and 10 mM tetrapolyphosphate were utilized to produce maximum stabilization). The percentage of aFGF thiols remaining in solution is determined after a 10-min incubation with cupric chloride. NP indicates experiment not performed.
[b]Data taken from Volkin *et al.* (1993).

Suramin also partially stabilizes aFGF against both thermal unfolding and autooxidation of cysteine residues, as shown by the same methodologies outlined above, with the T_m of aFGF increasing 5–10°C and approximately 80% protection of the protein's cysteine residues from copper-induced oxidation. These observations led to the conclusion that suramin interacts with aFGF at the protein's polyanion binding site. In fact, the ability of various ligands to displace suramin from the aFGF polyanion binding site was later utilized to screen a variety of compounds for stabilizing interactions with aFGF (Volkin *et al.*, 1992).

A combination of dynamic light scattering and gel filtration chromatography demonstrated that the binding of suramin to aFGF at its polyanion binding site induces reversible microaggregation, to at least the hexameric state, with a return to the monomeric state in the presence of excess polyanions including suramin itself. The bifunctional nature of suramin, along with the potential of multiple polyanion binding sites on aFGF, is the probable cause of suramin-induced microaggregation of the growth factor. As expected, high concentrations of suramin decrease the size of these complexes as all of the polyanion binding sites become occupied. Similar observations were recorded for other heparin binding growth factors including bFGF, PDGF, and IGF-1 (Middaugh et al., 1992). Although a direct testing of this hypothesis in vivo remains to be performed, it is likely that the inhibition of growth factor activity by suramin may be explained by the induction of small conformational changes and microaggregation of the protein by the binding of suramin to these protein's polyanion binding site. These observations also clearly demonstrate that stabilization per se does not qualify an agent as a potential aFGF formulation excipient since the corresponding aggregation in this case would reduce or eliminate the activity of the growth factor.

The mechanism of action of the antiulcer drug sucralfate, the aluminum salt of the disaccharide sucrose octasulfate, has been proposed to involve the stabilization of endogenous fibroblast growth factors from acid degradation in the stomach. This could then result in acceleration of healing by preserving the growth factor's angiogenic and mitogenic activities (Folkman et al., 1991). It has also been proposed that combination therapy employing both FGFs and sucralfate may overcome a natural loss of endogenous growth factors and thereby further accelerate the ulcer healing process. It was therefore of interest to systematically examine the interaction of aFGF with both the soluble potassium salt of sucrose octasulfate as well as its insoluble aluminum salt, sucralfate (Volkin et al., 1993b).

Similar to heparin, the soluble potassium salt of sucrose octasulfate (SOS) potentiates the mitogenic activity of aFGF by 20–50-fold as measured by stimulation of cell division in mouse fibroblast 3T3 cells. This enhancement of aFGF's biological activity is due at least in part to the conformational stabilization of the growth factor. SOS stabilizes aFGF against thermal unfolding with a 20–25°C increase in the T_m value compared to unliganded protein as measured by CD, fluorescence, and differential scanning calorimetry. Like other stabilizing polyanions, SOS also partially protects the cysteine residues of aFGF from copper-catalyzed oxidation. In the presence of a 40-fold molar excess of SOS to aFGF, urea-induced unfolding reveals that the free energy of stabilization of the native compared to the unfolded state is approximately 3.0 kcal/mole, a value similar to that obtained for aFGF–heparin complexes. SOS was also shown to bind at the aFGF polyanion binding site as determined by its ability to displace, in a concentration-dependent manner, protein from aFGF–heparin complexes (measured by a decrease in the size of these complexes by dynamic light scattering) and aFGF–suramin complexes (measured by a decrease in suramin fluorescence). Thus, due to its high charge density, SOS is essentially a heparin analogue that binds and stabilizes aFGF via interaction with the growth factor's polyanion binding site (Volkin et al., 1993b).

The conformation and stability of aFGF bound to the insoluble aluminum salt of

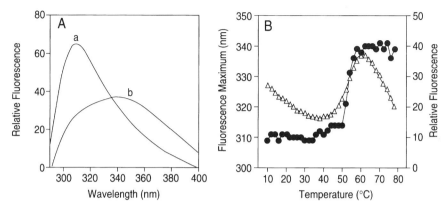

Figure 8. (A) Front-face fluorescence emission spectra of aFGF bound to the insoluble drug sucralfate (aluminum sucrose octasulfate) at (a) 10°C and (b) 70°C. The spectra (excitation 280 nm) are corrected for light scattering by subtraction. (B) Thermal unfolding of aFGF adsorbed to sucralfate as measured by front-face fluorescence spectroscopy. Experimental details in Volkin *et al.* (1993b) courtesy of Elsevier Science Publishing.

sucrose octasulfate (sucralfate) can be examined by front-face fluorescence. This technique allows one to directly measure the intrinsic fluorescence properties of proteins adsorbed to solids in the presence of excessive light scattering. As shown in Fig. 8A, front-face fluorescence measurements of aFGF bound to sucralfate show a tyrosine dominant emission spectrum indicative of native structure (as described in Section 2.1). For comparison, a tryptophan emission dominant spectra of aFGF bound to sucralfate after exposure of the complex to elevated temperatures (70°C) indicates the protein is significantly unfolded under these conditions. Figure 8B illustrates an entire thermal unfolding experiment in which the unfolding of aFGF adsorbed to sucralfate is followed by monitoring the fluorescence spectra every 2°C. It can be seen that a major conformational transition is observed at 53°C, implying that although sucralfate stabilizes aFGF (the unliganded protein unfolds at about 30°C), the effect of surface adsorption itself is destabilizing (the T_m of aFGF bound to soluble SOS is 58°C). Fluorescence spectroscopy also demonstrated that both SOS and sucralfate protect aFGF from acid-induced unfolding at low pH, thereby potentially allowing aFGF to remain biologically active in the low-pH gastric environment (Volkin *et al.*, 1993b).

Analogous to the sucralfate experiments, front-face fluorescence spectroscopy was also utilized to examine the conformation and stability of aFGF on a different type of polyanionic solid surface in the form of various chromatography resins. Fibroblast growth factors were originally isolated from tissue extracts by a combination of heparin affinity chromatography and reverse-phase chromatography (see reviews, Burgess, 1991; Burgess and Macaig, 1989). During the development of a large-scale isolation procedures for the preparation of clinical supplies of recombinant human aFGF from *E. coli*, a series of affinity and ion-exchange resins were examined. Front-face fluorescence spectroscopy and differential scanning calorimetry (DSC) were utilized to better understand the interaction of aFGF with these chromatography resins (Volkin *et al.*, manuscript in preparation). Comparisons of fluorescence spectra of aFGF adsorbed to various ion-exchange and heparin affinity resins show that increasing the hydrophobicity of the resin matrix leads to the destabilization of the protein. For example, although both carbohydrate and polymeric heparinized resins stabilized aFGF (T_m of ~50°C and ~45°C, respectively) compared to the unliganded protein in solution (T_m of 30°C), surface adsorption destabilized aFGF compared to the heparin bound protein in solution (T_m of 60°C). Similar data were recorded for a variety of ion exchange resins.

As final example of the relative nonspecificity of the interaction of the aFGF polyanion binding site with various polyanions, the ability of nucleotides to bind and stabilize aFGF was examined (Chavan *et al.*, 1994). Several nucleotide polyphosphates such as ATP and GTP are present at millimolar concentrations within cells and could potentially interact with and stabilize aFGF *in vivo*. Three categories of differentially phosphorylated compounds were examined, including inorganic phosphates, nucleotide polyphosphates, and dinucleotide polyphosphates. It was observed that increasing the phosphorylation state of the ligand resulted in enhanced aFGF thermal stability. For example, the T_m of aFGF (as measured by fluorescence and CD spectroscopy) increased by 10–20°C in the presence of tetrapolyphosphate, adenosine tetraphosphate, and diadenosine hexaphosphate compared to the unliganded protein. The specificity of these compounds for the polyanion binding site of aFGF was established by showing that they were displaced by heparin and that they inhibited the ability of DTNB (Ellman's reagent) to interact with the cysteine residues of aFGF. A more direct visualization of the amino acid residues of aFGF directly involved in the binding of nucleotide ligands was performed via photolabeling experiments with [^{32}P]-azido nucleotides. The radioactive ligand was incubated with aFGF and covalently linked to the protein via exposure to light. The photolabeled protein was then precipitated with perchloric acid, digested with trypsin, and resulting peptides were separated by Al^{3+} chromatography. Radioactive peaks were further purified by reverse-phase chromatography and then subjected to amino acid sequence analysis to determine the site of photoinsertion. From these experiments, eight different amino acid residues in aFGF were identified, all of them located on the perimeter of the presumptive aFGF polyanion binding site (Chavan *et al.*, 1994).

3.3. Structure of the aFGF Polyanion Binding Site

Although a high-resolution crystal or NMR structure of human aFGF complexed to heparin has not yet been reported, a wide variety of chemical and molecular biological studies have been performed that lend significant insight into the nature of this binding region so crucial to stabilization (and ultimately formulation) of the protein. Most importantly, crystallographic and NMR structures of both basic and acidic FGF from several animal sources containing various low-molecular-weight nonheparin polyanions have been solved. We will briefly summarize some of these studies.

The earliest clues to the location of the heparin binding site on the FGFs came from a combination of chemical modification, site-directed mutagenesis, and peptide competition studies (Harper and Lobb, 1988; Burgess et al., 1991; Burgess, 1991; Thompson et al., 1994; Li et al., 1994). This work led to the identification of several proximate basic residues (e.g., Lys-118, Arg-122) as well as other polar residues (Thompson et al., 1994) that appear to be present within the polyanion binding region. The extent of this site in both aFGF and bFGF has been explored by examining the interaction of these growth factors with heparin fragments of varying length as well as by polysaccharide protection experiments (see Volkin et al., 1993; Aviezer et al., 1994, and references therein). In the case of aFGF, it was clear that a tetrasaccharide was sufficient to functionally fill the heparin binding site. The situation is somewhat less obvious with bFGF where some experimental evidence suggests that the polyanion binding region may be somewhat more extensive (Ornitz et al., 1992; Walker et al., 1994). It is also now generally accepted that octasaccharides and above are required for completely effective functional interaction of the FGFs with their high-affinity receptor, perhaps reflecting the additional involvement of a polyanion binding site on the receptor itself which may be involved in formation of a tertiary complex (e.g., Pantoliano et al., 1994). Recently, the polyanion binding site on aFGF was directly mapped on human aFGF employing photoaffinity labeling with multiple phosphorylated nucleotides (Chavan et al., 1994) as described in the previous section. The extent of the region defined in these studies was consistent with tetrasaccharide dimensions, but also suggested significant nonspecificity in polyanion binding since the large region labeled could only be simply explained by multiple orientations of the bound polyanions. Some evidence for a second (or more expansive) binding site was suggested by these as well as several other of the studies, but this remains an unresolved issue.

The most definitive information about the localization of the polyanion binding site comes from X-ray crystallography and NMR studies of several different FGFs with low-molecular-weight polyanions bound. Both bovine (Zhu et al., 1991, 1993; Zhu, 1993) and human (Pineda-Lucena et al., 1994) aFGF as well as human bFGF (Zhu et al., 1991; Eriksson et al., 1991, 1993; Zhang et al., 1991; Ago et al., 1991) have been examined in these studies with sulfate, iridium hexachloride, selenate, sucrose octasulfate, and inositol hexasulfate employed as ligating anions. In general, all of these structural determinations have identified the same region in the FGFs as the most probable site of interaction with heparin. In the case of aFGF, this consists of a positively charged region in the C-terminal third of the protein. Four basic residues as well as several uncharged but polar side chains are identified as contact points with bound polyanions (Zhu *et al.*, 1993; Pineda-Lucena *et al.*, 1994). The NMR data are also consistent with a lack of specificity of the binding site and suggest that stabilization is induced by rigidifying a hairpin loop involving β-strands 10 and 11. Although definitive description of the heparin binding site must await crystal structure of FGFs with bound heparin fragments currently in progress (R. J. Linhardt, personal communication), the studies described above establish with some confidence the location of this critical region in the protein.

4. FORMULATION AND DELIVERY OF aFGF AS A WOUND-HEALING AGENT

4.1. *In Vitro* Stability Considerations: Conformational and Chemical Integrity of aFGF

The formulation of a protein pharmaceutical drug requires the development of a dosage form (liquid or lyophilized powder in a defined container) which maintains the protein's physicochemical properties and biological activity during storage. Typically, pharmaceutical drugs must be stable for 1 to 2 years under specified storage conditions. The development of a stable formulation for a protein drug requires a thorough understanding of the causes and mechanisms of inactivation, including both physical and chemical pathways. Furthermore, the effects of these changes on the biological activity of the protein must be elucidated. By understanding the degradative processes leading to protein inactivation, rational approaches to the design of the formulation can be utilized to minimize or prevent their occurrence. Based on the experience of pharmaceutical scientists working on protein formulation over the past decade, many of these degradative processes have been identified for both liquid and lyophilized dosage forms (Cleland and Langer, 1994; Ahern and Manning, 1992; Wang and Pearlman, 1992; Volkin and Middaugh, 1992; Volkin and Klibanov, 1989). Physical instability can occur due to denaturation, aggregation, and precipitation as well as adsorption of protein to container surfaces. Chemical instability can be most commonly caused by deamidation, racemization, hydrolysis, oxidation, beta-elimination, and disulfide exchange reactions as well as chemical interactions with pharmaceutical excipients.

4.1.1. CONFORMATIONAL STABILITY

The conformational instability of aFGF required a thorough understanding of the interaction of the growth factor with stabilizing polyanions. From the studies described above, it is clear that the native conformation of aFGF is inherently unstable with significant unfolding of the protein at temperatures at or below physio-

Table II. Biophysical and Biochemical Characterization of aFGF in the Presence of ~16-kDA Heparin Derived from Either Bovine Lung or Porcine Mucosa[a]

	Bovine	Porcine
1. Sulfur content (% S) of heparin molecules	13.3%	13.5%
2. Thermal unfolding ($T_m \pm 2°C$) as measured by		
• fluorescence	62°C	63°C
• circular dicroism	72°C	72°C
• differential scanning calorimetry	71°C	71°C
3. Urea-induced unfolding		
• [urea]1/2	3.6 ± 0.2 M	3.6 ± 0.2 M
• ΔG of N $\leftrightarrow$ U	8.9 ± 0.4 kcal/m	9.3 ± 0.3 kcal/m
• kinetics (unfolding rate in 4.4M urea)	$0.0068 \pm .001$ s^{-1}	$0.0077 \pm .001$ s^{-1}
4. Stoichiometry of raFGF–heparin complexes		
• Maximum number of aFGF molecules bound to a single heparin chain	13 ± 1	13 ± 1
• Molar ratio of heparin/raFGF required to displace suramin from raFGF	~ 0.1	~ 0.1
5. Percent raFGF thiol groups protected ($\pm 10\%$) from CuCl$_2$ oxidation (10 min, 30 min)	>99% 95%	97% 91%
6. Mitogenic activity in pg/ml ($\pm$ S.D.) (IC$_{50}$ value of an assay standard)	113 ± 20	91 ± 16

[a]Stability experiments contain 3X heparin (by weight) in a phosphate-buffered saline solution.

logical levels. In the presence of stabilizing polyanions, however, dramatic stabilization of the protein's native structure is observed with enhancement of the T_m value of aFGF by 25–30°C as measured by a variety of biophysical techniques. The stabilizing properties of heparin on aFGF are summarized in Table II. It can be seen that different animal sources of heparin (porcine mucosa versus bovine lung) are similar in their ability to physically interact and stabilize, as well as potentiate the biological activity, of aFGF. In addition, heparin is known to dramatically reduce the susceptibility of aFGF to proteolysis, presumably due to the maintenance of the protein's native state which is more protease resistant than partially unfolded forms (see references in reviews, Middaugh et al., 1993; Burgess, 1991; Burgess and Macaig, 1989).

Despite the effectiveness of heparin-induced stabilization of aFGF, this sulfated carbohydrate is an inherently heterogeneous material derived from animal sources and possesses well-known anticoagulant activity. The need for a chemically well-defined synthetic polyanion stabilizer is therefore apparent. Due to the relative nonspecificity of the aFGF polyanion binding site, several small-molecular-weight, synthetic ligands which stabilize aFGF to the same extent as heparin were identified as potential stabilizers for aFGF clinical formulations (as described in Section 3). The final choice of a stabilizing polyanion for clinical formulations of aFGF, however, requires considerations beyond the protein's stability, such as the safety and tolerability of the ligand as well as any effects the ligand may have on the biological efficacy of aFGF. These considerations are discussed in further detail in the following sections.

Even though the inclusion of a stabilizing polyanion in the formulation of aFGF dramatically enhances the conformational stability of the aFGF, storage conditions need to be optimized to take full advantage of this effect. For example, the optimum pH of the aFGF–heparin solution needs to be determined for maximum long-term stability and solubility. Acidification of aFGF solution below pH 4 leads to the partial unfolding of the protein as monitored by fluorescence spectroscopy (Copeland *et al.*, 1991). Although the addition of heparin inhibits the rate and extent of this pH induced conformational change, irreversible aggregation of the protein still occurs at low pH over time (Tsai *et al.*, 1993; Pineda-Lucena *et al.*, 1994). When aFGF–heparin solutions at various pH values are subjected to accelerated stability testing such as the turbidity assay described above, aFGF appears to be most stable at neutral-to-alkaline pH values (Fig. 9). However, alkaline pH accelerates certain chemical degradation processes such as cysteine oxidation and asparagine deamidation (next section). Therefore, selection of the optimum pH value for a formulation of aFGF is a balance between the conformational and chemical stability of the growth factor. Topical formulations for wound healing were therefore prepared at pH 7.0 to both maximize physicochemical stability of the protein and to minimize any pain from applying nonphysiological pH solutions to a wound site. The concentration of buffer salts also effects the stability of aFGF as determined by thermal unfolding experiments. For

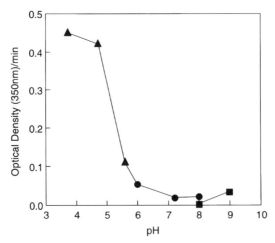

Figure 9. pH dependence of the heat-induced aggregation of aFGF in the presence of 0.33X heparin by weight at 55°C. Experiments were performed with 0.1 mg/ml protein in a citrate (triangles), phosphate (circles), or borate buffer (squares) containing 120 mM sodium chloride. Experimental details in Tsai *et al.* (1993) courtesy of Plenum Publishing.

example, as the concentration of sodium phosphate buffer is increased from 0.6 to 6.0 to 100 mM, the T_m of unliganded protein increased from 39 to 47 to 56°C, respectively, as measured by circular dichroism (Chavan *et al.*, 1994). Similarly, high concentrations of commonly used nonspecific agents such as sugars and amino acids (~1 M) increases the thermal unfolding temperature of polyanion-stabilized aFGF by an additional 6–12°C (Tsai *et al.*, 1993). However, the stabilizing effect of high concentrations of buffer salts and nonspecific agents must be balanced against the requirement of solution isotonicity for application to wound sites.

4.1.2. OXIDATION OF CYSTEINE RESIDUES

Human aFGF contains three cysteine residues (Cys-16, -83, -117). Two of these residues (Cys-16, -83) are highly conserved in the FGF family while Cys-117 is unique to human aFGF (Linemeyer *et al.*, 1990). A series of site-directed mutants of aFGF have been prepared in which one, two, or all three of the cysteine residues have been removed. The mutants were compared in terms of relative specific activity in an *in vitro* mitogenic assay and relative stability by prolonged incubation at 37°C prior to examining the mitogenic activity. The wild type and all three single mutants (Ser-16, -83, -117) are equally active in the presence of heparin. In the absence of heparin, however, the Ser-117 mutant is three times more active than the wild-type protein. The activity of the Ser-117 mutant is therefore less heparin dependent compared to wild-type protein (a 7-fold versus a 20-fold enhancement of mitogenic activity). Similarly, Ser-117 aFGF is more stable than the wild-type protein or any of the other single-mutant proteins (with a mitogenic activity half-life of 1.4 and 240 hr at 37°C in the absence and presence of heparin, respectively, compared to 0.08–0.62 and 12–26 hr for the other proteins under the same conditions; Ortega *et al.*, 1991). The triple mutant (Ser-16, -83, -117) was the most active and stable of the constructs with approximately 2.5 and 20 times the activity as well as 9 and 280 times more stable than wild-type protein in the presence and absence of heparin, respectively. From these experiments it can be concluded that none of the cysteine residues are absolutely required for biological activity and that Cys-117 appears to be chemically more sensitive than the other two thiolate residues.

Human aFGF (wild-type and certain single Cys to Ser mutants) can form either intra- and intermolecular disulfide bonds after oxidation by copper ions (Linemeyer *et al.*, 1990; Engleka and Maciag, 1992). The effect of intramolecular disulfide bond formation on the mitogenic activity of the Ser-117 mutant of aFGF is shown in Fig. 10. It can be seen that oxidation leads to the inactivation of aFGF which can be reversed by the addition of reducing agents such as dithiothreitol. Similar results have been observed for copper-induced intermolecular dimer formation with wildtype aFGF. Thus, oxidation of the reduced cysteine residues of aFGF leads to inactivation of the growth factor and therefore care must be taken when formulating the protein to protect these labile groups.

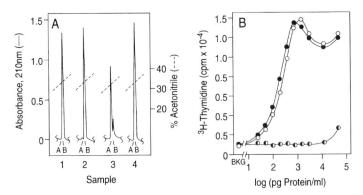

Figure 10. Reversible inactivation of a Cys → Ser-117 mutant aFGF by oxidation of cysteine residues to intramolecular disulfide bonds. (A) Separation of copper-ion-induced oxidized protein (A) from native protein (B) by reverse-phase HPLC. Sample 1 is untreated protein, sample 2 is air-oxidized protein, sample 3 is copper-oxidized protein, and sample 4 is copper-oxidized protein reduced with dithiothreitol. (B) Ability of aFGF to stimulate DNA synthesis in Balb/c 3T3 fibroblast cells as measured by incorporation of tritiated thymidine. Open symbol is native protein, half closed symbol is oxidized protein, and solid symbol is oxidized protein treated with the reducing agent dithiothreitol. Experimental details in Linemeyer *et al.* (1990) courtesy of Harwood Academic Publishers.

4.1.3. DEAMIDATION OF ASPARAGINE RESIDUES

The spontaneous, nonenzymatic deamidation of asparagine residues is one of the most frequently observed *in vitro* covalent modifications of protein molecules. Many papers have recently appeared describing examples of deamidation reactions occurring during either the isolation or storage of proteins (for review, see Clarke, 1992). The deamidation of aFGF can be induced by prolonged storage under accelerated conditions of temperature and pH. Ammonia evolution, a by-product of the deamidation reaction in which an Asn is converted to an Asp residue via a cyclic imide intermediate, can be used as a measure the deamidation reaction. The time course of ammonia release can be determined either by calculation from IEF gels or measured directly enzymatically (Volkin *et al.*, 1995). Figure 11, the average of three independent experiments, shows the kinetics of the deamidation reaction in polyanion-stabilized aFGF during prolonged storage. It can be estimated from these data that native, nondeamidated aFGF (complexed with heparin) has a half-life of 16 weeks at pH 7, 30°C and 4 weeks at pH 8, 40°C. These initial deamidation events have no significant effect on the protein's overall conformation, thermal stability, and interaction with heparin as determined by a combination of CD and fluorescence spectroscopy as well as affinity chromatography. In addition, deamidation of aFGF has no effect on the biological activity of the growth factor as evaluated by an *in vitro* mitogenic assay (Volkin *et al.*, 1995).

N-terminal protein sequencing of the first 21 amino acid residues of aFGF has

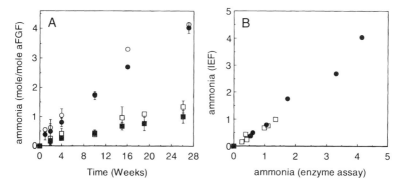

Figure 11. (A) Time course of deamidation of asparagine residues in aFGF as measured by the evolution of ammonia monitored by urea-IEF (closed symbols) and an enzymatic ammonia assay (open symbols). Samples were incubated at pH 7, 30°C (squares) and pH 8, 40°C (circles). (B) Correlation of ammonia evolution as measured by urea-IEF and ammonia assay at pH 7, 30°C (open squares) and pH 8, 40°C (closed circles). Experimental details in Volkin *et al.* (1995) courtesy of American Chemical Society.

identified one of the deamidation sites (Asn_8-Tyr_9) in a flexible, peptide-like region of the protein. In fact, the N-terminus region cannot be seen in the crystal structure of the FGFs, presumably due to high mobility (Zhu *et al.*, 1991; Eriksson *et al.*, 1991; Zhang *et al.*, 1991). Although the Asn-Tyr sequence is not an intrinsically labile deamidation sequence, increased flexibility is known to enhance the ability of the deamidation reaction to proceed in several other proteins (Clarke, 1992). Interestingly, an Asn_3-Leu_4 site did not deamidate under these storage conditions. In addition, the notoriously labile Asn-Gly sequence at position 19 did not undergo significant deamidation. This suggests no simple correlation exists between local amino acid sequence, conformational flexibility, and deamidation potential. The Asn_{19} residue is known from aFGF X-ray crystallography to be involved in the binding of the heparin analogue, sucrose octasulfate. Therefore, the labile Asn_{19}-Gly_{20} deamidation sequence may be protected from deamidation either sterically or by the conformational rigidity induced by the binding of aFGF to heparin.

4.2. Delivery of aFGF as a Topical Agent

The formulation of aFGF as a wound-healing agent requires considerations beyond maintaining physicochemical and biological activity during storage. Foremost, biologically active growth factor must be easily applied to the wound site in a clinical setting and successfully delivered to and maintained at the desired region of tissue. Application of the growth factor to skin can best be accomplished if the formulation produces a drop that does not bead and run off the site. To prevent run-off, a viscous preparation was considered appropriate provided it (1) does not interfere with bioactivity of the protein, (2) can withstand freezing at $-70°C$ without loss of viscous properties, (3) is compatible with buffer components, (4) retains bioactivity of the protein after drying on the treatment area, (5) does not interfere with bioanalytical capabilities, and (6) can withstand sterilization. A solution of hydroxyethyl cellulose (HEC) was found to meet all of these requirements while solutions containing a variety of other polymers such as xanthan gum and hydroxypropyl cellulose failed one or more of these criteria.

4.2.1. RELEASE AND BIOANALYTICAL CAPABILITIES

The release of aFGF from a 1% HEC solution was followed by measuring the rate of exchange of the protein from the viscous solution using a diffusion cell equilibrated at $32°C$ (Matuszewska *et al.*, 1994). A solution containing aFGF, heparin, and 1% HEC was spread on a polycarbonate membrane with a 0.4-micron pore diameter and the amount of protein passing through to the receptor side over time was measured. Approximately 98% of the aFGF but only 7% of the HEC passed through the membrane in 24 hr. This simple experiment demonstrates that aFGF can be released from the viscous solution in a controlled fashion over 24 hr and that there is minimal interaction between aFGF and the polymer. In addition, when this HEC formulation of aFGF with heparin was air-dried and then reconstituted with buffer, full recovery of mitogenic activity was achieved.

A critical aspect to the design of any protein formulation is the ability to retain bioanalytical capabilities including the determination of protein concentration and bioactivity. In addition, stability-indicating assays must be performed without interference from the formulation excipients. Although viscous in nature, a 1% HEC solution containing aFGF is optically clear, thus permitting spectroscopic analyses of the protein such as UV, fluorescence, and circular dichroism spectroscopies. In fact, it can be demonstrated by these techniques that aFGF maintains its native, folded conformation after formulation and that the presence of HEC does not affect the thermal unfolding temperature (T_m) of the protein. The addition of HEC to an aqueous solution of aFGF does not interfere with the mitogenic assay for aFGF bioactivity (*in vitro* stimulation of mitosis by BALB/c mouse fibroblast cells as measured by the uptake of tritiated thymidine) or the determination of the concentration of solution excipients such as heparin or the pH of the solution.

Determination of the concentration of aFGF in a viscous formulation containing stabilizing polyanions such as heparin required the development of a novel size-exclusion HPLC assay. Protein mass in a viscous (or nonviscous) formulation was quantitated using a Toso Haas G-3000 SWXL column with a 0.1 M phosphate buffer (pH 6.8) containing 0.5 M cesium chloride as a mobile phase. Cesium chloride was required to dissociate protein–ligand complexes and to reduce nonspecific interaction between the protein and the column matrix. This assay method had appropriate linearity, recovery, specificity, and reproducibility to determine the concentration of aFGF in a viscous 1% HEC solution and has been utilized in numerous stability studies (Bruner *et al.*, manuscript in preparation).

Stability-indicating assays must be developed to monitor the storage stability of formulated protein. Based on the physicochemical stability studies described above, several potential mechanisms of aFGF inactivation have been identified: conformational instability causing partial unfolding and/or aggregation, oxidation of the protein's three cysteine residues, and deamidation of asparagine residues. The challenges involved in identifying and developing stability-indicating assays for formulated aFGF include a low protein concentration (low dose formulations of 50 μg/ml are potentially employed), the presence of stabilizing polyanions, and the high viscosity of the solutions. Despite these difficulties, the following methodologies can be utilized to follow the accumulation of degradants during storage: SEC-HPLC to determine monomeric protein and soluble aggregates; fluorescence and UV spectroscopy to monitor formulations for partially unfolded protein and larger insoluble aggregates, respectively; SDS-PAGE to detect oxidized protein and any potential hydrolysis by-products; and urea-IEF to identify and quantify deamidation of asparagine residues as well as any other chemical modifications altering the overall charge of the protein. In addition, high-resolution checks of chemical integrity of formulated protein such as peptide mapping and matrix-assisted laser desorption time-of-flight mass spectroscopy appear to be promising approaches.

Despite extensive use of these sophisticated bioanalytical techniques to monitor the conformational and chemical stability of aFGF, a requirement to monitor the biological activity of the growth factor over time still remains since one can never rigorously exclude the possibility of a subtle, undetected change that might perturb the protein's activity. The mitogenic activity of aFGF is quantitated with a 6-day *in vitro* bioassay which measures the ability to stimulate DNA synthesis in the BALB/c 3T3 fibroblast cell line. The interaction of aFGF with its specific high-affinity receptor leads to a mitogenic signal through a series of still poorly defined molecular and cellular events which cause DNA synthesis and ultimately cell division. DNA synthesis is measured by incorporation of tritiated thymidine into the DNA of the stimulated cells which has been shown to correlate with cell division (Linemeyer *et al.*, 1990 and references therein). The concentration of aFGF required to achieve one-half the maximal response is designated the IC_{50} value. Test samples of aFGF are always compared to an internal aFGF reference standard whose IC_{50} value is defined as 4.2×10^6 units/mg (1 unit/ml = 100 pg/ml aFGF). Due to weekly variations in cell culture conditions and the difficulty in defining accurately the maximal and half-maximal activity in the dose response curve (on a log scale), the inter- and intra-day assay variability was determined to be about 20%. Validation tests show that a loss of about 25–50% of the protein mass is required before losses detected in the mitogenic assay are statistically significant. Nevertheless, based on experimental stability data collected over several years, detectable losses in the mitogenic activity of formulated aFGF almost always correlates with a loss in monomeric protein. Consideration of the conformational and chemical instability features of aFGF, described in detail above, argues that such a correlation is expected.

4.2.2. ACCELERATED AND REAL TIME STABILITY

By combining considerations of aFGF's physicochemical stability with the need for proper delivery of the growth factor at a wound site, several candidate topical formulations were designed, prepared, and stability-tested. Various concentrations of aFGF were combined with a stabilizing polyanionic ligand in a phosphate-buffered saline solution (pH 7.0) containing 1% hydroxyethyl cellulose (HEC). As shown in Table III (Part I), formulations containing 50 μg/ml aFGF and 3X heparin by weight are stable for at least 1 year at 5°C as measured by SEC-HPLC (% protein mass) and mitogenic activity (bioassay). When the same formulation is stored at accelerated temperatures such as 30°C, aFGF undergoes complete inactivation within 2 to 4 months. One approach to potentially enhance the storage stability of polyanion-stabilized aFGF is to add the chelating agent EDTA. This reagent has been shown to inhibit the aggregation of aFGF at high temperatures as judged by the turbidity assay, presumably by chelating trace metal ions involved in the autooxidation of aFGF's three cysteine residues (Volkin *et al.*, 1993; Tsai *et al.*, 1993). When 0.15 mM EDTA is added to the formulation (see Table III, Part II), equivalent storage stability is observed at 5°C with no significant loss in protein mass or bioactivity after one year. Greatly enhanced storage stability, however, is seen at higher temperatures (30°C) with over 70% of the protein mass remaining after 1 year. The effect of different stabilizing polyanions is also shown in Table III (Part III). Formulations of aFGF containing chemically well-defined polyanions such as sulfated β-cyclodextrin and sucrose octasulfate show equivalent stability to that recorded with heparin-containing formulations.

Degraded samples of formulated aFGF, as determined by loss of protein mass (SEC-HPLC) and bioactivity (mitogenic assay), were analyzed by the stability-indicating assays described above. Typically, UV spectroscopy revealed aggregated protein as determined by the increase in the light-scattering component of the spectrum while fluorescence spectroscopy showed the accumulation of some partially unfolded protein. SDS-PAGE analysis detected the accumulation of covalent dimers and higher-molecular-weight oligomers as compared to a suitability standard (a reference lot of aFGF ± copper-induced oxidation of cysteine residues). In addition, small amounts of deamidation were observed by IEF compared to another suitability standard (aFGF incubated for 6 months at 30°C, pH 7). As described above, however, the initial deamidation events do not result in a loss of biological activity. Based on these preliminary data, the predominant causes of aFGF inactivation during real-time storage in viscous formulations appear to be the same as those described earlier in the chapter for the unformulated protein: conformational instability and disulfide mediated oligomerization.

Table III. Storage Stability of aFGF in Viscous Formulations[a]

	Months	Mitogenic activity (units/mg $\times 10^6$)	% Initial protein mass (SEC-HPLC)
I. aFGF + 3X heparin			
at 5°C	0	3.2	100
	3	3.4	100
	6	2.5	98
	12	3.4	100
at 30°C	0	3.2	100
	1	2.0	N.P.
	2	0.3	56
	4	N.P.	0
II. aFGF + 3X heparin + 0.15 mM EDTA			
at 5°C	0	4.7	100
	3	4.2	110
	6	3.5	101
	12	2.6	99
at 30°C	0	4.7	100
	3	3.6	97
	6	2.6	83
	12	1.8	70
III. aFGF + 3X ligand + 0.15 mM EDTA at 5°C			
Sulfated β-cyclodextrin	0	3.4	100
	7	N.P.	100
	13	4.6	99
Dextran sulfate	0	2.9	100
	7	N.P.	98
	13	3.6	90
Pentosan polysulfate	0	3.2	100
	7	N.P.	102
	13	3.8	89
Sucrose octasulfate	0	3.1	100
	7	N.P.	101
	13	3.8	102
Heparin	0	3.2	100
	7	N.P.	103
	13	3.5	104

[a]Samples contained 50 μg/ml protein and 1% HEC in a phosphate-buffered saline solution (pH 7.0) plus the indicated polyanionic stablizer by weight. N.P., not performed.

Containers of different compositions and processed by different sterilization techniques were utilized at different times in the development of the formulation. In general, at high protein concentrations (see below), the container type did not have a significant influence on aFGF stability. The sterilization method could potentially, however, be an important consideration. Preliminary data suggest that γ-irradiation sterilization of certain types of plastic resins (prior to the addition of sterile filtered aFGF formulations) may have a detrimental effect on aFGF during long-term storage at 5°C.

Stability studies similar to those described in Table III were carried out with higher concentrations of aFGF (stabilized with heparin) such as 250, 500, and 800 μg/ml protein (data not shown). Some of these viscous aFGF formulations are stable during storage at 5°C for up to 36 months. In general, higher concentrations of protein (250–800 μg/ml) were observed to be more stable than the low dose formulations (50 μg/ml). Experiments were carried out to determine the effect of low protein concentration on the stability of aFGF in various containers (Burke *et al.*, 1992). Protein solutions containing 1–20 μg/ml aFGF were incubated overnight in eight different containers (untreated glass, siliconized glass, sulfur-treated glass, Purcoat glass, polyester, polypropylene, and nylon). Protein adsorption to the container surface was observed at concentrations below 10 μg/ml. For example, adsorptive losses at 1 μg/ml aFGF in the various containers were in the range of 20–40% or 0.2–0.8 μg protein/cm^2 container.

4.2.3. POTENTIAL FOR A LYOPHILIZED FORMULATION

During the development of clinical formulations of aFGF, the effect of lyophilization on the storage stability of aFGF was examined in hopes of developing a room-temperature stable product. Several approaches were undertaken to develop a freeze-dried formulation of aFGF both in the presence and absence of the viscosity enhancing agent HEC (Bondi *et al.*, 1992). When a phosphate-buffered saline (PBS) solution containing aFGF and heparin (100 μg/ml protein and 33 μg/ml heparin) is lyophilized, the recovery of monomeric protein is poor (<80%) due to extensive aggregation. If a 20-fold diluted PBS solution containing aFGF and heparin (100 μg/ml protein and 33 μg/ml heparin) is freeze-dried, the recovery of monomeric, biologically active protein is much better (>95%) indicating that removal of salt helps to minimize aggregation during drying. However, the room-temperature stability of this formulation is poor with only ~60% of monomeric protein remaining after 3 months. When lyoprotectants such as sucrose are added at 2% by weight to this aFGF–heparin solution (with a PBS buffer adjusted to maintain isotonicity of solution), good recovery and storage stability are obtained with full retention of monomeric protein and mitogenic activity after storage for 1 year at 25°C. Interestingly, when the same lyophilization experiment is repeated with 2% dextrose as the lyoprotectant, full recovery of monomeric protein is observed after 6-months storage at 25°C, but mitogenic activity is completely lost. This is a rare example when loss of aFGF mitogenic activity does not correlate with the amount of monomeric protein in solution. Preliminary analysis of this biologically inactive material showed a significant decrease in the titratable amino groups of aFGF, as measured by colorimetric titration with picrylsulfonic acid (TNBS), suggesting that dextrose (a monosaccharide containing a reducing end) may be forming a Schiff's base adduct with the lysine residues of aFGF (i.e., the Maillard reaction) in the solid state during storage, leading to loss of biological activity. Recently, it has been demonstrated that the *in vitro* incubation of bFGF with various reducing sugars leads to protein glycation with concomitant loss in the growth factor's mitogenic activity (Giardino *et al.*, 1994).

When lyophilization of aFGF–heparin in a PBS solution is performed in the presence of 1% HEC, full recovery of monomeric protein is observed, thereby demonstrating the lyoprotectant properties of the polymer. However, the time required for reconstitution of the viscous aFGF formulation is unacceptably long (>3 hr). Upon addition of 2% sucrose to this mixture, followed by lyophilization, good recovery of both monomeric protein and mitogenic activity is seen with a concomitant reduction of the time required for reconstitution to less than 5 min. This lyophilized formulation, possessing the appropriate viscosity upon reconstitution, had good stability for at least 6 months at 25°C as measured by retention of protein mass (SEC-HPLC) and bioactivity (mitogenic assay). These preliminary experiments demonstrate the feasibility of developing a room-temperature stable, viscous or nonviscous, formulation of aFGF (Bondi *et al.*, 1992). Further studies are required to more fully understand the role of the protein powder's water content and the lyophilization processing parameters on the recovery and storage stability of aFGF formulations containing various stabilizing polyanions.

4.3. *In Vivo* Mouse Model Studies to Support Formulation Development

The db/db diabetic mouse has become a standard impaired healing model to measure the beneficial effect of wound-healing agents such as growth factors. Wounds in the diabetic mouse exhibit significant delay in closure and healing times (Greenhalgh *et al.*, 1990). The ability of aFGF to accelerate wound healing in this model has been recently established (Matuszewska *et al.*, 1994; Mellin *et al.*, 1995). For example, treatment with aFGF after injury shortens the mean time at which 50% of the wounds are completely healed (wound closure) by 30 days, i.e., from 45 to 15 days (Mellin *et al.*, 1995). Moreover, dose titration studies with aFGF have identified optimal acceleration of wound healing at a dose of 3.0 μg/cm^2 (compared to the corresponding vehicle). Histological examination of the healing sites shows that aFGF induces a three- to fivefold enhancement of reepithelialization and granulation tissue formation by 10 days after injury compared to the vehicle alone (Mellin *et al.*, 1995).

In vivo evaluation of viscous formulations of aFGF have also been examined in the db/db mouse (Tsai *et al.*, 1993; Matuszewska *et al.*, 1994). Topical formulations containing aFGF stabilized by either heparin, inositol hexasulfate, or sulfated

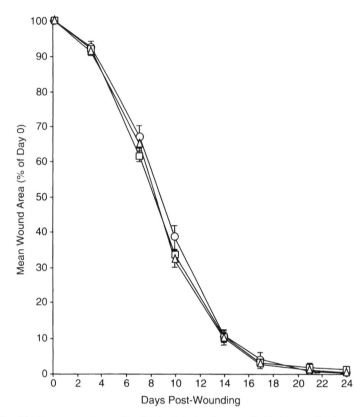

Figure 12.   The time course of wound healing in diabetic mice treated with three applications of 3 µg/cm²
aFGF formulated with heparin (circle), sulfated β-cyclodextrin (square), or inositol hexasulfate (triangle)
in a phosphate-buffered saline solution containing 1% hydroxyethyl cellulose. Values are shown as a
percentage of original wound area (mean ± standard deviation). Experimental details in Tsai *et al.* (1993)
courtesy of Plenum Publishing.

β-cyclodextrin in PBS containing 1% HEC and 0.2 mM EDTA (in the latter two
formulations) were applied to 2 cm² wounds on day 0, 3, and 7 at a concentration of
3 µg/cm². The decrease in the mean wound area for full-thickness wounds treated
with active formulations is shown in Fig. 12. It can be seen that all three formulations
are equivalent in their ability to accelerate wound healing. Comparisons of these
three aFGF formulations to their corresponding placebos showed statistically significant differences in the time required for 70% and 90% healing (Tsai *et al.*, 1993).
Thus, lower-molecular-weight polyanions such as sulfated β-cyclodextrin and inositol hexasulfate may be potential substitutes for heparin in viscous aFGF formulations.

5. CONCLUSIONS

The preformulation and formulation studies with aFGF described in this chapter are of particular interest because of the requirement for a polyanion to enhance the stability and bioactivity of this inherently labile protein. Therefore, in contrast to most protein formulations which primarily require an identification and understanding of the types of artificial formulation excipients that result in optimized storage stability, formulations of aFGF must also include a detailed characterization of the interaction of aFGF with its natural ligand(s) as well as synthetic analogues. These considerations are of critical importance to both the structure, stability, and bioactivity of aFGF. Our approach was to attempt to understand in as much detail as possible the interaction of aFGF with its natural ligand heparin. These studies quantitatively determined the stoichiometry and affinity of this interaction as well as the structural requirements needed for heparin to stabilize aFGF against both conformational and chemical degradation. Based on this understanding, synthetic analogues of heparin were semiempirically identified and evaluated. It was determined that many of these analogues can stabilize aFGF to the same extent as heparin itself. Concomitantly, protein preformulation work was performed to identify the optimum environmental conditions and formulation excipients to both stabilize aFGF–polyanion complexes and deliver them topically to the wound site. This formulation process required an understanding of the causes and mechanisms of aFGF inactivation which were determined to be predominantly conformational instability leading to aggregation and the oligomerization of the protein due at least partially to oxidation of aFGF's cysteine residues. This approach may have general utility for the formulation of heparin binding growth factors since a similar successful formulation strategy has been recently described for keratinocyte growth factor (Chen *et al.*, 1994). Critical differences will be found for each growth factor, however, as described for bFGF in another chapter in this volume.

Although formulation development of protein pharmaceuticals must emphasize the physicochemical properties and *in vitro* stability of a protein, the effects of formulation on the safety and *in vivo* efficacy of a drug are of utmost importance. In the case of aFGF, the type of polyanion used to stabilize the protein has the potential to affect the biological activity since the *in vitro* mitogenic activity of aFGF is potentiated 20-fold by heparin. We showed that a variety of well-defined polyanions also potentiate the mitogenic activity of aFGF as well as maintain its ability to accelerate *in vivo* wound healing as measured in a diabetic mouse model. Note that this does not directly imply the involvement of such artificial polyanions in the formation of biologically active aFGF/receptor/polyanion ternary complexes since the growth factors may rapidly exchange onto natural polyanionic substrates *in situ*. Nonetheless, the safety profile and current regulatory status of each potential stabilizing polyanion must be considered in addition to the above considerations before the final formulation choice can be made.

Preparation of topical formulations of aFGF for use as a wound-healing agent required a balance between physicochemical properties of the growth factor to ensure storage stability and delivery of the growth factor to the wound site. Second-generation formulations could be developed to enhance both the stability and delivery of aFGF. Site-directed mutants of aFGF have been identified with enhanced stability and/or activity. For example, the replacement of certain cysteine residues in aFGF with serine (Linemeyer *et al.*, 1990; Ortega *et al.*, 1991) as well as a particular surface exposed histidine residue with alanine (Arakawa *et al.*, 1993) have been described. Alternative delivery vehicles could be developed if, for example, the controlled release of the growth factor or incorporation of aFGF into standard wound dressings or plaster of Paris enhanced the efficacy of the drug (Rosenblum *et al.*, 1993; Finetti and Farina, 1992). Several preliminary studies have been undertaken with FGFs to explore the use of alternative delivery vehicles such as microspheres (Edelman *et al.*, 1991), hydrogels (Tefft *et al.*, 1992), and collagen-based matrices (Marks *et al.*, 1991; McPherson, 1992). An optimal topical wound-healing formulation will probably ultimately be a form of combination therapy containing multiple growth factors and perhaps other chemotactic agents, each physiochemically stabilized and delivered in a controlled manner at the site of injury. This idealized formulation would deliver the optimum amount of each one of the required growth mediators in a predetermined temporal and spatial sequence to maximize the complex wound-healing process at the site of injury. A more complete understanding of the molecular and cellular biology of the normal wound-healing process as well as further developments in formulation and delivery technology for protein drugs will be required to make this optimized therapy for wounds a medical reality.

REFERENCES

Ago, H., Kitagawa, Y., Fujishima, A., Matsuura, Y., and Katsube, Y., 1991, Crystal structure of basic fibroblast growth factor at 1.6 A resolution, *J. Biochem.* **110**:360–363.

Ahern, T. J., and Manning, M. C. (eds.), 1992, *Stability of Protein Pharmaceuticals. Part A. Chemical and Physical Pathways of Protein Degradation*, Plenum Press, New York.

Arakawa, T., Horan, T. P., Narhi, L. O., Rees, D. C., Schiffer, S. G., Holst, P. L., Prestrelski, S. J., Tsai, L. B., and Fox, G. M., 1993, Production and characterization of an analog of acidic fibroblast growth factor with enhanced stability and biological activity, *Protein Eng.* **6**:541–546.

Aviezer, D., Levy, E., Safran, M., Svahn, C., Buddecke, E., Schmidt, A., David, G., Vlodavsky, I., and Yayon, A., 1994, Differential structural requirements of heparin and heparan sulfate proteoglycans that promote binding of basic fibroblast growth factor to its receptor, *J. Biol. Chem.* **269**:114–121.

Bondi, J., Henley, M. W., and Matuszewska, B., 1992, Lyophilized acidic fibroblast growth factor, European Patent Application 92309544.2.

Burgess, W. H., 1991, Structure-function studies of acidic fibroblast growth factor, *Ann. N.Y. Acad. Sci.* **638**:89–97.

Burgess, W. H., and Macaig, T., 1989, The heparin-binding (fibroblast) growth factor family of proteins, *Ann. Rev. Biochem.* **58**:575–606.

Burgess, W. H., Shaheen, A. M., Hampton, B., Donohue, P. J., and Winkles, J. A., 1991, Structure-function studies of heparin-binding (acidic fibroblast) growth factor-1 using site-directed mutagenesis, *J. Cell. Biochem.* **45:**131–138.

Burke, C. J., Steadman, B. L., Volkin, D. B., Tsai, P. K., Bruner, M. W., and Middaugh, C. R., 1992, The adsorption of proteins to container surfaces, *Int. J. Pharm.* **86:**89–93.

Burke, C. J., Volkin, D. B., Mach, H., and Middaugh, C. R., 1993, Effect of polyanions on the unfolding of acidic fibroblast growth factor, *Biochemistry* **32:**6419–6426.

Castellot, Jr., J. J., Choay, J. Lormeau, J. C., Petitou, M., Sache, E., and Karnovsky, M. J., 1986, Structural determinants of the capacity of heparin to inhibit the proliferation of vascular smooth muscles. II. Evidence for a pentasaccharide sequence that contains a 3-*O*-sulfate group, *J. Cell Biol.* **102:**1979–1984.

Chavan, A. J., Haley, B. E., Volkin, D. B., Marfia, K. E., Verticelli, A. M., Bruner, M. W., Draper, J. P., Burke, C. J., and Middaugh, C. R., 1994, Interactions of nucleotides with acidic fibroblast growth factor (FGF-1), *Biochemistry* **33:**7193–7202.

Chen, B.-L., Arakawa, T., Morris, C. F., Kenney, W. C., Wells, C. M., and Pitt, C. G., 1994, Aggregation pathway of recombinant human keratinocyte growth factor and its stabilization, *Pharm. Res.* **11:**1581–1587.

Clarke, S., Stephenson, R. C., and Lowenson, J. D., 1992, Lability of asparagine and aspartic acid residues in proteins and peptides, in: *Stability of Protein Pharmaceuticals. Part A. Chemical and Physical Pathways of Protein Degradation* (T. J. Ahern and M. C. Manning, eds.), Plenum Press, New York, pp. 1–29.

Cleland, J. and Langer, R. (Eds.), 1994, *Formulation and Delivery of Proteins and Peptides*, American Chemical Society, Washington, DC.

Copeland, R. A., Ji, H., Halfpenny, A. J., Williams, R. W., Thompson, K. C., Herber, W. K., Thomas, K. A., Bruner, M. W., Ryan, J. A., Marquis-Omer, D., Sanyal, G., Sitrin, R. D., Yamazaki, S., and Middaugh, C. R., 1991, The structure of human acidic fibroblast growth factor and its interaction with heparin, *Arch. Biochem. Biophys.* **289:**53–61.

Dabora, J. M., Sanyal, G., and Middaugh, C. R., 1991, Effects of polyanions on the refolding of human acidic fibroblast growth factor, *J. Biol. Chem.* **266:**23637–23640.

Edelman, E. R., Mathiowitz, E., Langer, R., and Klagsbrun, M., 1991, Controlled and modulated release of basic fibroblast growth factor, *Biomaterials* **12:**619–626.

Engleka, K. A., and Maciag, T., 1992, Inactivation of human fibroblast growth factor-1 (FGF-1) activity by interaction with copper ions involves FGF-1 dimer formation induced by copper-catalyzed oxidation, *J. Biol. Chem.* **267:**11307–11315.

Eriksson, A. E., Cousens, L. S., and Matthews, B. W., 1993, Refinement of the structure of human basic fibroblast growth factor at 1.6 Å resolution and analysis of presumed heparin binding sites by selenate substitution, *Protein Sci.* **2:**1274–1284.

Eriksson, A. E., Cousens, L. S., Weaver, L. H., and Matthews, B. W., 1991, Three-dimensional structure of human basic fibroblast growth factor, *Proc. Natl. Acad. Sci. USA* **88:**3441–3445.

Finetti, G., and Farina, M., 1992, Recombinant human basic fibroblast growth factor: different medical dressings for clinical application in wound healing, *IL Farmaco* **47:**967–978.

Folkman, J., Szabo, S., Strovroff, M., McNeil, P., Li, W., and Shing, Y., 1991, Duodenal ulcer. Discovery of a new mechanism and development of angiogenic therapy that accelerates healing, *Ann. Surg.* **214:**414–427.

Giardino, I., Edelstein, D., and Brownlee, M., 1994, Nonenzymatic glycosylation *in vitro* and in bovine endothelial cells alters basic fibroblast growth factor activity: A model for intracellular glycosylation in diabetes, *J. Clin. Invest.* **94:**110–117.

Greenhalgh, D. G., Strugel, K. H., Murray, M. J., and Ross, R., 1990, PDGF and FGF stimulate wound healing in the genetically diabetic mouse, *Am. J. Pathol.* **163:**1235–1246.

Harper, J. W., and Lobb, Roy R., 1988, Reductive methylation of lysine residues in acidic fibroblast growth factor: Effect on mitogenic activity and heparin affinity, *Biochemistry* **27:**671–678.

Jans, D. A., 1994, Nuclear signaling pathways for polypeptide ligands and their membrane receptors?, *FASEB J.* **8:**841–847.

Kan, M., Wang, F., Xu, J., Crabb, J. W., Hon, J., and McKeehan, W. L., 1993, An essential heparin-binding domain in the fibroblast growth factor receptor kinase, *Science* **259:**1918–1921.

Li, L.-Y., Safran, M., Aviezer, D., Böhlen, P., Seddon, A. P., and Yayon, A., 1994, Diminished heparin binding of a basic fibroblast growth factor mutant is associated with reduced receptor binding, mitogenesis, plasminogen activator induction, and *in vitro* angiogenesis, *Biochemistry* **33:**10999–11007.

Linemeyer, D. L., Menke, J. G., Kelly, L. J., DiSalvo, J., Soderman, D., Schaeffer, M.-T., Ortega, S., Giménez-Gallego, G., and Thomas, K. A., 1990, Disulfide bonds are neither required, present, nor compatible with full activity of human recombinant acidic fibroblast growth factor, *Growth Factors* **3:**287–298.

Linhardt, R. J., 1991, Heparin: an important drug enters its seventh decade, *Chem. Ind.* **21:**45–50.

Mach, H., Burke, C. J., Volkin, D. B., Dabora, J. M., Sanyal, G., and Middaugh, C. R., 1992, Effect of polyanions on the folding and unfolding of acidic fibroblast growth factor, in: *Harnessing Biotechnology for the 21st Century* (M.R. Ladish and A. Bose, eds.), American Chemical Society, Washington, DC, pp. 290–293.

Mach, H., and Middaugh, C. R., 1994, Probing protein-ligand affinity by unfolding kinetics: Interaction of acidic fibroblast growth factor with polyanions, *Arch. Biochem. Biophys.* **309:**36–42.

Mach, H., and Middaugh, C. R., 1995, Interaction of partially unfolded states of acidic fibroblast growth factor with phospholipid membranes, *Biochemistry*, in press.

Mach, H., Ryan, J. A., Burke, C. J., Volkin, D. B., and Middaugh, C. R., 1993b, Partially structured self-associating states of acidic fibroblast growth factor, *Biochemistry* **32:**7703–7711.

Mach, H., Volkin, D. B., Burke, C. J., Middaugh, C. R., Linhardt, R. J., Fromm, J. R., Loganathan, D., and Mattsson, L., 1993, Nature of the interaction of heparin with acidic fibroblast growth factor, *Biochemistry* **32:**5480–5489.

Marks, M. G., Doillon, C., and Silver, F. H., 1991, Effect of fibroblasts and basic fibroblast growth factor on facilitation of dermal wound healing by type I collagen matrices, *J. Biomed. Mater. Res.* **25:** 683–696.

Matuszewska, B., Keogan, M., Fisher, D. M., Soper, K. A., Hoe, C. M., Huber, A. C., and Bondi, J. V., 1994, Acidic fibroblast growth factor: evaluation of topical formulations in a diabetic mouse wound healing model, *Pharm. Res.* **11:**65–71.

McKeehan, W. L., and Kan, M., 1994, Heparan sulfate fibroblast growth factor receptor complex; structure-function relationships, *Mol. Reprod. Dev.* **39:**69–82.

McPherson, J. M., 1992, The utility of collagen-based vehicles in delivery of growth factors for hard and soft tissue wound repair, *Clin. Mater.* **9:**225–234.

Mellin, T. N., Cashen, D. E., Ronan, J. J., Murphy, B. S., DiSalvo, J., and Thomas, K. A., 1995, Acidic fibroblast growth factor accelerates dermal wound healing in diabetic mice, *J. Invest. Dermatol.* **104:**850–855.

Middaugh, C. R., Mach, H., Burke, C. J., Volkin, D. B., Dabora, J. M., Tsai, P. K., Bruner, M. W., Ryan, J. A., and Marfia, K. E., 1992, Molecular basis of the anti-growth factor activity of suramin, *Biochemistry* **31:**9016–9024.

Middaugh, C. R., Volkin, D. B., and Thomas, K. A., 1993, Acidic and basic fibroblast growth factor, *Curr. Opin. Invest. Drugs* **2:**991–1005.

Nachtmann, F., Atzl, G., and Roth, W. D., 1983, Heparin sodium, in: *Analytical Profiles of Drug Substances*, Vol. 12 (K. Florey, ed.), Academic Press, pp. 215–263.

Ornitz, D. M., Yayon, A., Flanagan, J. G., Svahn, C. M., Levi, E., and Leder, P., 1992, Heparin is required for cell-free binding of basic fibroblast growth factor to a soluble receptor and for mitogenesis in whole cells, *Mol. Cell. Biol.* **12:**240–247.

Ortega, S., Schaeffer, M.-T., Soderman, D., DiSalvo, J., Linemeyer, D. L., Giménez-Gallego, G., and Thomas, K. A., 1991, Conversion of cysteine to serine residues alters the activity, stability, and heparin dependence of acidic fibroblast growth factor, *J. Biol. Chem.* **266:**5842–5846.

Pantoliano, M. W., Horlick, R. A., Springer, B. A., Van Dyk, D. E., Tobery, T., Wetmore, D. R., Lear, J. D., Nahapetian, A. T., Bradley, J. D., and Sisk, W. P., 1994, Multivalent ligand-receptor binding interactions in the fibroblast growth factor system produce a cooperative growth factor and heparin mechanism for receptor dimerization, *Biochemistry* **33**:10229–10248.

Pineda-Lucena, A., Jiménez, M. A., Nieto, J. L., Santoro, J., Rico, M., and Giménez-Gallego, G., 1994, ^{1}H-NMR assignment and solution structure of human acidic fibroblast growth factor activated by inositol hexasulfate, *J. Mol. Biol.* **242**:81–98.

Pineda-Lucena, A., Núñez De Castro, I., Lozano, R. M., Muñoz-Willery, I., Zazo, M., and Giménez-Gallego, G., 1994, Effect of low pH and heparin on the structure of acidic fibroblast growth factor, *Eur. J. Biochem.* **222**:425–431.

Rosenblum, S. F., Frenkel, S., Ricci, J. R., and Alexander, H., 1993, Diffusion of fibroblast growth factor from a plaster of paris carrier, *J. Appl. Biomater.* **4**:67–72.

Tefft, J., Roskos, K. V., and Heller, J., 1992, Development of hydrogel containing stabilized basic fibroblast growth factors for wound treatment, Proc. Int. Symp. Control. Rel. Bioact. Mater. **19**:371–372.

Thompson, L. D., Pantoliano, M. W., and Springer, B. A., 1994, Energetic characterization of the basic fibroblast growth factor-heparin interaction: Identification of the heparin binding domain, *Biochemistry* **33**:3831–3840.

Tsai, P. K., Volkin, D. B., Dabora, J. M., Thompson, K. C., Bruner, M. W., Gress, J. O., Matuszewska, B., Keogan, M., Bondi, J. V., and Middaugh, C. R., 1993, Formulation design of an acidic fibroblast growth factor, *Pharm. Res.* **10**:649–659.

Volkin, D. B., and Klibanov, A. M., 1989, Minimizing protein inactivation, in: *Protein Function: A Practical Approach* (T.E. Creighton, ed.), Oxford Press, Oxford, England, pp. 1–24.

Volkin, D. B., and Middaugh, C. R., 1992, The effect of temperature on protein structure, in: *Stability of Protein Pharmaceuticals. Part A. Chemical and Physical Pathways of Protein Degradation* (T. M. Ahern and M. C. Manning, eds.), Plenum Press, New York, pp. 215–247.

Volkin, D. B., Tsai, P. K., Dabora, J. M., Gress, J. O., Burke, C. J., Linhardt, R. J., and Middaugh, C. R., 1993a, Physical stabilization of acidic fibroblast growth factor by polyanions, *Arch. Biochem. Biophys.* **300**:30–41.

Volkin, D. B., Tsai, P. K., Dabora, J. M., and Middaugh, C. R., 1991, The effect of polyanions on the stabilization of acidic fibroblast growth factor, in: *Harnessing Biotechnology for the 21st Century* (M. R. Ladish and A. Bose, eds.), American Chemical Society, Washington, DC, pp. 298–302.

Volkin, D. B., Verticelli, A. M., Bruner, M. W., Marfia, K. E., Tsai, P. K., Sardana, M. K., and Middaugh, C. R., 1995, Deamidation of polyanion-stabilized acidic fibroblast growth factor, *J. Pharm. Sci.* **84**:7–11.

Volkin, D. B., Verticelli, A. M., Marfia, K. E., Burke, C. J., Mach, H., and Middaugh, C. R., 1993b, Sucralfate and soluble sucrose octasulfate bind and stabilize acidic fibroblast growth factor, *Biochim. Biophys. Acta* **1203**:18–26.

Walker, A., Turnbull, J. E., and Gallagher, J. T., 1994, Specific heparan sulfate saccharides mediate the activity of basic fibroblast growth factor, *Biochemistry* **33**:10229–10248.

Wang, Y. J., and Pearlman, R., 1992, *Stability and Characterization of Protein Drugs: Case Histories I*, Plenum Press, New York.

Wiedlocha, A., Madshus, I. H., Mach, H., Middaugh, C. R., and Olsnes, S., 1992, Tight folding of acidic fibroblast growth factor prevents its translocation to the cytosol with diphtheria toxin as vector, *EMBO J.* **11**:4835–4842.

Wu, J., Yang, J. T., and Wu, C. C. S., 1992, β-II conformation of all β-proteins can be distinguished from unordered structure by circular dichroism, *Anal. Biochem.* **200**:359–364.

Zhang, J., Cousens, L. S., Barr, P. J., and Sprang, S. R., 1991, Three-dimensional structure of human basic fibroblast growth factor, a structural homolog of interleukin 1β, *Proc. Natl. Acad. Sci. USA* **88**:3446–3450.

Zhu, X., 1993, Structure-function studies of fibroblast growth factors (FGFs), Ph.D. thesis, California Institute of Technology, Pasadena, CA.

Zhu, X., Hsu, B. T., and Rees, D. C., 1993, Structural studies of the binding of the anti-ulcer drug sucrose octasulfate to acidic fibroblast growth factor, *Structure* **1**:27–34.

Zhu, X., Komiya, H., Chirino, A., Faham, S., Fox, G. M., Arakawa, T., Hsu, B. T., and Rees, D. C., 1991, Three-dimensional structures of acidic and basic fibroblast growth factors, *Science* **251**:90–93.

4

Stability, Characterization, Formulation, and Delivery System Development for Transforming Growth Factor-Beta₁

Wayne R. Gombotz, Susan C. Pankey,
Lisa S. Bouchard, Duke H. Phan,
and Alan P. MacKenzie

1. INTRODUCTION

1.1. The TGF-β Family of Proteins

During the past decade, research on growth factors and their actions in the regulation of cell growth has played an important role in the development of modern cell biology. Several families of growth factors have been discovered, but none appear to play such a broad multifunctional role as the transforming growth factor-beta (TGF-β) family of proteins. Transforming growth factor-beta₁ (TGF-β₁), one member of the TGF-β family, was first identified by its ability to cause a phenotypic transformation of rat fibroblasts (Roberts *et al.*, 1981). The protein has since been shown to have numerous regulatory actions on both normal and neoplastic cells. Almost all cell types have a specific high-affinity receptor for TGF-β (Massague

Wayne R. Gombotz • Department of Drug Delivery and Formulation, Immunex Corporation, Seattle, Washington 98101. *Susan C. Pankey, Lisa S. Bouchard, and Duke H. Phan* • Pharmaceutical Research Institute, Bristol-Myers Squibb, Seattle, Washington 98101. *Alan P. MacKenzie* • Mercer Island, Washington 98040.

Formulation, Characterization, and Stability of Protein Drugs, Rodney Pearlman and Y. John Wang, eds., Plenum Press, New York, 1996.

et al., 1985; Frolik *et al.*, 1984; Tucker *et al.*, 1984) and many different cells synthesize the protein (Anzano *et al.*, 1985; Roberts *et al.*, 1981). TGF-β is therefore a fundamental regulatory molecule that can elicit its effects by both autocrine and paracrine mechanisms (Sporn *et al.*, 1986).

1.2. *In Vitro* Activities of TGF-β

The biologic activities of TGF-β are variable and depend on the cell type, on the culture conditions, and on the presence of other substances such as other growth factors. The main effects of TGF-β can be described in terms of its regulation of cell growth (activation and adhesion), of cell behavior (adhesion and migration), of cell differentiation, and its effects on the extracellular matrix (Piez and Sporn, 1990).

TGF-β has been shown to stimulate the growth of some fibroblasts as well as some mesenchymal, endothelial, and transformed cells. The original studies involved in the discovery of TGF-β measured its ability to stimulate proliferation of normal rat kidney (NRK) fibroblasts in soft agar (Roberts *et al.*, 1981). TGF-β was then shown to inhibit NRK growth in monolayer cultures by an autocrine mechanism (Roberts *et al.*, 1985; Assoian *et al.*, 1983). Subsequent studies showed that TGF-β exerted inhibitory effects on many cell lines, both neoplastic and nonneoplastic, in both monolayer and soft agar (Moses *et al.*, 1985; Roberts *et al.*, 1985; Tucker *et al.*, 1984). TGF-β is a strong inhibitor of proliferation in many primary and secondary cultures including embryo fibroblasts, hepatocytes, T and B lymphocytes, bronchial epithelial cells, and keratinocytes (Sporn *et al.*, 1986). In cells derived from mesenchymal origin, the stimulation or inhibition of TGF-β depends on the presence or absence of other growth factors (Roberts *et al.*, 1985).

TGF-β also modulates the differentiation of many different cell types. For example, it has been shown to stimulate differentiation of human bronchial epithelial cells (Masui *et al.*, 1986) and intestinal crypt epithelial cells (Kurokawa *et al.*, 1987). In contrast, it inhibits the differentiation of keratinocytes (Reiss and Sartorelli, 1987) and adipocytes (Ignotz and Massague, 1985).

Many *in vitro* studies indicate that the action of TGF-β depends on the presence or absence of a particular cell type or specific molecules in the extracellular matrix. For example, the effects of TGF-β on isolated endothelial cells have been shown to be influenced by the extracellular matrix (Madri *et al.*, 1988). TGF-β has been shown to enhance the accumulation of extracellular matrix components by fibroblasts through (i) the stimulation of the production of collagens, fibronectins, thrombospondin, and tenascin, (ii) an increase in the synthesis of receptors for cell attachment factors, matrix proteoglycans, and glycosaminoglycans and (iii) inhibition of the effects of proteolytic enzymes on matrix proteins (Puolakkainen and Twardzik, 1993).

1.3. *In Vivo* Activities of TGF-β

The TGF-βs have been suggested to play a central role in numerous *in vivo* processes, including embryogenesis, immunoregulation, bone and cartilage remodeling, wound healing, cardiac function, and carcinogenesis. Mesenchymal cell development during embryogenesis has been shown to require TGF-β as evidenced by the high levels of expression in the larynx, cardiac valves, teeth, hair follicle, bones, and cartilage (Heine *et al.*, 1987). TGF-β is a potent supressor of interleukine 1–induced T-lymphocyte proliferation and of antibody production in B cells. It also depresses the cytolytic activity of natural killer cells and inhibits the production of cytotoxic T cells and lymphokine-activated killer cells (Roberts and Sporn, 1990). When TGF-β is administered to mice that have experimentally induced autoimmune diseases, it has been shown to exhibit immunosuppressive properties (Kuruvilla *et al.*, 1991).

The TGF-βs may play an important role in bone growth and remodeling due to its stimulatory effects on the synthesis of matrix components. TGF-β has been shown to stimulate the differentiation of rat muscle mesenchymal cells and their subsequent production of cartilage-specific macromolecules (Seyedin *et al.*, 1986) as well as to stimulate the formation of periosteal bones in rat calvaria (Noda and Camilliere, 1989). Injection of TGF-β has also been shown to initiate or stimulate subperiosteal chondrogenesis and osteogenesis (Joyce *et al.*, 1990), intramedullary woven bone formation (Marcelli *et al.*, 1990), and subperiosteal bone formation (Tanaka *et al.*, 1993; Mackie and Trechsel, 1990; Marcelli *et al.*, 1990).

When TGF-β is injected subcutaneously in mice, it causes the formation of granulation tissue (induction of angiogenesis and activation of fibroblasts to produce collagen) at the site of injection (Roberts *et al.*, 1986). These data suggest that TGF-β may play an important role in soft tissue repair. Although large amounts of TGF-β have been found in cardiac myocytes, its role in normal cardiac function is unknown. It has been shown to exhibit cardioprotective effects in ischemic cardiac injury (Lefer *et al.*, 1990).

TGF-β is known to interact with a variety of other growth factors, including platelet derived growth factor, epidermal growth factor, insulin-like growth factor, and fibroblast growth factor (Nilsen-Hamilton, 1990). Because of these numerous interactions, it has been suggested that the primary role of TGF-β is that of a general mediator of regulation in the cell, and its primary mechanism of action is to modify and regulate the effects of other growth factors.

1.4. Potential Clinical Applications

Because of the multiple actions that the TGF-βs exhibit on many different cell types, they have potential for therapeutic use in several common clinical conditions for which there are currently no adequate pharmacological agents. Descriptions of some of the different types of delivery systems that have been investigated for the administration of TGF-β_1 can be found at the end of this chapter.

Since TGF-β appears to act as a brake of the immune system in order to arrest its excessive proliferation when activated by antigen stimulation, it may have potential as an immunosuppressive agent in patients undergoing organ transplants (Sporn and Roberts, 1989).

The ability of TGF-β to stimulate the formation of granulation tissue suggests that it may have practical applications in the repair of wounds caused by trauma, burns, surgery, or debility in the aged (Sporn *et al.*, 1986). TGF-β has been shown to enhance wound healing in several animal models (Schultz *et al.*, 1992; Jones *et al.*, 1991; Amman *et al.*, 1990; Beck *et al.*, 1990; Mustoe, *et al.*, 1987) and recently it has been tested in humans.

The first human clinical trial involving TGF-β studied the effects of TGF-β_2 on the treatment of macular defects (Smiddy *et al.*, 1993; Glaser *et al.*, 1992). The product known as BetaKine is made by Celtrix Pharmaceuticals. Idiopathic macular holes, which are nontraumatic wounds of the eye, occur in the central region of the retina and cause a severe loss of visual acuity in 70% to 100% of patients. The loss is related to the size of the hole and the surrounding cuff of subretinal fluid. About 10,000 cases of macular holes occur in the United States annually. Preclinical studies in rabbits showed that TGF-β_2 could stimulate the formation of a chorioretinal adhesion when applied to a surgically induced retinal tear (Smiddy *et al.*, 1989). This work provided impetus to look at the ability of TGF-β_2 to heal macular defects in humans. The clinical study showed that a single intraocular application of TGF-β_2 had a statistically significant beneficial effect on resolution of the subretinal fluid cuff surrounding a macular hole when used in conjunction with standard vitrectomy for full-thickness macular holes.

Since the TGF-βs have the ability to induce or enhance bone formation they offer a potential treatment for many clinical indications in which the bony repair process is impaired. These include complications in which there is too much bone loss for the bone to regenerate, such as skeletal deformations caused by trauma, malformation, cancer, or reconstructive surgeries. In addition, the TGF-βs may have potential in the promotion of bone growth into orthopoedic implants.

2. STRUCTURE AND PROPERTIES OF TGF-β_1

2.1. The TGF-β Superfamily

The importance of TGF-β as a fundamental regulatory molecule is emphasized by the fact that its amino acid sequence is identical in man, monkeys, cows, pigs, and chickens (Sporn and Roberts, 1989). TGF-β_1 is a member of a growing superfamily of related dimeric proteins that exists in at least five distinct isoforms (TGF-β₁₋₅). Family members have 66% to 80% amino acid sequence identity and nine strictly conserved cysteines (Daopin *et al.*, 1992; Marquardt *et al.*, 1987). Other proteins in the TGF-β superfamily include inhibins (Mason *et al.*, 1985), activins (Ling *et al.*, 1986), Mullerian inhibitory substances (Cate *et al.*, 1986), and bone morphogenetic proteins (Wozney *et al.*, 1988). The unifying properties of these proteins are their structural similarities and their ability to regulate development and cell differentiation.

2.2. Structure

Mature TGF-β₁ consists of two identical peptide chains, each containing 112 amino acids. The mature homodimeric protein which has a molecular weight of 24 kDa contains a total of nine disulfide bonds, one of which links the monomeric subunits (Assoian *et al.*, 1983). Upon reduction it yields two identical peptides of approximately 12 kDa. The nonreduced homodimer is known to be the biologically active form of the molecule. The primary structure of the monomeric subunit of TGF-β₁ is shown in Fig. 1. Although the crystal structure of TGF-β₁ is not known, it has been determined for TGF-β₂ (Daopin *et al.*, 1992). Since the amino acid sequence of TGF-β₁ shares 71% homology with TGF-β₂ (Seyedin *et al.*, 1987), it is probable that they also share some structural homology. It was determined that TGF-β₂ lacks a well-defined hydrophobic core but displays an unusual elongated nonglobular fold. The fold is approximately 60 Å by 20 Å by 15 Å. Sequence analysis

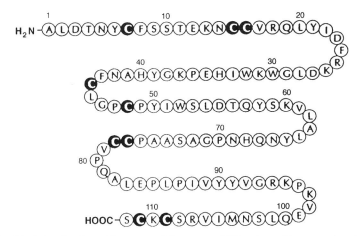

Figure 1. The deduced amino acid sequence of the processed 112-amino-acid monomeric unit of human TGF-β (Puolakkainen and Twardzik, 1993).

of other members of the TGF-β superfamily imply that they also adopt this unique fold. Eight of the cysteines form four intrachain disulfide bonds, which are clustered in a core region. The dimer is stabilized by the ninth cysteine, which forms an interchain disulfide bond and two identical hydrophobic interfaces.

2.3. Latency

It appears that most cell lines and tissues synthesize TGF-β_1 as part of a larger, latent protein complex that is unable to bind to cellular receptors (Miyazono *et al.*, 1988; Pircher *et al.*, 1986). The latent complex fractionates as a 130-kDa species upon size-exclusion chromatography at neutral conditions (Lioubin *et al.*, 1991). Mature active TGF-β_1 is produced only after cleavage. This implies that cells must have a mechanism of activating TGF-β_1 such that active growth factor can become available when and where it is needed. In healing wounds for example, the acidic microenvironment and the production of proteases by activated macrophages could contribute to activation of latent TGF-β. The exact sequence of events in the processing of TGF-β_1 *in vivo* is uncertain but appears to include cleavage of a 29-amino-acid signal sequence, glycosylation, and mannose 6-phosphorylation of the precursor, cleavage of the C-terminal 112-amino-acid monomer (12 kDa) from the 390-amino-acid precursor and disulfide isomerization (Fig. 2) (Gentry *et al.*, 1988; Purchio *et al.*, 1988). It has been hypothesized that cleavage may occur either during or after the translational process concomitant with interchain disulfide bond formation (Sharples *et al.*, 1987). This cleavage is characteristic of all the TGF-β family members (Miller *et al.*, 1990).

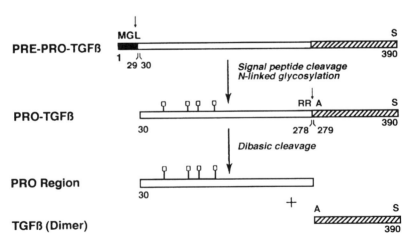

Figure 2. Processing events of TGF-β precursor protein in transfected CHO cells (Puolakkainen and Twardzik, 1993).

The *in vitro* activation of TGF-β_1 can be accomplished by acid treatment (pH <4) (Lawrence *et al.*, 1985), by alkalinization (pH >9), by protease treatment with plasmin or cathepsin D (Lyons *et al.*, 1988; Keski-Oja *et al.*, 1987), or by exposure to denaturing agents such as urea and by γ-interferon (Twardzik *et al.*, 1990; Miyazono *et al.*, 1988; Wakefield *et al.*, 1988).

3. ANALYTICAL CHARACTERIZATION

3.1. Reversed-Phase High-Performance Liquid Chromatography (RP-HPLC)

The integrity of TGF-β_1 can be analyzed by RP-HPLC which can separate TGF-β_1 and its derivatives based on the difference in partitioning between hydrophobic column packing and the relatively hydrophilic mobile phase. This assay is performed on a .46 cm ID × 25 cm Vydac C4 column with a 5-μm particle size packing (Rainnin, Emeryville, CA). The solvents, set at a flow rate of 1.0 ml/min, consist of 0.1% trifluoroacetic acid in water in reservoir A and 0.1% trifluoroacetic acid in acetonitrile in reservoir B. The gradient goes from 28% to 34% solvent B in 35 min, then increases to 90% solvent B over the next 5 min. The flow rate is then increased to 1.5 ml/min and solvent B is decreased to the 28% starting concentration over the next 3 min. Samples are injected in volumes ranging from 20 to 200 μl to obtain protein loads ranging from 15 to 25 μg and detected by absorbance at 214 nm. A typical RP-HPLC chromatogram is shown in Fig. 3. The main peak is flanked on either side by ascending and descending shoulders which are biologically inactive forms of the protein.

3.2. Sodium Dodecylsulfate Polyacrylamide Gel Electrophoresis (SDS-PAGE), Native PAGE, and Western Blot Analysis

SDS-PAGE is commonly used to analyze TGF-β_1 for aggregation and degradation. In a typical assay, samples are electrophoresed in precast 10–20% Tricine, SDS-PAGE gels at a concentration of 2 μg per lane. SDS denatures and binds to the proteins giving them similar shape and net negative charge. When current is applied, the proteins migrate through the gel toward the anode. Separation occurs primarily according to molecular weight. In the presence of SDS, covalent aggregates will stay intact, but noncovalent aggregates may, or may not, dissociate depending on the nature and strength of the bonding between molecules. The addition of a reducing agent, such as 2-mercaptoethanol, can be used to fragment the molecule at the covalent disulfide bond sites. Native PAGE is run without denaturant and surfactant such as SDS. Therefore, protein separation is influenced not only by size but by configuration and inherent net charge, and aggregates stay intact. Figure 4 shows a typical SDS-PAGE (reduced and nonreduced) of TGF-β_1 stained with Coomassie

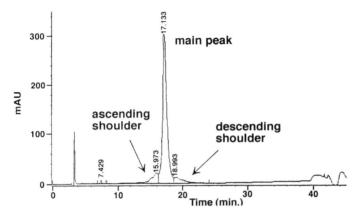

Figure 3. Reversed phase HPLC of TGF-β_1. Some resolution of denatured species, exhibited as ascending and descending shoulders on the main TGF-β_1 peak, is achieved using a Vydac C4 (.46 × 25 cm) column with 5-μm particle size. The mobile phase consists of a gradient achieved over 35 min of 28% to 34% 0.1% trifluoroacetic acid (TFA)/acetonitrile in 0.1% TFA/water at a flow rate of 1 ml/min. Injection volumes range from 20 to 200 μl to deliver 15 to 25 μg of protein detected at 214 nm.

Blue R-250. Mature TGF-β_1 migrates as a single 24-kDa species under non-reducing conditions. Under reducing conditions, a single 12-kDa species is observed which results from the reduction of the disulfide bond that covalently links the two monomeric components of the protein.

Western blot analysis is performed by electrophoresing 2 μg TGF-β_1 then

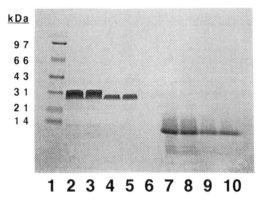

Figure 4. SDS-PAGE of TGF-β_1. TGF-β_1 samples are run on 10–20% Tricine polyacrylamide gels stained with Coomassie Blue R250 to visualize all bands. Lanes 2, 3, 7, and 8 containing 8 μg protein each are overloaded in an attempt to pick up trace amounts of contaminants or degradants. This could contribute to incomplete SDS treatment, causing the smearing of the homodimeric band in lanes 2 and 3. Lanes 4, 5, 9, and 10 contain the optimal 2 μg protein. Nonreducing conditions in Lanes 1–5 exhibit the 24-kDa intact homodimeric molecule. Reducing conditions with the addition of 2-mercaptoethanol in Lanes 7–10 reveal the 12-kDa monomeric subunits.

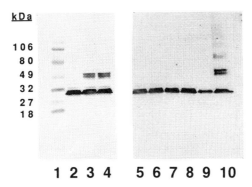

Figure 5. Western blot of TGF-β_1 samples after a freeze/thaw stability study in different buffers. Samples were electrophoresed using nonreducing SDS-PAGE, electroblotted onto nitrocellulose, and probed with antibody specific to TGF-β_1 to visualize the bands. Two formulations were evaluated: (a) TGF-β_1 in 5 mM HCl, pH 2.5 after 0 (Lane 2), 1 (Lane 3), and 6 (Lane 4) $-70°$C freeze/thaw cycles, and TGF-β_1 in 30 mM citric acid and 30 mg/ml mannitol, pH 2.5, after 0 (Lane 5), 1 (Lane 6), and 6 (Lane 7) $-70°$C freeze/thaws. Additional samples include TGF-β_1 lyophilized in the citric acid/mannitol buffer and reconstituted after 3 months storage at 4°C (Lane 8), and a lot of TGF-β_1 in 5 mM HCl stored at 2–8°C (Lane 9) and at $-70°$C (Lane 10) for 2 years. Results reveal SDS-stabile multimeric aggregates appearing in the samples frozen in 5 mM HCl, pH 2.5, and no aggregation or breakdown products appearing in samples frozen or lyophilized in 30 mM citric acid and 30 mg/ml mannitol, pH 2.5.

transferring the TGF-β_1 from the SDS-PAGE gel to a nitrocellulose membrane. The membrane is then exposed to a TGF-β_1-specific antibody probe. A secondary antibody–alkaline phosphatase conjugate reactive to the probe is applied onto the blot. The labeled TGF-β_1 bands are then visualized by the addition of alkaline phosphatase substrate, 5-bromo-4-chloro-3-indoyl phosphate/nitro blue tetrazolium salt (BCIP/NBT), which produces an insoluble blue chromophore. A Western blot showing the labeled TGF-β_1 is shown in Fig. 5.

3.3. Enzyme-Linked Immunosorbent Assay (ELISA)

An ELISA has been developed to quantitate the amount of TGF-β_1 in solution. The ELISA is based on the specific binding of a mouse anti-TGF-β_1 monoclonal antibody to the TGF-β_1 molecule. Monoclonal antibody coated on 96-well microtiter plates captures TGF-β_1 from the applied sample and standard solutions. Captured TGF-β_1 is then probed by a rabbit polyclonal anti-TGF-β_1 antibody, which in turn is bound by goat antirabbit IgG–horse radish peroxidase conjugate. A color reaction occurs by adding the chromophore/substrate solution of 3,3',5,5'-tetramethylbenzidine (TMB) in citrate/phosphate buffer containing hydrogen peroxide. The reaction is stopped with the addition of 1 N sulfuric acid and the absorbances at 450 nm are determined by a microtiter plate reader using a 630-nm reference filter. Concentrations of the unknown samples are quantified relative to a TGF-β_1 standard curve run on the same plate.

3.4. Cell Growth Inhibition Assay (GIA)

A GIA is used to determine the bioactivity of the TGF-β_1. The GIA measures the ability of TGF-β_1 to inhibit the growth of mink lung epithelial cells (ATCC #CCL64) (Ikeda *et al.*, 1987). The activity of the growth factor is determined by the inhibitory response of the cells to different concentrations of TGF-β_1. Cell viability is based on the enzymatic cleavage by metabolically active cells of a tetrazolium salt into an orange/red formazan product. Prior to the assay cells are trypsinized and plated in a 96-well flat-bottomed plate at a concentration of 1000 cells/well. After allowing the cells to attach, samples containing the TGF-β_1 and a reference standard are diluted to concentrations ranging from 1000 to 1.95 pg/ml and added to the wells. The cells are incubated for 4 days after which time a 100 μL solution containing 25 μg of sodium 3'-[1-(phenylamino)-carbonyl]-3,4-tetrazolium]-bis(4-methoxy-6-nitro) benzene sulfonic acid hydrate and 5 mM phenazine methosulfate in media was added to each well. The cells are then incubated for 7 hr and the plates read on a microplate reader at an absorbance of 450 nm with a 630-nm reference filter. The specific activity of a sample is calculated relative to the reference material.

3.5. Cell Proliferation Assay

The cell proliferation assay is based on the ability of TGF-β_1 to stimulate the growth of C3H-10T$_{1/2}$ mouse embryo fibroblasts (Reznikoff *et al.*, 1973). These normal mouse fibroblasts exhibit a well-defined density-dependent growth arrest. This characteristic contact inhibition facilitates the staging of a uniform cell population in the G$_0$ phase of the cell cycle, thus achieving a steady state. Addition of TGF-β_1 to a monolayer of staged cells triggers the reinitiation of a synchronous cell population to enter and progress through the G$_1$ phase into the S phase of the cell cycle. In the S phase, DNA replication occurs and can be measured by the incorporation of tritiated thymidine into newly synthesized DNA.

4. STABILITY OF TGF-β_1

4.1. Stability in Solution

Human recombinant TGF-β_1 (Bristol-Myers Squibb Pharmaceutical Research Institute, Seattle, WA) produced from transfected CHO cells was used for these studies. The pI of TGF-β_1 is 9.82, which is also the pH region of its least solubility. Initial preformulation studies on TGF-β_1 indicated that the protein was most soluble and stable at relatively low pH and aggregated in buffers at pHs approaching and above neutrality. This was determined when the TGF-β_1 was formulated in buffers that ranged in pH from 2.0 to 8.0 at a concentration of 1 mg/ml. At a pH of 4.5 or greater the protein formed a small amount of visible aggregates. The aggregation was exacerbated as the pH was increased to 7.0. As the pH was decreased to less than 4.5, the aggregates became solubilized and a clear solution resulted at a pH of 2.5. A pilot stability study was therefore initiated at 4°C in 5 mM HCl, pH 2.5, with a TGF-β_1 concentration of 1.0 mg/ml. At regular time intervals the sample was assayed by RP-HPLC, SDS-PAGE, ELISA and GIA. After approximately 6 months the ascending shoulder became a discrete peak on the RP-HPLC chromatogram and was increasing in size (Fig. 6) while the descending shoulder remained unchanged. The peak area continued to increase throughout the stability study with some lots of material increasing from 5% at the beginning of the study to greater than 15% after 2 years. When the ascending peak was fractionated and evaluated by the GIA, no bioactivity was detected.

Efforts were next directed at determining the mechanism behind the ascending peak formation. Analysis by native gels indicated that the degradant had the same molecular weight as the TGF-β_1 molecule (data not shown). Thus, aggregation was not the cause of the ascending peak formation. We hypothesized that the TGF-β_1 was undergoing a chemical rearrangement. Since the protein has nine disulfide bonds, it was possible that an intramolecular disulfide bond rearrangement was occurring. Experiments were next carried in an attempt to accelerate the disulfide bond exchange. Zale and Klibanov (1986) showed that the addition of free thiols to aqueous

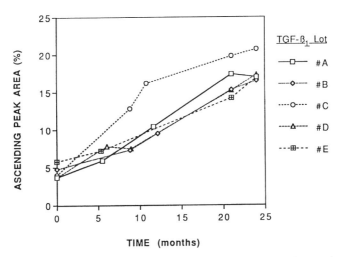

Figure 6. The change of ascending shoulder peak area % over time of five development lots of TGF-β_1 stored in 5 mM HCl, pH 2.5, at 2–8°C as determined by reversed phase HPLC. Each lot shows a continuous increase in ascending peak area over 2 years time.

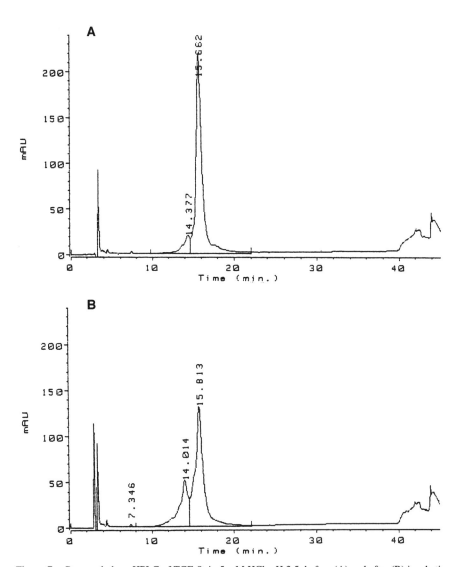

Figure 7.   Reversed phase HPLC of TGF-β_1 in 5 mM HCl, pH 2.5, before (A) and after (B) incubation with 1 mM L-cysteine at 37°C for 5 days to encourage inter and intramolecular disulfide bond rearrangement. The increase in the ascending peak area and corresponding decrease in the main peak area (B) indicate that the ascending peak could be due to disulfide bond rearrangement.

solutions of ribonuclease could accelerate the disulfide exchange reaction and that the process could be eliminated by adding thiol inhibitors. When the thiol, L-cysteine, was added to a 5 mM HCl solution containing 1 mg/ml of TGF-β_1 and heated to 37°C for 5 days, a significant increase in the size of the ascending peak was observed (Fig. 7A,B). This increase in peak size was not seen when the free-thiol inhibitors, ethylmaleimide or $CuCl_2$, were added. Reports in the literature also suggest that disulfide exchange reactions are catalyzed by HCl under acidic conditions (Ryle and Sanger, 1955). When we exposed TGF-β_1 to increasing concentrations of HCl at 50°C, the ascending peak area also increased in size. Preliminary peptide mapping studies using a lys-c digest have been carried out on both main and ascending peak fractions of TGF-β_1 (data not shown). Nonreduced peptide maps indicate that the two fractions differ in the cysteine containing portions of the molecule, suggesting differences in disulfide bonding. These experiments support the hypothesis that the TGF-β_1 is undergoing a disulfide bond rearrangement in 5 mM HCl at 4°C.

Many therapeutic proteins which undergo chemical rearrangements upon storage in liquid formulations have been successfully stabilized by lyophilization (Pikal et al., 1991; Geigert, 1989). Although freeze-drying cannot completely eliminate these reactions from occurring, they can be slowed down considerably. Our efforts were therefore directed toward the development of a lyophilized formulation for TGF-β_1 with the goal of stopping the formation of the ascending peak seen on reverse-phase HPLC while retaining the bioactivity of the protein.

4.2. Prelyophilization Stability Studies

Before freeze-drying of the TGF-β_1 was undertaken, a series of prelyophilization stability studies were carried out with candidate formulations. Since the protein was less prone to aggregation at low pH, a citric acid buffer was chosen. This buffer provided a low pH for the TGF-β_1 and formed a glass upon freeze-drying (Chang and Randall, 1992). The glass can be utilized as a matrix which protects the protein and eliminates the need to add other glass forming sugars as protecting agents. Mannitol was also included in the formulation as a cake-forming agent and for adjustment of the osmolality.

The TGF-β_1 was buffer exchanged from 5 mM HCl, pH 2.5, into 30 mM citric acid, pH 2.5 with 20 mg/ml mannitol. TGF-β_1 was also exchanged into the same buffer with no mannitol. The buffer exchange process was done by adding 0.5-ml aliquots of TGF-β_1 into 2.0-ml Centricon-10's. Each device was filled to volume with the desired formulation and centrifuged at 5000 g for 40 minutes in a refrigerated centrifuge. The filtrate was discarded and fresh buffer was added to the retentate before the next spin. Each sample went through four exchanges. The concentrations of TGF-β_1 were determined by their absorbances at 280 nm (ϵ = 2.21) and diluted to 1.0 mg/ml with the appropriate buffer. The samples were exposed to various treatments, including storage at 4°C, and multiple freeze-thaw cycles at −70°C and analyzed using the techniques of Section 3.

Little to no loss of TGF-β_1 was seen in the 30 mM citric acid buffer, pH 2.5, throughout the buffer exchange process as determined by absorbance at 280 nm. The GIA revealed that there was no loss in activity when compared to the same concentration of control TGF-β_1 in 5 mM HCl. RP-HPLC analysis of samples stored in the citrate buffer, pH 2.5 at 4°C for 30 days revealed that there was no change in the ascending peak area. After 30 days, however, the sample with no mannitol had an increase in peak size from about 9% to 12.5% while the mannitol containing sample did not change (Fig. 8). After 60 days the mannitol containing sample also began to degrade.

The freeze-thawed samples exhibited no increase in ascending peak size when compared to the controls. The Western blot analysis of the freeze-thawed samples (Fig. 5) indicated that no TGF-β_1 aggregation or degradation occurred in the 30 mM citric acid, 30 mg/ml mannitol, pH 2.5, formulation even after six freeze-thaw cycles (Lanes 5, 6, and 7). The TGF-β_1 in the 5 mM HCl (Lanes 2, 3, and 4), on the other hand, had significant aggregation present after one and six freeze-thaws. A sample stored frozen for 2 years at −70°C in 5 mM HCl (Lane 10) also had several different molecular-weight aggregates present.

The fact that TGF-β_1 aggregates are still present after running the sample on an unreduced SDS gel gives us some insight into the nature of the aggregates. SDS will usually dissociate weak noncovalent aggregates. Since the TGF-β_1 aggregates are still present after SDS treatment, the aggregates are either covalently bound or

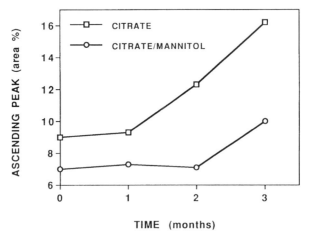

Figure 8. Ascending shoulder peak area % determined by reversed-phase HPLC of prelyophilized TGF-β_1 stored in 30 mM citric acid, pH 2.5, with or without 30 mg/ml mannitol, for 3 months. Results show some extended liquid stability of TGF-β_1 in this buffer in the presence of mannitol.

associated by very strong noncovalent interactions. One or six freeze-thaw cycles in 5 mM HCl induced some aggregation, while long-term storage at $-70°C$ caused severe aggregation. The aggregation may be due to a freeze-concentration of the TGF-β_1 combined with the physical state of HCl at this temperature. HCl freezes at $-114.8°C$ and is in a liquid state at $-70°C$. Aqueous HCl in the presence of ice will therefore obviously be in a liquid state at $-70°C$. TGF-β_1 samples stored at $-70°C$ are thus exposed to a highly concentrated HCl solution within a frozen-ice matrix. The TGF-β_1 may have been exposed to very high HCl concentrations during freezing which could ultimately have led to increased intra- and intermolecular disulfide bond exchanges and aggregation.

Although the primary purpose of the mannitol in the formulation was to serve as cake-forming agent during lyophilization, it appeared to have a stabilizing effect on the TGF-β_1 when stored at $4°C$ or during repeated freeze-thaw cycles. The use of polyols (which are defined as any substance with multiple-hydroxyl groups, including polyhydric alcohols such as mannitol, sorbitol, and glycerol or carbohydrates) have been shown to stabilize proteins in solution (Wang and Hanson, 1988), yet much is still unknown about the mechanism of this stabilization. Several theories have been proposed in an attempt to explain the observed effects of polyols on protein stability. Polyols are known to increase the surface tension and viscosity of a solution, thus lowering the potential for protein aggregation (Schein, 1990). Timasheff and co-workers have suggested that the polyols cause preferential hydration of the protein which can increase the stability of proteins in aqueous solutions—the volume exclusion mechanism (Arakawa and Timasheff, 1982). In our formulation, the mannitol appears to stabilize the TGF-β_1 against aggregation during freeze-thawing. This may be due to an enhanced water structure created around the protein which sterically excludes the protein molecules from contacting one another. The mannitol also reduces the rate of ascending peak formation in the TGF-β_1 during storage at $4°C$. The volume exclusion mechanism could lead to a more tightly packed and stable protein structure which would be less likely to unfold and form intermolecular disulfide bonds.

We concluded from these studies that the TGF-β_1 was stable for 2 months at $4°C$ in the solution containing 30 mM citric acid, 30 mg/ml mannitol, pH 2.5. The sample could also be repeatedly freeze-thawed at $-70°C$ without aggregation or degradation. Even in this formulation, however, the TGF-β_1 should not be stored longer than 60 days at $4°C$. Freezing the TGF-β_1 in 5 mM HCl should be avoided since it causes significant protein aggregation.

4.3. Container Adsorption Study

Since TGF-β_1 is known to have a high affinity for glass, a study was done to determine the stability of TGF-β_1 in siliconized and nonsiliconized glass vials. Sterile glass vials were filled with Sigmacote (Sigma), drained, and air-dried. An approximately 1 μg/ml solution of TGF-β_1 was prepared in 30 mM citric acid containing 30 mg/ml mannitol, pH 2.5. To a portion of the preparation was added 0.01% Tween 80. One milliliter aliquots of each preparation (with and without Tween 80) were placed in each of the following: (i) sterile polypropylene Nunc vials, (ii) sterile uncoated glass vials, and (iii) sterile siliconized glass vials. The vials were capped with siliconized rubber stoppers and stored upright at 4°C for 11 days. The amount of TGF-β_1 present in the containers was evaluated by the specific ELISA.

The results of the vial study are shown Table I. Not one of the samples was at the target concentration of 1 μg/ml, which could be due to either a dilution error or protein adsorption to the containers. Some significant observations, however, were apparent. There was much greater recovery of TGF-β_1 in all containers when 0.01% Tween 80 was present in the formulation. The highest concentration of TGF-β_1 was recovered from polypropylene containers. Furthermore, the siliconized glass containers were more compatible with TGF-β_1 than uncoated glass. The siliconization alone was not sufficient to achieve complete recovery, and the addition of Tween 80 increased the concentration approximately twofold in both the glass and polypropylene. Therefore, TGF-β_1 stored in 30 mM citric acid with 30 mg/ml mannitol, pH 2.5, is less prone to adsorption to siliconized glass when compared to uncoated glass. The addition of 0.01% Tween 80 can further reduce protein adsorption to the vials.

4.4. Stability in the Lyophilized State

A variety of formulations were evaluated in the lyophilization study, all of which were based on the 30 mM citric acid buffer (Table II). The samples were buffer-exchanged as described above for the prelyophilization studies, the only difference being that Centriprep 10's (Amicon, Beverly, MA) were used instead of Centricon 10's for the filtration. These devices hold a total volume of 15 ml and were

Table I. Effect of Vial Type and Formulation on TGF-β_1 Recovery Determined by ELISA[a]

Vial	With 0.01% Tween 80		Without Tween 80	
	Mean (μg/ml)	SD	Mean (μg/ml)	SD
($n = 1$) Polypropylene	0.74	—	0.39	—
($n = 3$) Glass	0.49	0.055	<0.10	—
($n = 3$) Siliconized glass	0.70	0.046	0.37	0.15

[a]Initial TGF-β_1 concentration was approximately 1.0 μg/ml. Samples were stored in 30 mM citric acid, 20 mg/ml mannitol, pH 2.5, at 4°C for 11 days.

**Table II. Formulations Used
in the TFG-β_1 Lyophilization Study**[a]

TGF-β (μg/ml)	Formulation
	30 mM citric acid +
1000	20 mg/ml mannitol
1000	30 mg/ml mannitol
1000	40 mg/ml mannitol
250	20 mg/ml mannitol
250	30 mg/ml mannitol
250	40 mg/ml mannitol
100	20 mg/ml mannitol
100	30 mg/ml mannitol
100	40 mg/ml mannitol
100[b]	30 mg/ml mannitol
1	20 mg/ml mannitol
1	30 mg/ml mannitol
1	40 mg/ml mannitol
	30 mg/ml mannitol
1	+ 0.01% Tween 80
1	+ 6 mg/ml HSA
1	+ 6 mg/ml HSA
	+ 0.01% Tween 80
1	+ 6 mg/ml gelatin

[a]All samples were prepared in 30 mM citric acid, pH 2.5.
Citric acid, human serum albumin, fraction V (HSA),
gelatin, Type B from bovine skin, and Tween 80 were
obtained from Sigma; D-mannitol was obtained from
Fluka.
[b]TGF-β_1 further purified by ion-exchange HPLC.

centrifuged at 1500 g. After samples were exchanged into the appropriate formulation and diluted to the correct concentration they were 0.2 μm sterile filtered, aseptically pipetted into 2-ml glass vials in 1-ml volumes, and lyophilized. A portion of each pre-lyophilized sample (termed prefill) was retained in polypropylene vials for analysis.

The concentrations of TGF-β_1 used were 1000, 250, 100, and 1 μg/ml. The amount of mannitol was also varied in concentrations of 20, 30, and 40 mg/ml. Since the concentration of the 1 μg/ml TGF-β_1 samples was very low, the possibility existed that some of the protein could be lost due to adsorption to the vial's surface or denaturation at the aqueous–air interface. To prevent this potential loss, additional formulations were prepared with 30 mg/ml mannitol that contained 6 mg/ml of human serum albumin (HSA) $\pm$ 0.01% Tween 80, 6 mg/ml gelatin alone, and 0.01% Tween 80 alone.

A TGF-β_1 sample further fractionated by cation-exchange HPLC to contain reduced amounts of ascending peak was also prepared for lyophilization. The ratio-

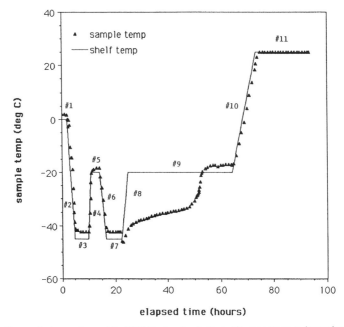

Figure 9.   Freeze-drying cycle used for TGF-β_1 showing both shelf temperature and sample temperature.

nale was to remove or reduce the contaminant peak and see if the lyophilization process could retard its re-formation.

The lyophilization was done with a Virtis 10 SRC-X lyophilizer. The entire cycle consisted on 11 segments each of which could be defined in terms of time and shelf temperature (Fig. 9). The first segment was isothermal during which the filled, half-stoppered vials were loaded into the lyophilizer. During Segment 2 the shelf temperature was lowered at a constant rate. Segment 3 was a second isothermal that allowed the sample material to achieve a constant low temperature. Segments 4, 5, and 6 consisted of a thermal treatment which was done to guarantee crystallization of the mannitol. Segment 7 was an additional isothermal treatment at the end of which time the vacuum pump was started. The samples were warmed (Segment 8) and exposed to another isothermal treatment during which the sublimation of ice was completed (Segment 9). Segment 10 was a deliberately slow warming segment followed by a final isothermal treatment (Segment 11) which continually reduced the residual moisture in the product. Segments 8 through 11 of the cycle was run at a chamber pressure of 25 μm Hg (25 milli Torr) and the vials were stoppered under a 0.9 atm of argon.

The temperature of the sample material was followed throughout the freeze-drying with the aid of thermal probes (30 gauge copper-constantan, Type T, thermocouples, made from 10 mil, i.e., 0.25-mm-diameter wires) placed in each of six representative sample vials. Thermocouple readings were printed to furnish six separate thermal histories.

The sample temperature shown in Fig. 9 is a mean of six thermocouple readings. The primary drying of the sample started at about 20 hr and was finished after 60 hr. The sudden increase in temperature at about 50 hr is attributed to the end of evaporative cooling that is associated with the sublimation of ice (i.e., the sublimation of ice is completed).

This cycle was designed to allow ample times for sample cooling, heating, and drying and reflects a generally conservative approach. There are places where the cycle could possibly be shortened, thus, careful comparative studies should be run to determine if this is feasible.

Visual analysis indicated that the freeze-dried products were formed in well-structured cakes which were observed to retain the dimensions and the general appearance of the frozen, "thermally treated" material (i.e., they were not reduced in volume, nor were they macroscopically "collapsed"). This was equally true of all formulations (i.e., those containing mannitol and citric acid buffer only and those with added HSA, gelatin, and Tween 80).

Stability of the TGF-β_1 at concentrations of greater than 100 μg/ml can be analyzed by RP-HPLC. None of the lyophilized samples exhibited an increase in ascending peak area after being stored for 24 months at 4°C. The sample containing the fractionated main peak had a much smaller ascending peak to begin with, which also did not increase in size over time. Thus, lyophilization of TGF-β_1 in 30 mM citric acid with mannitol, pH 2.5, prevented additional ascending peak formation in samples stored at 4°C for at least 24 months. This experiment demonstrates that it would be possible to reprocess TGF-β_1 to reduce the amounts of ascending peak prior to lyophilization, although considerable effort would have to be devoted to scaling up the reprocessing method.

ELISA was used to determine the concentrations of TGF-β_1 in the lyophilized and prefill samples. All of the samples with TGF-β_1 concentrations of 100 μg/ml or greater retained the initial concentration that was determined for the prefill solutions.

The unlyophilized and reconstituted concentrations of TGF-β_1 lyophilized at a concentration of 1.0 μg/ml are shown in Table III. The samples that contained only mannitol in 30 mM citric acid all underwent significant reductions in TGF-β_1 concentration. This decrease was also observed in the one prefill vial that was assayed. Thus, the decrease of TGF-β_1 occurs prior to the lyophilization and is probably due to adsorption of the protein to the vial and not the lyophilization process.

When HSA ± 0.01% Tween 80 or gelatin were included in the formulation at a concentration of 6 mg/ml, much less TGF-β_1 was lost. When these samples were reconstituted after 6 months of storage at 4°C (24 months for the HSA sample without Tween 80), almost complete recovery of the protein was achieved (i.e., between 0.9 and 1.2 μg/ml). The addition of 0.01% Tween 80 by itself improved the recovery

**Table III. TGF-β_1 (μg/ml) Determined by ELISA
of Prelyophilized Solutions and Reconstituted Samples[a]**

Formulation: 30 mM citric acid, pH 2.5 +				Reconstituted samples		
Mannitol (mg/ml)	Tween-80 (0.01%)	Protein (6 mg/ml)	Prelyo	Dry:3.5 Mo.	Dry:6.5 Mo.	Dry:24 Mo.
20	—	—	ND	ND	0.19	ND
30	—	—	<0.10	ND	0.29	ND
40	—	—	ND	ND	0.18	ND
30	+	—	0.59	0.58	0.63	ND
30	+	HSA	ND	ND	0.97	ND
30	—	HSA	ND	0.99	0.97	1.2
30	—	Gelatin	ND	ND	0.90	ND

[a]Initial TGF-β_1 concentration of all samples was approximately 1.0 μg/ml.

when compared to samples with no Tween, but was less effective than the HSA or gelatin additives. These proteins may stabilize the TGF-β by competing for adsorption sites on the surface of the vials.

Western blot analysis of the 1000-μg/ml sample lyophilized in 30 mg/ml mannitol showed that the TGF-β_1 was not aggregated or degraded after storage for 3 months at 4°C (Lane 8, Fig. 5).

Growth inhibitory assays were performed on several of the lyophilized samples and the bioactivity was compared with a known concentration of TGF-β_1 reference material (data not shown). All of the samples tested retained complete bioactivity for at least 24 months of storage at 4°C. Some of the lyophilized material after storage for over 3 months at 4°C was evaluated by the cell proliferation assay. The results of the assay are shown in Table IV. There is essentially no loss in activity in these samples when compared to the controls.

The water content of the TGF-β_1 sample was 2.98 ± 0.45%. This number represents the amount of water in a sample that had been stored for 6 months at 4°C and is probably not representative of the initial moisture content in the sample immediately after lyophilization. Pikal *et al.* (1991) has shown that the water content in lyophilized hGH formulations increased upon storage and was due to absorption of water from the stopper. It will be useful in future studies to determine the moisture content of the sample immediately after lyophilization and after storage time intervals.

These studies demonstrate that TGF-β_1 can be stabilized by lyophilization in a citric acid/mannitol buffer system. At TGF-β_1 concentrations of 1.0 μg/ml the addition of HSA or gelatin to the formulation is necessaary to prevent adsorption of the protein to the glass vial.

Table IV. TGF-β_1 Activity Determined by the Cell Proliferation Assay on Lyophilized, Prelyophilized, and Control Samples[a]

TGF-β_1 (μg/ml)	Mannitol (mg/ml)	Tween 80 (0.01%)	HSA (6 mg/ml)	Calculated activity (μg/ml)	S.D. ($N = 3$)	Percent activity remaining	S.D. ($N = 3$)
1100[b]	–	–	–	1175	43	107	4
1000[b]	–	–	–	994	98	99	10
100[c]	30	–	–	107	13	98	12
100	20	–	–	88	4	88	4
100	30	–	–	106	16	106	16
100	40	–	–	100	8	100	8
1	30	–	+	1.21	0.23	121	23
1	30	+	+	0.84	0.11	84	11

Formulation: 30 mM citric acid, pH 2.5 + ... Proliferation assay results

[a]Lyophilized samples were reconstituted after storage for 3 months at 4°C.
[b]Control samples stored at 4°C in 5 mM HCl, unlyophilized.
[c]Prelyophilized sample.

5. USE OF TGF-β_1 IN CONTROLLED RELEASE SYSTEMS

Because of the multifunctional nature of TGF-β_1, it is probable that desirable clinical results will be obtained only with the appropriate dose, administration rate and site of administration. For this reason, several different controlled release systems have been evaluated to study the *in vivo* effects of TGF-β_1 in various preclinical models.

5.1. Bone Regeneration

In the area of bone regeneration, TGF-β_1 has been put into several different types of delivery systems ranging from water-soluble gels to ceramic implants. Beck *et al.* (1991) used a 3% methylcellulose gel containing 20 mM sodium acetate buffer at a pH of 5.0 as a vehicle to deliver TGF-β_1 to skull defects in rabbits. In the study, a single application of TGF-β_1 induced a dose-dependent increase in intramembranous bone formation, and complete bony bridging occurred within 28 days. Sites treated with vehicle alone did not heal with bone formation but contained dense fibrous connective tissue between the defect margins.

TGF-β_1 has been incorporated into demineralized bone matrix (DBM) (Kibblewhite *et al.*, 1993; Toriumi *et al.*, 1991), DBM/poly(lactic-*co*-glycolic) acid (PLGA) composites (Gombotz *et al.*, 1994 and 1993), and calcium sulfate ceramic implants (Gombotz *et al.*, 1994). The DBM implants containing TGF-β_1 showed an increase in bone formation in a rabbit facial augmentation model and the calcium sulfate implants containing TGF-β_1 increased bone formation in a rat critical skull defect model when compared to control implants. The composite DMB/PLGA implants, however, when tested in the rat critical defect model, induced little to no bone formation and caused a significant inflammatory response. The TGF-β_1 was shown to be released *in vitro* from the implants in an active form. Since the lack of bone growth was seen in composite implants with or without TGF-β_1, it was suggested that the acidic degradation products of the PLGA could be responsible for the detrimental response.

In a study designed to determine if TGF-β_1 could stimulate bone ingrowth into orthopoedic devices, TGF-β_1 was physically adsorbed from a citric acid buffer onto the surface of hydroxyapatite/tricalcium phosphate (HA/TCP) coated titanium implants and then lyophilized (Sumner *et al.*, in press). The strong ionic interaction between the positively charged TGF-β_1 molecules and the negatively charged HA/TCP resulted in a high affinity of TGF-β_1 for the surface of the implant. When implanted into the proximal humeri of dogs, the implants that contained 120 μg of TGF-β_1 showed a threefold higher amount of bone ingrowth than the untreated control implants.

5.2. Dermal Wound Healing

Although it has been shown that TGF-β_1 may play an important role in soft-tissue healing, the precise amount and duration of time that the TGF-β_1 is present at a wound site are unknown. Several different types of vehicles have therefore been evaluated for the topical delivery of TGF-β_1 in wound-healing applications. A 3% methyl cellulose preparation containing TGF-β_1 was effectively used to promote healing of full-thickness wounds in rabbit (Beck *et al.*, 1991, 1990) and swine (Beck *et al.*, 1990) models. TGF-β has also been mixed with collagen formulations and used to accelerate wound healing in a rat model (Curtsinger *et al.*, 1989; Brown *et al.*, 1988; Mustoe *et al.*, 1987). TGF-β_2 incorporated into a collagen/heparin sponge was shown to accelerate dermal wound healing in guinea pigs (Mustoe *et al.*, 1987). In one study, several types of delivery systems designed to release TGF-β_1 over different time durations were evaluated in a full-thickness wound model in rats (Puolakkainen *et al.*, 1995). The carriers included a Pluronic gel, DuoDERM hydroactive paste, a polyethylene oxide hydrogel and phosphate-buffered saline. The Pluronic gel, which provided the slowest sustained release of TGF-β_1 *in vitro*, was found to be the most effective formulation for the enhancement of wound healing.

5.3. Localized Delivery to Gastrointestinal Tract

The ability of TGF-β_1 to inhibit the growth of intestinal epithelial cells is believed to be of potential therapeutic benefit as an enterocyte protectant during intensive chemotherapy. TGF-β_1 was incorporated into alginate microbeads and administered orally to rats in an attempt to target the growth factor to the luminal side of the small intestine (Mumper *et al.*, 1994; Puolakkainen *et al.*, 1994). In initial studies the TGF-β_1 had a very high affinity for the alginate and lost much of its bioactivity upon release from the microspheres. The addition of poly(acrylic acid) to the alginate/TGF-β_1 solution was found to stablize the growth factor *in vitro*. *In vivo* studies showed that the TGF-β_1 treated animals had a decreased villus height in the intestinal mucosa and significantly reduced proliferating and mitotic indices compared to control animals.

6. CONCLUSIONS

This chapter has reviewed the multifunctional role that the TGF-βs play with diverse proliferative and suppressive effects on many different cell types. The various *in vitro* and *in vivo* effects of TGF-β was discussed with emphasis on the therapeutic potential of this growth factor in areas such as wound healing and bone regeneration. The structure and properties of TGF-β were presented, followed by a more detailed description of the characterization and stabilization of TGF-β_1 in both the liquid and lyophilized state. The chapter concluded with a review of some of the different controlled release systems that have been utilized for the delivery of TGF-β_1 to various preclinical models. Clearly the therapeutic potential for TGF-β_1 is great. Both the formulation and delivery of this growth factor will play an important role in its eventual clinical success.

ACKNOWLEDGMENTS. The authors would like thank Dr. Kirk Leister and Linda Kozik of Bristol-Myers Squibb for their assistance with the cell proliferation assay.

REFERENCES

Amman, A. J., Beck, L. S., DeGuzman, L., Hirabayashi, S. E., Lee, W. P., McFatridge, L., Nguyen, T., Xu, Y., and Mustoe, T. A., 1990, Transforming growth factor beta. Effect on soft tissue repair, *Ann. N.Y. Acad. Sci.* **593**:124–134.

Anzano, M. A., Roberts, A. B., De Larco, J. E., Wakefield, L. M., Assoian, R. K., Roche, N. S., Smith, J. M., Lazarus, J. E., and Sporn, M. B., 1985, Increased secretion of type beta transforming growth factor accompanies viral transformation of cells, *Mol. Cell. Biol.* **5**:242–247.

Arakawa, T., and Timasheff, S. N., 1982, Stabilization of protein structure by sugars, *Biochemistry* **26**: 7813–7818.

Assoian, R. K., Komoriya, A., Meyers, C. A., Miller, D. M., and Sporn, M. B., 1983, Transforming growth factor beta in human platelets. Identification of a major storage site, purification and characterization, *J. Biol. Chem.* **258**:7155–7160.

Beck, S. L., Chen, T. L., Hirabayashi, S. E., Deguzman, L., Lee, W. P., McFatridge, L. A., Xu, Y., Bates, R. L., and Ammann, A. J., 1990a, Accelerated healing of ulcer wounds in the rabbit ear by recombinant human transforming growth factor beta 1, *Growth Factors* **2**:273–282.

Beck, S. L., Chen, T. L., Mikalauski, P., and Ammann, A. J., 1990b, Recombinant human transforming growth factor beta 1 (rhTGF-β_1) enhances healing and strength of granulation skin wounds, *Growth Factors* **3**:267–275.

Beck, S. L., Deguzman, L., Lee, W. P., Xu, Y., McFatridge, L. L., and Amento, E. P., 1991a, TGF-β_1 accelerates wound healing: Reversal of steroid-impaired healing in rats and rabbits, *Growth Factors* **6**:295–304.

Beck, S. L., Deguzman, L., Lee, W. P., McFatridge, L. L., Gillett, N. A., and Amento, E. P., 1991b, TGF-β_1 induces bone closure of skull defects, *J. Bone Miner. Res.* **6**:1257–1265.

Brown, G. L., Curtsinger, L. J., White, M., Mitchell, R. O., Pietsch, J., Nordquist, R., vonFraunhofer, A., and Schultz, G. S., 1988, Acceleration of tensile strength of incisions treated with EGF and TGF-β, *Ann. Surg.* **208**:788–793.

Cate, R. L., Mattaliano, R. J., Hession, C., Tizard, R., Farber, N. M., Cheung, A., Ninfa, E. G., Frey, A. Z., Gash, D. J., and Chow, E. P., 1986, Isolation of the bovine and human genes for Mullerian inhibiting substance and expression of the human gene in animal cells, *Cell* **45**:685–698.

Chang, B. S., and Randall, C. S., 1992, Use of subambient thermal analysis to optimize protein lyophilization, *Cryobiology* **29**:632–656.

Curtsinger, L. J., Pietsch, J. D., Brown, G. L., von Fraunhofer, A., Ackerman, D., Polk, H. C., and Schultz, G. S., 1989, Reversal of adriamycin-impaired wound healing by transforming growth factor-beta, *Surg., Gynecol. Obstet.* **168**:517–522.

Daopin, S., Piez, K. A., Ogawa, Y., and Davies, D. R., 1992, Crystal structure of transforming growth factor-β_2: An unusual fold for the superfamily, *Science* **257**:369–373.

Frolik, C. A., Wakefield, L. M., Smith, D. M., and Sporn, M. B., 1984, Characterization of a membrane receptor for transforming growth factor-beta in normal rat kidney fibroblasts, *J. Biol. Chem.* **259**:10995–11000.

Geigert, J., 1989, Overview of the stability and handling of recombinant protein drugs, *J. Parent. Sci. Technol.* **43**:220–224.

Gentry, L. E., Lioubin, M. N., Purchio, A. F., and Marquardt, H., 1988, Molecular events in the processing of recombinant type 1 pre-pro-transforming growth factor beta to the mature polypeptide, *Mol. Cell. Biol.* **8**:4162–4168.

Glaser, B. M., Michels, R. G., and Kuppermann, B. D., 1992, Transforming growth factor-2 for the treatment of full-thickness macular holes. A prospective randomized study, *Opthamology* **99**:1162–1173.

Gombotz, W. R., Pankey, S. C., Bouchard, L. S., Phan, D. H., and Puolakkainen, P. A., 1994, Stimulation of bone healing by transforming growth factor-beta$_1$ released from polymeric or ceramic implants, *J. Appl. Biomater.* **5**:141–150.

Gombotz, W. R., Pankey, S. C., Bouchard, L. S., Ranchalis, J., and Puolakkainen, P., 1993, Controlled release of TGF-β_1 from a biodegradable matrix for bone regeneration, *J. Biomater. Sci. Polym. Ed.* **5**:49–63.

Heine, U. I., Munoz, E. F., Flanders, K. C., Ellingsworth, L. R., Lam, H. Y., Thompson, N. L., Roberts, A. B., and Sporn, M. B., 1987, Role of transforming growth factor beta in the development of the mouse embryo, *J. Cell Biol.* **105**:2861–2876.

Ignotz, R. A., and Massague, J., 1985, Type beta transforming growth factor controls the adipogenic differentiation of 3T3 fibroblasts, *Proc. Natl. Acad. Sci.* **82**:8530–8534.

Ikeda, T., Lioubin, M. N., and Marquardt, H., 1987, Human transforming growth factor type 2: Production by a prostatic adenocarcinoma cell line, purification and initial Characterization, *Biochemistry* **26**:2406–2410.

Jones, S. C., Curtsinger, L. J., Whalen, J. D., Pietsch, J. D., Ackerman, D., Brown, G. L., and Schultz, G. S., 1991, Effect of topical recombinant TGF-β on healing of partial thickness injuries, *J. Surg. Res.* **51**:344–352.

Joyce, M. E., Roberts, A. B., Sporn, M. B., and Bolander, M. E., 1990, Transforming growth factor- and the initiation of chondrogenesis and osteogenesis in the rat femur, *J. Cell Biol.* **110**:2195–2207.

Keski-Oja, J., Lyons, R. M., and Moses, H. L., 1987, Inactive secreted form(s) of transforming growth factor-β (TGFβ): Activation by proteolysis, *J. Cell. Biochem. (Suppl.)* **11A**:60.

Kibblewhite, D. J., Bruce, A. G., Strong, D. M., Ott, S. M., Purchio, A. F., and Larrabee, W. F., 1993, Transforming growth factor-beta accelerates osteoinduction in a craniofacial onlay model, *Growth Factors* **9**:185–193.

Kurokawa, M., Lynch, K., and Podolsky, D. K., 1987, Effects of growth factors on an intestinal epithelial cell line: Transforming growth factor beta inhibits proliferation and stimulates differentiation, *Biochem. Biophys. Res. Commun.* **142**:775–782.

Kuruvilla, A. P., Shah, R., Hochwald, G. M., Liggitt, H. D., Palladino, M. A., and Thorbecke, G. J., 1991, Protective effect of transforming growth factor 1 on experimental autoimmune diseases in mice, *Proc. Natl. Acad. Sci.* **88**:2918–2921.

Lawrence, D. A., Pircher, R., and Jullien, P., 1985, Conversion of a high molecular weight latent beta-TGF from chicken embryo fibroblasts into a low molecular weight active beta-TGF under acidic conditions, *Biochem. Biophys. Res. Commun.* **133**:1026–1034.

Lefer, A. M., Tsao, P., Aoki, N., and Palladino, M. A., 1990, Mediation of cardioprotection by transforming growth factor-beta, *Science* **249**:61–64.

Ling, N., Ying, S. Y., Ueno, N., Shimasaki, S., Esch, F., Hotta, M., and Guillemin, R., 1986, Pituitary FSH is released by a heterodimer of the beta-subunits from the two forms of inhibin, *Nature* **321**:779–782.

Lioubin, M. N., Madisen, L., and Marquardt, H., 1991, Characterization of latent recombinant TGF-β_2 produced by Chinese hamster ovary cells, *J. Cell. Biochem.* **45**:112–121.

Lyons, R. M., Keski-Oja, J., and Moses, H. L., 1988, Proteolytic activation of latent transforming growth factor-beta from fibroblast-conditioned medium, *J. Cell. Biol.* **106**:1659–1665.

Mackie, E. J., and Trechsel, U., 1990, Stimulation of bone formation *in vivo* by transforming growth factor-β: remodeling of woven bone and lack of inhibition by indomethacin, *Bone* **11**:295–300.

Madri, J. A., Pratt, B. M., and Tucker, A., 1988, Phenotypic modulation of endothelial cells by transforming growth factor-β depends upon the composition and organization of the extracellular matrix, *J. Cell Biol.* **106**:1375–1384.

Marcelli, C., Yates, A. J., and Mundy, G. R., 1990, *in vivo* effects of human recombinant transforming growth factor β on bone turnover in normal mice, *J. Bone Miner. Res.* **5**:1087–1096.

Marquardt, H., Lioubin, M. N., and Ikeda, T., 1987, Complete amino acid sequence of human transforming growth factor type β_2, *J. Biol. Chem.* **262**:12127–12131.

Mason, A. J., Hayflick, J. S., Ling, N., Esch, F., Ueno, N., Ying, S. Y., Guillemin, R., Niall, H., and Seeburg, P. H., 1985, Complementary DNA sequences of ovarian follicular inhibin show precursor structure and homology with transforming growth factor-beta, *Nature* **318**:659–663.

Massague, J., 1985, Subunit structure of a high-affinity receptor for type beta-transforming growth factor. Evidence for a disulfide-linked glycosylated receptor complex, *J. Biol. Chem.* **260**:7059–7066.

Masui, T., Wakefield, L. M., Lechner, J. F., LaVeck, M. A., Sporn, M. B., and Harris, C. C., 1986, Type beta transforming growth factor is the primary differentiation-inducing serum factor for normal human bronchial epithelial cells, *Proc. Natl. Acad. Sci.* **83**:2438–2442.

Miller, D. A., Pelton, R. W., Derynk, R., and Moses, H. A., 1990, Transforming growth factor-β a family of growth regulatory proteins, *Ann. N.Y. Acad. Sci.* **593**:208–217.

Miyazono, K., Hellman, U., Wernstedt, C., and Helin, C. H., 1988, Latent high molecular weight complex of transforming growth factor beta 1. Purification from human platelets and structural characterization, *J. Biol. Chem.* **263**:6407–6415.

Moses, H. L., Tucker, R. F., Leof, E. B., Coffey, R. J., Halper, J., and Shipley, G. D., 1985, Type-β transforming growth factor is a growth stimulator and growth inhibitor, *Cancer Cells* **3**:65–71.

Mumper, R. J., Hoffman, A. S., Puolakkainen, P. A., Bouchard, L. S., and Gombotz, W. R., 1994, Calcium-alginate beads for the oral delivery of transforming growth factor-β_1 (TGF-β_1); stabilization of TGF-β_1 by the addition of polyacrylic acid within acid-treated beads, *J. Control. Rel.* **30**:241–251.

Mustoe, T. A., Pierce, G. F., Thomason, A., Gramates, P., Sporn, M. B., and Deuel, T. F., 1987, Accelerated healing of incisional wounds in rats induced by transforming growth factor β, *Science* **237**:1333–1336.

Nilsen-Hamilton, M., 1990, Transforming growth factor beta and its actions on cellular growth and differentiation, *Curr. Top. Dev. Biol.* **24**:95–136.

Noda, M., and Camilliere, J. J., 1989, *In vivo* stimulation of bone formation by transforming growth factor-β, *Endocrinology* **124:**2991–2995.

Piez, K. A., and Sporn, M. B., 1990, Transforming growth factor-βs, chemistry, biology and therapeutics, *Ann. N.Y. Acad. Sci.* **593.**

Pikal, M. J., Dellerman, K. M., Roy, M. L., and Riggin, R. M., 1991, The effects of formulation variables on the stability of freeze-dried human growth hormone, *Pharm. Res.* **8:**427–436.

Pircher, R., Jullien, P., and Lawrence, D. A., 1986, Beta-transforming growth factor is stored in human blood platelets as a latent high molecular weight complex, *Biochem. Biophys. Res. Commun.* **136:** 30–37.

Puolakkainen, P. A., Ranchalis, J. E., Gombotz, W. R., Hoffman, A. S., Mumper, R. J., and Twardzik, D. R., 1994, Novel delivery system for inducing quiescence in intestinal stem cells in rats by transforming growth factor β₁, *Gastroenterology* **107:**1319–1326.

Puolakkainen, P., and Twardzik, D. R., 1993, Transforming growth factors alpha and beta, in: *Neurotrophic Factors* (S. E. Loughlin and J. H. Fallon, eds.), Academic Press, San Diego, pp. 359–389.

Puolakkainen, P. A., Twardzik, D. R., Ranchalis, J. E., Pankey, S. C., Reed, M. J., and Gombotz, W. R., 1995, The enhancement in wound healing by transforming growth factor beta 1 (TGF-β₁) depends on the topical delivery system, *J. Surg. Res.* **58:**321–329.

Purchio, A. F., Cooper, J. A., Brunner, A. M., Lioubin, M. N., Gentry, L. E., Kovacine, K. S., Roth, R. A., and Marquardt, H., 1988, Identification of mannose 6-phosphate in two asparagine-linked sugar chains of recombinant transforming growth factor beta 1 precursor, *J. Biol. Chem.* **263:**14211–14215.

Reiss, M., and Sartorelli, A. C., 1987, Regulation of growth and differentiation of human keratinocytes by type beta transforming growth factor and epidermal growth factor, *Cancer Res.* **47:**6705–6709.

Reznikoff, C. A., Brankow, D. W., and Heidelberger, C., 1973, Establishment and characterization of a cloned line of C3H mouse embryo cells sensitive to postconfluence inhibition of division, *Cancer Res.* **33:**3231–3238.

Roberts, A. B., Anzano, M. A., Lamb, L. C., Smith, J. M., and Sporn, M. B., 1981, New class of transforming growth factors potentiated by epidermal growth factor: Isolation from nonneoplastic tissues, *Proc. Natl. Acad. Sci.* **78:**5339–5343.

Roberts, A. B., Anzano, M. A., Wakefield, L. M., Roche, N. S., Stern, D. F., and Sporn, M. B., 1985, Type beta transforming growth factor: a bifunctional regulator of cellular growth, *Proc. Natl. Acad. Sci.* **82:**119–123.

Roberts, A. B., and Sporn, M. B., 1990, Transforming growth factor-βs, in: *Handbook of Experimental Pharmacology*, Vol. 95, Springer-Verlag, Berlin, pp. 419–472.

Roberts, A. B., Sporn, M. B., Assoianm, R. K., Smoth, J. M., Roche, N. S., Wakefield, L. M., Heine, U. I., Liotta, L. A., Falanga, V., Kehrl, J. H., and Fauci, A. S., 1986, Transforming growth factor type β: Rapid induction of fibrosis and angiogenesis *in vivo* and stimulation of collagen formation *in vitro*, *Proc. Natl. Acad. Sci.* **83:**4167–4171.

Ryle, A. P., and Sanger, F., 1955, Disulfide interchange reactions, *Biochem. J.* **60:**535–540.

Schein, C. H., 1990, Solubility as a function of protein structure and solvent components, *Biotechnology* **8:**308–317.

Schultz, G., Chegini, N., Grant, M., Khaw, P., and MacKay, S., 1992, Effects of growth factors on corneal wound healing, *Acta Ophthalmol.*, Suppl. 70, pp. 60–66.

Seyedin, S. M., Segarini, P. R., and Rosen, D. M., 1987, Cartilage inducing factor-β₂ is a unique protein structurally and functionally related to transforming growth factor-beta, *J. Biol. Chem.* **262:**1946–1949.

Seyedin, S. M., Thompson, A.Y., Bentz, H., Rosen, D. M., McPherson, J. M., Conti, A., Siegel, N. R., Galluppi, G. R., and Piez, K. A., 1986, Cartilage-inducing factor-A. Apparent identity to transforming growth factor-beta, *J. Biol. Chem.* **261:**5693–5695.

Sharples, K., Plowman, G. D., Rose, T. M., Twardzik, D. R., and Purchio, A. F., 1987, Cloning and sequence analysis of simian transforming growth factor-β cDNA, *DNA* **6:**239–244.

Smiddy, W. E., Glaser, B. M., and Green, W. R., 1989, Transforming growth factor beta. A biologic chorioretinal glue, *Arch. Opthalmol.* **107:**577–580.

Smiddy, W. E., Glaser, B. M., Thommepson, J. T., Sjaarda, R. N., Flynn, H. W., Hanham, A., and Murphy, R. P., 1993, Transforming growth factor-β_2 significantly enhances the ability to flatten the rim of subretinal fluid surrounding macular holes, *Retina* **13**:296–301.

Sporn, M. B., and Roberts, A. B., 1989, Transforming growth factor-beta. Multiple actions and potential clinical applications, *JAMA* **262**:938–941.

Sporn, M. B., Roberts. A. B., Wakefield, L. M., and Assoian, R. K., 1986, Transforming growth factor-β: Biological function and chemical structure, *Science* **233**:532–534.

Sumner, D. R., Turner, T. M., Purchio, A. F., Gombotz, W. R., Urban, R. M., and Galante, J. O., Enhancement of bone ingrowth by transforming growth factor beta, *J. Bone Joint Surg.*, in press.

Tanaka, T., Taniguchi, Y., Gotoh, K., Satoh, R., Inazu, M., and Ozawa, H., 1993, Morphological study of recombinant human transforming growth factor β_1-induced intramembranous ossification in neonatal rat parietal bone, *Bone* **14**:117–123.

Toriumi, D. M., East, C. A., and Larrabee, W. F., 1991, Osteoinductive biomaterials for medical implantation, *J. Long Term Effects Med. Implants* **1**:53077.

Tucker, R. F., Branum, E. L., Shipley, G. D., Ryan, R. J., and Moses, H. L., 1984, Specific binding to cultured cells of ¹²⁵I-labeled type beta transforming growth factor from human platelets, *Proc. Natl. Acad. Sci.* **81**:6757–6761.

Tucker, R. F., Shipley, G. D., Moses, H. L., and Holley, R. W., 1984, Growth inhibitor from BSC-1 cells closely related to platelet type beta transforming growth factor, *Science* **226**:705–707.

Twardzik, D. R., Mikovits, J. A., Ranchalis, J. E., Purchio, A. F., and Ellingsworth, L., 1990, Interferon activation of latent transforming growth factor-β by human monocytes, *Ann. N.Y. Acad. Sci.* **593**: 276–284.

Wakefield, L. M., Smith, D. M., Flanders, K. C., and Sporn, M. B., 1988, Latent transforming growth factor-beta from human platelets. A high molecular weight complex containing precursor sequences, *J. Biol. Chem.* **263**:7646–7654.

Wang, Y. J., and Hanson, M. A., 1988, Parenteral formulations of proteins and peptides: Stability and stabilizers, *J. Parent. Sci. Tech. Suppl.* **42**:S3–S26.

Wozney, J. M., Rosen, V., Celeste, A. J., Mitsock, L. M., Whitters, M. J., Kriz, R. W., Hewick, R. M., and Wang, E. A., 1988, Novel regulators of bone formation: Molecular clones and activities, *Science* **242**: 1528–1534.

Zale, S. E., and Klibanov, A. M., 1986, Why does ribonuclease irreversibly inactivate at high temperatures?, *Biochemistry* **25**:5432–5444.

5

Stability and Characterization of Recombinant Human Relaxin

Tue H. Nguyen and Steven J. Shire

1. BACKGROUND

1.1. Isolation and Purification of Human Relaxin

Relaxin is a protein hormone primarily known for its role in the reproductive biology of various species (Bryant-Greenwood, 1982; Kemp and Niall, 1984; Sherwood, 1993; Bryant-Greenwood and Schwabe, 1994). This protein generates changes in organ structure during pregnancy and parturition by modulating the restructuring of connective tissues in target organs. Relaxin regulates a number of biological responses of reproductive tissues in pregnant animals, as discussed in more detail in subsequent sections. Some of the potential important roles for relaxin as a therapeutic agent include inhibition of premature labor and induction of cervical ripening prior to parturition. Many early, poorly controlled human clinical trials were performed using porcine relaxin isolated from corpus lutea and ovaries (MacLennan *et al.*, 1981, 1986b; Evans *et al.*, 1983). The identification of the human genes responsible for the expression of human relaxin (Hudson *et al.*, 1983, 1984) made it possible to clone and express a recombinant DNA-derived human relaxin that is active in a cyclic AMP response bioassay using human endometrial cells (Fei *et al.*, 1990).

Relaxin consists of two polypeptide chains that are linked by inter- and intra-chain disulfide bonds in a similar fashion to insulin. The protein is naturally derived

Tue H. Nguyen and Steven J. Shire • Department of Pharmaceutical Research and Development, Genentech, Inc., South San Francisco, California 94080.

Formulation, Characterization, and Stability of Protein Drugs, Rodney Pearlman and Y. John Wang, eds., Plenum Press, New York, 1996.

from a single polypeptide prohormone in which a C-peptide portion is removed to produce the mature two-chain protein. Although the amino acid sequence homology between relaxin and insulin is low (Fig. 1), there are several important homologies between these protein hormones. The positions of the disulfide links are similar in both proteins and there is a conservation of the glycine residues immediately adjacent to the cysteine residues in the B chain (Sherwood, 1988). The individual A and B chains of human relaxin were expressed in *E. coli*, and purified by a combination of gel permeation, ion-exchange and reversed-phase chromatography to >90% purity as judged by analytical reversed-phase high-performance liquid chromatography (RP-HPLC). The purified A and B chains were then combined to form human relaxin that was purified by ion-exchange and reversed-phase chromatographic techniques. The final product is greater than 95% homogeneous as determined by RP-HPLC.

1.2. Pharmacology and Pharmacokinetics of Relaxin

1.2.1. PHARMACOLOGY

The pharmacological effects of relaxin include its inhibition of myometrial contraction and its effects on the structure of connective tissues. Porcine relaxin and recombinant human relaxin injected intramuscularly induced the elongation of collagen-rich interpubic ligament in mice (Hisaw, 1926; Steinetz *et al.*, 1982). This activity of the molecule is the basis of a well-established mouse pubic symphysis bioassay (Ferraiolo *et al.*, 1989). When injected subcutaneously, relaxin caused an increase in pelvic area, cervical dilatation, and a reduction in calving intervals in dairy heifers (Frieden and Hisaw, 1953; Musah *et al.*, 1986; Bagna *et al.*, 1991). These observations led to early speculations that relaxin may be used clinically to induce uterine quiescence and cervical ripening to assist the parturition process (Eichner *et al.*, 1958; MacLennan *et al.*, 1986a).

More recent data indicate that there are differences in relaxin activity among the species. While exogenous porcine and human relaxins rapidly inhibit the contraction of the myometrium in pigs and mice, these hormones have minimal effect on myometrial tissues obtained from pregnant and nonpregnant women *in vitro* (MacLennan *et al.*, 1986b; MacLennan and Grant, 1991). On the other hand, the contraction of human cervical smooth muscle tissues, particularly at term, was effectively inhibited by porcine and recombinant human relaxin (rhRlx) (Norstrom *et al.*, 1984). In rats and pigs, the blood level of relaxin increases prior to parturition and drops to baseline levels after delivery (Sherwood *et al.*, 1993a). The surge in circulating relaxin occurs in the first trimester of pregnancy in the human, but there is no apparent correlation between systemic relaxin and activities leading to parturition (Bell *et al.*, 1988; Peterson *et al.*, 1992). Recent literature suggests that relaxin may

A chain:

| | 1 | | | | 5 | | | | | 10 | | | | | 15 | | | | | 20 | | | | | 25 |
human relaxin: gln leu tyr ser ala leu ala asn lys cys cys his val gly cys thr lys arg ser leu ala arg phe cys
porcine relaxin: arg met thr leu ser glu lys cys cys gln val gly cys ile arg lys asp ile ala arg leu cys
porcine insulin: gly ile val glu gln cys cys thr ser ile cys ser leu tyr gln leu glu asn tyr cys asn

B chain:

| 1 | | | | 5 | | | | | 10 | | | | | 15 | | | | | 20 | | | | | 25 | | | | | 30 | | | | | 35 |
human relaxin: asp ser trp met glu val ile lys leu cys gly arg glu leu val arg ala gln ile ala ile cys gly met ser thr trp ser
porcine relaxin: gln ser thr asn asp phe ile lys ala cys gly arg glu leu val arg leu trp val glu ile cys gly ser val ser trp gly arg thr ala leu
porcine insulin: phe val asn gln his leu cys gly ser his leu val glu ala leu tyr leu val cys gly glu arg gly phe phe tyr thr pro lys ala

Figure 1. Amino acid sequence homology of A and B chains from porcine and human relaxins and porcine insulin. (Reproduced by permission from Cipolla and Shire, 1991.)

exert its effect both as an endocrine hormone as well as an autocrine or paracrine hormone (Evans, 1983; Bryant-Greenwood, 1991a,b, 1992). Thus, local administration of the hormone may be more desirable in some applications. In a limited clinical trial, porcine relaxin was administered intracervically as a topical gel. It induced ripening of the cervix and onset of labor (Evans *et al.*, 1983; MacLennan *et al.*, 1986a). Recombinant human relaxin was also tested in a small phase I clinical trial and shown to be safe at doses up to 6.0 mg (Bell *et al.*, 1993) when delivered topically to the cervical area. Cervical ripening was observed in some subjects, but a larger study is needed to obtain a statistically significant conclusion on the effect of the protein.

The collagenolysis activity of relaxin was explored as a treatment for scleroderma; a disease in which collagen is overexpressed and accumulates under the the skin and in various internal organs. Casten and Boucek (1958) treated their patients with porcine relaxin and reported marked improvement of symptoms. The basis of this approach was demonstrated recently with recombinant human relaxin in *in vitro* cell culture experiments of both normal and abnormal human skin fibroblasts obtained from the patients (Unemori and Amento, 1990; Unemori *et al.*, 1992). Continuous infusion of rhRlx induced a decrease in subdermal collagen accumulation in mice and rats (Unemori *et al.*, 1993) and an increase in skin expansion in the pig (Kibblewhite *et al.*, 1992).

The primary source of circulating relaxin is the ovary. Relaxin is also expressed in the myometrium, cervical tissues, and mammary gland of nonpregnant women (Bongers-Binder *et al.*, 1991) and apparently exerts its effect locally (Bongers-Binder *et al.*, 1991). Relaxin produced in the breast tissue of rats and pigs promotes growth in the mammary gland and adipose tissue and changes the lactating duct structure in preparation for lactation (Hwang *et al.*, 1991; Sherwood *et al.*, 1993). In the male, relaxin is produced by the prostate and released into the seminal fluid (Weiss, 1989; Winslow *et al.*, 1992) implying a potential role for the protein in sperm motility and ovum fertilization (Lessing *et al.*, 1985; Harris *et al.*, 1988; Neuwinger *et al.*, 1990). More recently, using autoradiography relaxin was shown to bind to rat brain regions implicated in the regulation of blood pressure and fluid balance (Osheroff and Phillips, 1991). *In vitro* experiments demonstrated chronotropic and ionotropic activities in the rat heart (Ward *et al.*, 1992; Han *et al.*, 1994). Chronic systemic administration of relaxin induces a sustained decrease in blood pressure in hypertensive rats suggesting a role for the hormone in the modulation of blood pressure and fluid balance (Kakouris *et al.*, 1993; Han *et al.*, 1994), although short-term infusion of rhRlx did not affect the blood pressure of pregnant monkeys (Golub *et al.*, 1994).

1.2.2. PHARMACOKINETICS

The pharmacokinetic parameters of recombinant human relaxin after intravenous injection have been determined in nonpregnant rabbit, rhesus monkeys, and

Table I. Pharmacokinetic Parameters for Recombinant
Human Relaxin in Nonpregnant Female Rabbits and Rhesus
Monkeys after Intravenous Bolus Administration
of 0.1 mg/kg, and in Nonpregnant Women after Intravenous
Administration of 0.01 mg/kg (mean ± SD)

Parameter	Rabbits ($n = 6$)	Rhesus monkeys ($n = 5$)	Women ($n = 25$)
Weight (kg)	3.1 ± 0.1	5.2 ± 1.0	Not available
V1/W (ml/kg)	57 ± 9	78 ± 25	78 ± 40
Vss min/w (ml/kg)	240 ± 20	690 ± 220	280 ± 100
Vss max/W (ml/kg)	2000 ± 400	1600 ± 200	1300 ± 400
Cl/W (ml/min/kg)	5.9 ± 0.4	4.1 ± 0.6	170 ± 50
$t_{1/2}11$ (min)	4.0 ± 0.4	2.0 ± 0.5	5.4 ± 2.1
	(58% AUC)	(13% AUC)	(20% AUC)
$t_{1/2}\alpha$ (min)	54 ± 4	24 ± 7	43 ± 7.2
	(39% AUC)	(44% AUC)	(65% AUC)
$t_{1/2}\beta$ (min)	180 ± 50	250 ± 50	276 ± 72
	(3% AUC)	(43% AUC)	(15% AUC)
T1 (min)	9.6 ± 1.2	19 ± 7	27 ± 9.6
Ω 1 (min)	42 ± 3	180 ± 80	96 ± 18
Ω body max (min)	350 ± 70	410 ± 70	468 ± 108

humans (Table I). Rabbits and rhesus monkeys were injected intravenously with 0.1 mg/kg. Blood samples were collected for 14 hr, and data were analyzed by noncompartmental modeling (Chen *et al.*, 1992; Cossum *et al.*, 1992, 1993). The relaxin serum concentration versus time profile was best described by triexponential equations. The normalized initial volume of distribution (V1/W) was approximately equal to the weight-normalized plasma volume of the animals. The weight-normalized volume of distribution at steady state was equivalent to the extracellular fluid. Recombinant human relaxin was eliminated quickly with a $t_{1/2\alpha}$ and $t_{1/2\beta}$ of 4 min and 54 min, respectively, for the rabbit and 2 min and 24 min, respectively, for the monkey. Studies performed in rats suggested that the kidney and liver are the primary clearing sites of the protein.

In the human trial, nonpregnant women were administered 0.01 mg/kg of recombinant human relaxin as a rapid bolus injection. Blood sampling was carried out for 24 hr and the data were analyzed as described earlier (Chen *et al.*, 1993). The overall pharmacokinetic profile of relaxin in women followed closely the profile obtained in rats, rabbits, and monkeys. After intravenous injection, the protein distributed primarily into the central compartment then into the extracellular space. It is cleared rapidly with $t_{1/2\alpha}$ and $t_{1/2\beta}$ of 5.4 min and 43 min, respectively, accounting for 85% of the area under the serum concentration versus time curve.

Relaxin was also applied intravaginally as a topical preparation to the rabbits and rhesus monkeys (Chen *et al.*, 1992). Table II is a summary of the pharmacokinetic

**Table II. Pharmacokinetic Parameters for Recombinant
Human Relaxin in Nonpregnant Female Animals
after Intravaginal Administration (mean ± SD)**

Species	Dose (mg/kg)	T_{max} (hr)	C_{max} (pg/ml)	Fraction absorbed
Rabbit ($n = 5$)	0.1	6–48	217–862	1.6%–4.7%
Rabbit ($n = 5$)	0.5	0.25–28	560–1981	0.5%–1.2%
Rhesus monkey ($n = 6$)	0.1	2.0–24	51–1475	0.2%–1.4%

parameters after intravaginal administration. The serum concentration data indicated low and variable absorption with estimated relative bioavailability ranging from 0.5 to 4.7% for the rabbits and 0.2 to 1.4% in the monkeys. It should be noted that the rabbit vaginal lining consists primarily of cuboidal or columnar epithelial cells while monkeys have a stratified squamous epithelium similar to human tissue. In the phase I clinical trial the same topical formulation was administered intravaginally and intra-cervically to nonpregnant women. The relaxin total dose initially administered was 0.75 mg, but eventually was increased to 6.0 mg. Irrespective of the dose, the systemic absorption of relaxin following intravaginal administration was minimal with 35% to 45% of the women exhibiting a detectable level of relaxin (20–200 pg/ml). However, the same number of subjects also showed a similar endogenous relaxin level after placebo treatment. Intracervical application induced detectable systemic levels of relaxin in 90% of the women (Chen *et al.*, 1993). As discussed earlier, topical administration of porcine relaxin induced cervical ripening and onset of labor in pregnant women. It is plausible that these effects result from the activity of relaxin on the local tissue and that systemic serum levels may not be relevant in predicting pharmacological response in this situation.

2. STRUCTURE AND PROPERTIES OF RECOMBINANT HUMAN RELAXIN

2.1. Primary Structure—Peptide Map

Chemical characterization of recombinant human relaxin and native relaxin isolated from corpus luteum of ectopic pregnancy was performed by a combination of tryptic peptide mapping (Fig. 2) and mass spectroscopy (Stults *et al.*, 1990; Canova-Davis *et al.*, 1991). The small amounts of native material that were obtained precluded either an extensive chemical characterization of its sequence or a mass determination of the intact relaxin molecule. As an alternative strategy, the masses

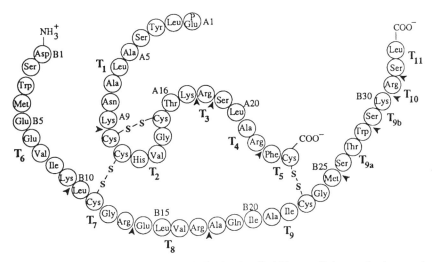

Figure 2. Structural schematic of human relaxin showing disulfide cross links, tryptic cleavage sites marked by arrows, and the corresponding labeled tryptic peptides.

of the individual A and B chains following reduction were determined. The mass of the isolated native A chain was in agreement with the expected mass based on the cDNA-derived primary structure after taking into account that the A chain has a pyroglutamic acid amino terminus. The actual size of the B chain was difficult to determine from the expected sequence because of the uncertainty of the proteolytic processing sites within the prorelaxin sequence. The expected mass of the 33-amino-acid B chain of 3798.6 was based on the proteolytic processing sites that were postulated by analogy to the processing sites of porcine and rat preprorelaxins (Canova-Davis *et al.*, 1990a). The observed mass of the isolated natural 29-amino-acid B chain was considerably smaller at 3319.9. Great care was taken to quickly freeze the excised tissue for relaxin isolation as well as to include protease inhibitors in the extraction solvents (Stults *et al.*, 1990; Canova-Davis *et al.*, 1991). Therefore, the observed B chain mass differences are believed to be genuine and not due to proteolysis during the isolation of human relaxin from tissue. Accordingly, on the basis of these studies, the expression vector for B-chain recombinant DNA synthesis was designed to produce a 29-amino-acid polypeptide chain. Hence, with the use of this recombinant human relaxin molecule it was now possible to characterize the hormone in detail and, especially, to assign the disulfide bonds unequivocally (Fig. 2). The isolation and mass analysis of the tryptic peptides (all within 0.3 Dalton) were in excellent agreement with that expected from the theoretical amino acid sequence. The disulfide bond arrangement was also shown by tandem mass spectrometry to match that of insulin as was expected (Stults *et al.*, 1990).

2.2. Secondary and Tertiary Structures

As mentioned there are significant structural homologies between insulin and relaxin, especially regarding the relative placement of the disulfide bonds. Previously reported estimations of secondary structure content from circular dichroism measurements in the far-UV region suggested that porcine relaxin and bovine zinc-free insulin had similar secondary structure content (~30% α-helix and 15–19% β-sheet) (Rawitch et al., 1980). The far-UV circular dichroism spectra for porcine relaxin and recombinant human relaxin are shown in Figs. 3A and 3B, respectively. Estimates of secondary structure were obtained from data collected in the far-UV range using the method of either Provencher (Provencher and Glockner, 1981) or Yang and co-workers (Chang et al., 1978). The bold solid lines in the figure are a result of an analysis using the Provencher fitting algorithm, and estimates of secondary structure from this analysis are included in Table III. Although both proteins exhibit a CD spectrum that is typical of the α-helix conformation, they differ significantly in regard to the position of the minimum near 209–211 nm and the maximum near 190–200 nm. The analysis using Provencher's algorithm suggests that there is little difference between the human and porcine relaxin secondary structures, whereas an analysis using the algorithm of Yang suggests that human relaxin has a 50% α-helix content compared to 37% for porcine (Table III). The values obtained for the latter analysis is consistent with that reported by previous workers for porcine relaxin using the Yang algorithm (Rawitch et al., 1980). However, this result should be interpreted with caution. The fit of the data using the Yang algorithm is shown as the solid lines in Figs. 3A and B. Although the fit to the human data is very close to that provided by the Provencher analysis, it is not nearly as good for the analysis of the porcine data. The estimation of 50% α-helix for human relaxin from far-UV CD measurements is further supported by an estimation of 58% α-helix from the X-ray structure of human relaxin at 1.5 Å resolution (Eigenbrot et al., 1991). The comparison of the relaxin crystal structure with that of bovine zinc-free insulin also shows that the overall tertiary structure of the two molecules is very similar.

2.3. Dimerization of Recombinant Human Relaxin

Human relaxin, as does insulin, crystallizes as a dimer, but the orientation of the dimers is completely different in the two molecules. In particular, a 146° rotation and translation is required to superimpose the relaxin/insulin pair after superimposition of the first pair. Although human relaxin crystallizes as a dimer, this protein chromatographs using size-exclusion chromatography essentially as a monomer with a molecular weight of ~6000 (Canova-Davis et al., 1990a). These results could suggest that the formation of a dimer upon crystallization is due to molecular packing rather than self-association in solution. Alternatively, if the association in solution is not very tight then the typical dilution encountered during gel-sizing chromatography

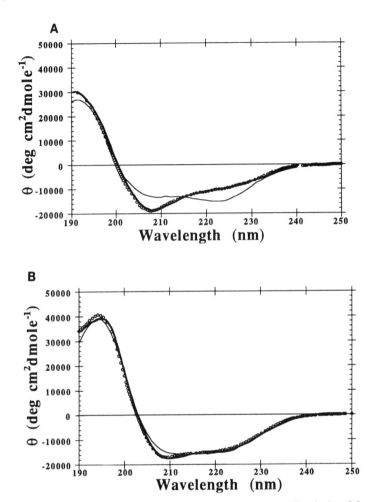

Figure 3. Far-UV circular dichroism of porcine (panel A) and human (panel B) relaxin at 0.5 mg/ml in a thermostated 0.01-cm cylindrical cuvette maintained at 20°C. Open circles are the result of an average of three scans using an average time for each single data point collection of 5 s. Data were collected at 0.2-nm intervals at a spectral bandwidth of 1.5 nm. Some data points are not shown for clarity. The bold solid line is a result of a fit using Provencher's algorithm, and the thin solid line is a result of a fit using Yang's algorithm. The estimated secondary structure from these analyses are presented in Table I. (Adapted by permission from Shire *et al.*, 1991.)

could result in dissociation, predominantly to monomer. This hypothesis was confirmed by sedimentation equilibrium analytical ultracentrifugation and circular dichroism spectroscopy (Shire *et al.*, 1991). The human relaxin ultracentrifuge data were adequately defined by a monomer–dimer self-association model with an association constant of ~6×10^5 M^{-1}, whereas porcine relaxin was essentially monomeric

Table III. Far-UV Circular Dichroism Parameters and Secondary Structure Estimations for Human Relaxin, Relaxin, and Bovine Insulin

Protein	$\Theta_{195}/\Theta_{208}$	$\Theta_{208}/\Theta_{222}$	% α-helix	% β-sheet	% remainder
Procine relaxin	1.54[a]	1.65–1.71[a,b]	29[c,f]	19[c,f]	—
Porcine relaxin[d]	1.16	1.86	50[e]	50[e]	0[e]
			37[f]	30[f]	32[f]
Human relaxin[d]	2.44	1.18	53[e]	47[e]	0[e]
			50[f]	50[f]	0[f]
Bovine insulin[g] zinc free	2.05[a]	1.38[a]	30[c,f]	15[c,f]	—

[a]Schwabe and Harmon (1978).
[b]Du et al. (1982).
[c]Rawitch et al. (1980).
[d]Shire et al. (1991).
[e]Provencher analysis.
[f]Yang analysis.
[g]Wood et al. (1975).

in solution. The monomer–dimer rhRlx association constant determined by analytical ultracentrifugation shows that dilution of the protein from 5 mg/ml to 10 μg/ml leads to an almost fivefold increase in the weight fraction of monomer. However, this large increase in monomeric rhRlx does not alter the far-UV CD spectrum of human relaxin (Fig. 4A), whereas the near-UV CD (Fig. 4B) does show a significant change in the region usually assigned to tyrosine residues. On the other hand, the environment of the tryptophans probably does not change greatly upon dissociation of the dimer since there are no changes in the broad band near 295 nm. (Fig. 4B). This suggests that upon dissociation to the monomer the lone tyrosine environment is altered sufficiently to allow for greater mobility of the tyrosine residue and hence a decrease in CD signal strength. This observation is further supported by the deter-

→

Figure 4.   Far-UV circular dichroism of human relaxin (panel A) at 0.5 mg/ml (bold solid line) and 10 μg/ml (open circles). The 0.5-mg/ml data were collected as described in Fig. 2. The CD data for relaxin at 10 μg/ml were obtained in a 1-cm thermostated cylindrical cuvette, and are the result of an average of 10 scans using an average time for each single data point collection of 10 s. The weight fraction of monomer estimated from the association constant determined by analytical ultracentrifugation is 0.13 at 0.5 mg/ml and 0.62 at 10 μg/ml. The far-UV CD for porcine relaxin is also shown as the thin solid line. Near-UV circular dichroism of human relaxin (panel B) at 0.5 mg/ml (solid line) and 20 μg/ml (thin line). Relaxin at 0.5 mg/ml was thermostated at 20°C in a 1-cm cell, whereas relaxin at 20 μg/ml was in an unthermostated 10-cm cylindrical cuvette. The temperature in the sample compartment was at ~27°C during the data collection process. The CD data were collected at 0.25-nm intervals at a spectral bandwidth of 0.5 nm and are the result of an average of three scans using an average time for each single data point collection of 5 s for the 0.5-mg/ml samples and the result of an average of 10 scans using an average time for each single data point collection of 10 s for the 20-μg/ml sample. The weight fraction of human relaxin monomer estimated from the determined association constant by analytical ultracentrifugation is 0.13 at 0.5 mg/ml and 0.50 at 20 μg/ml. (Adapted by permission from Shire et al., 1991.)

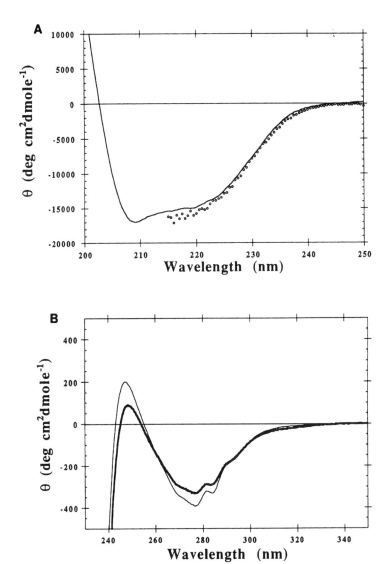

mination of the crystal structure of human relaxin (Eigenbrot *et al.*, 1991). This protein crystallizes as a dimer, and the lone tyrosine residue is centered at the dimer interface. In contrast to the near-UV CD, the fact that the far UV signal does not change upon dilution of the rhRlx suggests that the dissociation of the human relaxin dimer is accompanied by little overall change in secondary structure.

2.4. Solubility

Physically stable aqueous solutions of recombinant human relaxin can be prepared in the pH range from 3.0 to 9.0 at concentrations up to 1 mg/ml. Although a complete solubility versus pH profile is not available, the solubility behavior of rhRlx at pH 5.0 was studied in detail. This pH is the pH of maximum stability for rhRlx as will be shown in later sections describing the stability of the molecule in solution.

Recombinant human relaxin crystallized out following prolonged storage at 5°C of a solution containing 2.0 mg/ml protein, 10 mM citrate, pH 5.0, and 150 mM NaCl. The solubility behavior of rhRlx in various buffers is illustrated in Table IV. Solutions containing approximately 10 to 12 mg/ml of rhRlx in 10 mM acetate, 10 mM succinate at pH 5.0 with and without NaCl were prepared by concentrating 1.0 mg/ml solutions to the desired concentration by ultracentrifugation using Amicon microconcentrators (Microcon) with 5-kD molecular-weight cutoff. The concentration of NaCl was calculated such that the ionic strength of all solutions is around 0.155 M. The solution in 10 mM citrate was prepared with NaCl since human relaxin cannot be concentrated by ultracentrifugation in the absence of salt. A solution in 0.154 M NaCl was also prepared in which the pH was adjusted by trace amounts of 0.1 N HCl. Small crystals of rhRlx were then introduced into each of the solutions which were then stored at 5°C. The concentration of rhRlx was monitored periodically by UV spec-

Table IV. Effect of NaCl and Buffer Species on the Solubility of Recombinant Human Relaxin at pH 5.0, 5°C[a]

	1	2	3	4	5	6
Acetate	10 mM	10 mM				
Succinate			10 mM	10 mM		
Citrate					10 mM	
NaCl		147 mM		150 mM	124 mM	154 mM
pH	5.2	5.0	5.1	5.0	5.1	5.2
	rhRlx concentration (mg/mL)					
Before seeding	12.1	11.3	12.2	8.7	11.1	12.1
	(0.3)	(0.5)	(0.2)	(0.2)	(0.2)	(0.4)
After seeding	14.2	1.81	13.2	2.3	2.18	1.66
	(0.21)	(0.03)	(0.12)	(0.03)	(0.04)	(0.02)

[a]Concentrations are the mean values of triplicate; numbers in parentheses are standard deviations.

troscopy and by HPLC before and after the introduction of the crystals until equilibrium was reached. All test solutions started at 11 to 12 mg/ml. In the absence of NaCl, the amounts of rhRlx dissolved in 10 mM acetate and 10 mM succinate were 14.2 and 13.2 mg/ml, respectively, after rhRlx crystals were introduced into the solution. The slight increases in concentration at the end of the experiment were due to the dissolution of the relaxin crystals. Conversely, in all solutions in which NaCl was present, there was a drop in rhRlx concentration in the solution accompanied by clear growth of the rhRlx crystals. The solubility of rhRlx in these solutions ranges between 1.7 to 2.3 mg/ml. Thus, NaCl significantly depressed the solubility of rhRlx. The data available are not sufficient to demonstrate whether this effect was a specific salt effect or a general ionic strength phenomenon.

3. STABILITY CHARACTERIZATION

3.1. Assay Methodology

The structural identity of recombinant human relaxin has been characterized thoroughly using standard biophysical (Shire *et al.*, 1991) and analytical techniques (Canova-Davis *et al.*, 1990a, 1991). In this section, stability-indicating assays used in formulation development and shelf-life determination are described.

Chromatographic methods separate native rhRlx from trace impurities or its degradation products based on their charge, size, and hydrophobicity. Isoelectric focusing gel electrophoresis using precast LKB gel with pH range from 3.5 to 9.5 has been used to assess the purity of rhRlx (Canova-Davis *et al.*, 1991). However, the pI of relaxin computed from its amino acid composition is around 9.8, and it is difficult to maintain a reproducible pH in this range on the IEF gel. Due to its relatively small size, SDS PAGE analysis of relaxin was carried out on a 10% to 25% polyacrylamide gradient gel with 5% bis-acrylamide cross-linker and tris(hydroxymethyl) methylglycine was used in place of glycine in the electrode buffer.

3.1.1. REVERSED-PHASE HPLC

The preferred analytical method to follow relaxin stability is reversed-phase chromatography. There are several versions of the assay reported in the literature. These methods differ slightly on the mobile phase gradient and column temperature. These modifications were necessary to compensate for slight differences between columns. All of these assays offer baseline separation of the major relaxin degradation products. A typical chromatogram is shown in Fig. 5. The assay was performed on a Hewlett–Packard 1090L HPLC system. Samples containing from 5 to 20 μg of protein were injected onto a Vydac C-4 reversed-phase column equilibrated at 40°C. Mobile phase A consists of 0.1% aqueous trifluoroacetic acid; mobile phase B

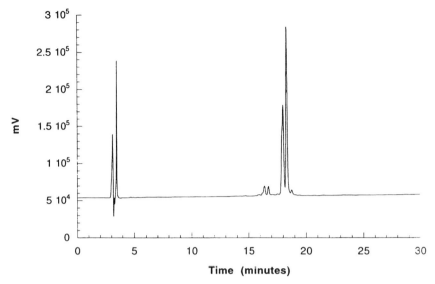

Figure 5.   Reversed-phase HPLC of recombinant human relaxin at pH 2.9 stored for 4 weeks at 40°C.

consists of 0.1% TFA in 1:9 (v/v) water:acetonitrile. The mobile phase flow rate was 1 ml/min and detection was at 214 nm. The separation was achieved with a linear gradient from 20% B to 50% B in 30 min. Under these conditions Met B(4) sulfoxide relaxin, Met B(25) sulfoxide relaxin and intact relaxin eluted at 16.5, 17.0, and 18.5 min, respectively. The other major degradation product, des-asp relaxin resulting from a cleavage of the N-terminal aspartic acid of the B chain (Canova-Davis *et al.*, 1990b), eluted at approximately 18.0 min.

Combination of reversed-phase HPLC with mass spectrometry and amino acid sequencing has been extensively used to identify the various degradation pathways for relaxin (Canova-Davis *et al.*, 1990b; Cipolla and Shire, 1991). Peaks resulting from the RP-HPLC analysis were collected, dried and dissolved in a 50:50 (v/v) water:methanol solution containing 0.1% formic acid. Mass spectral data were collected using a Sciex API III triple quadrupole instrument fitted with an ion-spray (nebulized-assisted electrospray) ion source and molecular masses were calculated and analyzed by the Hypermass software.

3.1.2. CYCLIC ADENOSINE MONOPHOSPHATE (cAMP) PRODUCTION ASSAY

A cell-based bioassay was developed for routine lot release and stability studies. Normal human uterine endometrial cells were seeded in nine-well tissue-culture plates and incubated for 24 hr at 37°C. Relaxin standard and samples were diluted into assay buffer containing 2 mM forskolin and 100 mM 3-isobutyl-1-methyl xanthine to a concentration between 3.2 and 1.6 ng/ml and incubated at 37°C for 30 min. The incubation medium is then discarded and intracellular cAMP was extracted with 200 ml of 0.1 N HCl for 30 min. Following neutralization by 0.1 N NaOH, intracellular cAMP released into the solution was quantitated by radioimmunoassay and expressed as pmol/ml. The concentration of active relaxin was determined by interpolation on the standard curve where the concentration of relaxin was plotted versus the amount of intracellular cAMP produced (Fei *et al.*, 1990).

3.1.3. MOUSE PUBIC SYMPHYSIS ASSAY

This assay is the original bioassay for relaxin (Steinetz *et al.*, 1969). Female albino CFW mice were primed with subcutaneous injection of 5 mg of estradiol 17β-cyclopentyl propionate in 0.2 mL of peanut oil. Seven days later the mice were dosed with 0.2 ml of samples containing from 0 to 12 mg/ml of relaxin in 1% benzopurpurine-4B. The animals were sacrificed after approximately 24 hr and the interpubic ligaments were exposed and measured with a calibrated caliper (Ferraiolo *et al.*, 1989).

Cipolla and Shire (1991) and Nguyen *et al.* (1993) have examined the correlation between the bioassay results and changes observed by RP-HPLC. The data indicate that even under harsh conditions where most of the native protein was oxidized to its various Met sulfoxide forms, relaxin still retains its *in vitro* and *in vivo* bioactivity. Consequently, RP-HPLC detects chemical alterations in the molecule during storage that do not result in decreased biopotency.

3.2. Stability in Solution

3.2.1. pH-DEGRADATION RATE PROFILE

The stability of relaxin as a function of pH was studied in the pH range of 3.0 to 9.0. Relaxin concentration was 1 mg/ml. Solutions at pH 3.0 were buffered with 10 mM sodium glycolate, pH 4.0 and 5.0 with 10 mM sodium acetate, pH 6.0 with 10 mM histidine, pH 6.5 and 7.0 with sodium phosphate, and pH 9.0 with 10 mM Tris. Sodium chloride was added to all samples to keep the ionic strength constant at 150 mM.

At 35°C the degradation rate in solution can be satisfactorily described by first-order kinetics. The slope of the semilog plot of the area under the peak for intact relaxin versus time was used to construct the pH-rate profile (Fig. 6). The degradation of relaxin is catalyzed by acid and based as evident from the V-shaped profile. The pH of maximum stability is around pH 5.0. In the acidic region below pH 4.0, the dominant degradation pathway is cleavage of the aspartic acid residue at the N-ter-

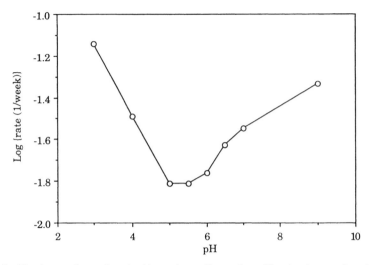

Figure 6.   The change of ascending shoulder peak area % over time of five development lots of TGF-β_1 stored in 5 mM HCl, pH 2.5, at 2–8°C as determined by reversed phase HPLC. Each lot shows a continuous increase in ascending peak area over 2 years time.

minus of the B chain. Methionine oxidation occurs at either Met B(4) and Met B(25), and there is no evidence of the formation of Met B(4), Met B(25) disulfoxide relaxin. In the basic pH range above pH 7.5, the chromatogram exhibited two additional peaks eluting between the Met sulfoxide relaxin and the des-Asp relaxin peaks. The proteins collected from these peaks have the same mass by mass spectrometry and have the exact same amino acid composition as the intact molecule. These species were tentatively designated as relaxin with various forms of scrambled disulfide bridges. As a note of caution, oxidation occurs because of the presence of very small quantities of oxidants or catalysts in the solution. The amount of these impurities can vary significantly from batch to batch, depending on the source of raw materials, the container closure systems, and the manufacturing process. Thus, it is not uncommon to see large variations in the rate of oxidation between batches and even between samples.

3.2.2.   TEMPERATURE-DEGRADATION RATE PROFILE

The stability of relaxin in solution at pH 5.0, 6.0, and 7.0 was followed in the temperature range between 35 and 5°C. The Arrhenius plot of the data is shown in Fig. 7. There is an apparent linear relationship between 5 and 25°C. The activation energy of the reaction calculated from the slope of the line was approximately 6.0

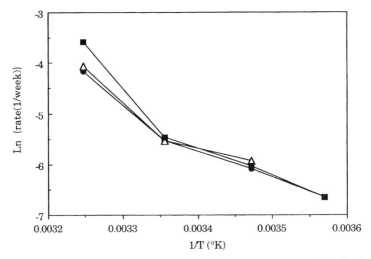

Figure 7. Arrhenius plot of the rate of degradation of recombinant human relaxin in buffered solutions:
(●) pH 5.0, (△) pH 6.0, (■) pH 7.0.

kcal per mole. The point corresponding to the degradation rate at 35°C deviates from linearity. Assuming that the relationship is also linear between 25 and 35°C the activation energy in this temperature range is estimated to be around 17.0 kcal per mole. These data indicate that there are a least two major degradation pathways. At temperatures above 25°C, the reaction with higher E_a dominates. As storage temperature was lowered, the reaction with lower E_a is dominant as it is the least temperature sensitive of the two. Indeed the chromatograms of samples formulated in pH 6.0 exhibit a degradation profile shifting from aspartic acid cleavage to methionine oxidation as the storage temperature was lowered from 35 to 5°C.

3.2.3. OXIDATION BY HYDROGEN PEROXIDE

Relaxin oxidizes readily in the presence of trace amounts of peroxide. In aqueous solution at pH 5.0, hydrogen peroxide-induced oxidation at the two methionine residues on the B chain (Nguyen *et al.*, 1993) results in Met B(4), Met B(25) disulfoxide relaxin as the end product. Figure 8 is a typical plot of the degradation of relaxin in the presence of a 2000-fold molar excess H_2O_2. Intact relaxin disappearance followed first-order kinetics with the concomitant appearance of Met B(4) sulfoxide relaxin, Met B(25) sulfoxide relaxin, and Met B(4), Met B(25) disulfoxide relaxin. The kinetics parameters of the different reactions are summarized in Table V. The rate of oxidation at Met B(25) is equivalent to the rate of oxidation of free

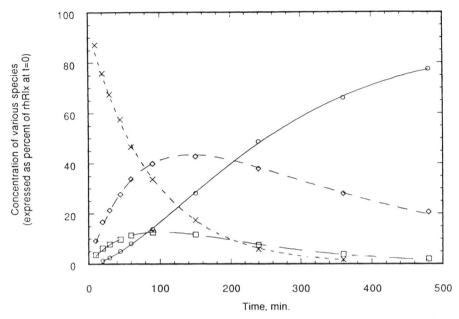

Figure 8.   Oxidation of recombinant human relaxin (1.7×10^{-5} M) by hydrogen peroxide (1.7×10^{-2} M) at room temperature at pH 5. Plot of the concentration of different species versus time. Point are experimental data; solid lines are generated from the kinetic model: (○) Met B(4), Met B(25) disulfoxide rhRlx; (□) Met B(4) sulfoxide rhRlx; (◇) Met B(25) sulfoxide rhRlx, (×) native rhRlx.

methionine or methionine on linear peptides. These results are in agreement with three-dimensional structure data indicating that Met B(25) is exposed to solvent and fully accessible to H_2O_2. Met B(4) oxidizes approximately 2.5 times more slowly although the crystal structure indicates that this residue is also located on the surface of the molecule. Local steric hindrance may be the origin of the small difference in reactivity between the two methionine residues.

3.2.4. METAL-CATALYZED OXIDATION

Metal ions such as Fe^{2+} or Cu^{2+} catalyzes rapid oxidation of relaxin in the presence of a pro-oxidant such as ascorbic acid. Oxidation of relaxin under these conditions was accompanied by a pH-dependent precipitation of the molecule, less evident at low pH values and more pronounced in the basic pH range (Li *et al.*, 1995). The data also suggested that, in addition to the oxidation of the B-chain methionine residues, oxidation also occurred at His A(10). This alteration apparently may have led to a slight change in the tertiary structure of relaxin which was followed by formation of noncovalently linked aggregates and precipitation.

Table V. Bimolecular Rate Constants for the Oxidation of Methionine Residues in 10 mM Acetate, pH 5.0, $T = 22$–$24°C$.

Reaction	Bimolecular rate constant $k'_i \times 10^{-2}$ $(s^{-1}\ M^{-1})$
rhR1x → Met B(25) sulfoxide rhR1x (k'_1)	0.85 ± 0.04
rhR1x → Met B(4) sulfoxide rhR1x (k'_3)	0.34 ± 0.02
Met B(25) sulfoxide rhR1x → Met B(4), Met B(25) disulfoxide rhR1x (k'_2)	0.38 ± 0.07
Met B(4) sulfoxide rhR1x → Met (B4), Met (B25) disulfoxide rhR1x (k'_4)	0.83 ± 0.10
AcSer-Trp-Met-Glu-GluNH$_2$	1.07 ± 0.03
AcCysNH$_2$-S-S-AcCys-Gly-Met-Ser-ThrNH$_2$	1.00 ± 0.02
Methionine	0.93 ± 0.16

3.2.5. OXIDATION IN THE PRESENCE OF LIGHT

The major route of degradation of human relaxin with a B chain of 33-amino-acid length during exposure to intense light has been investigated by reversed-phase HPLC and mass spectroscopy (Cipolla and Shire, 1991). After 17 days exposure to 3600 foot-candles of light, reversed-phase HPLC analysis revealed that >91% of the relaxin had been altered (Fig. 9). Tryptic peptide analysis of relaxin before and after exposure to intense light showed that the T6 and T9 tryptic peptides were altered (Fig. 10). Fast atom bombardment (FAB) mass spectroscopic analysis of the altered tryptic peptides was consistent with the formation of methionine sulfoxide (Table VI). Further confirmation was obtained by tandem mass spectrometric analysis of tryptic digests of the degraded protein that definitively showed an increase of 16 Daltons at the B25 and B4 methionine amino acid residues, respectively. The methionine B25 residue is more easily oxidized by exposure to light than the B4 residue as was the case for oxidation of methionine by hydrogen peroxide (Nguyen et al., 1993). Full activity after photooxidation of methionine residues was retained in both the mouse pubic symphysis bioassay and the cyclic AMP bioassay. Although there was no evidence of tryptophan oxidation, there were many small reversed-phase HPLC peaks which were not collected which may be due to tryptophan oxidation products or other as yet undetermined degradation products (Fig. 9).

3.3. Stability in Methylcellulose Gel

Relaxin was formulated as a hydrophilic gel for topical administration to the cervical area. The formulation consists of relaxin in 10 mM sodium citrate, pH 5.0, and 3% methylcellulose. As shown in Fig. 11 the stability of relaxin in the gel varied

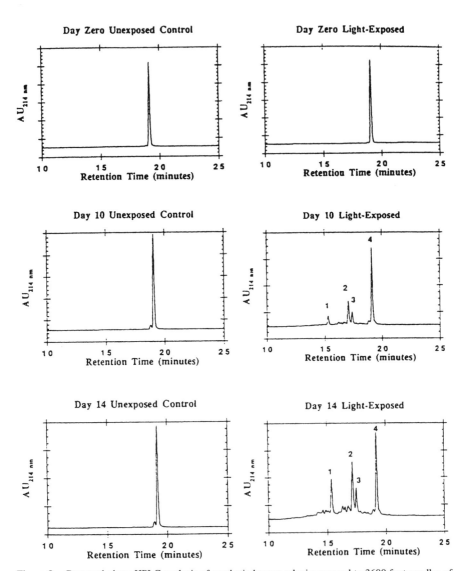

Figure 9.   Reversed-phase HPLC analysis of synthetic human relaxin exposed to 3600 foot-candles of light for 0, 10, and 14 days. The ordinate is an arbitrary scale, and each chromatogram is adjusted for full-scale expansion in order to clearly show all peaks. The four labeled fractions were prep-collected for further analysis. The percent of total area for each peak is as follows: peak 1 is 6% at day 10 and 12.8% at day 14; peak 2 is 17.4% at day 10 and 15.3% at day 14; peak 3 is 9.3% at day 10 and 7.9% at day 14; peak 4 is 50.3% at day 10 and 22% at day 14. The unexposed control sample was wrapped in foil to shield it from light. (Reproduced by permission from Cipolla and Shire, 1991.)

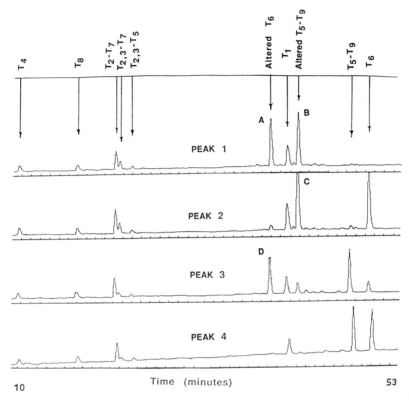

Figure 10. Reversed-phase HPLC analysis of tryptic digests of collected peaks 1–4 shown in Fig. 9. The four labeled components, A, B, C, and D, were collected for amino acid and mass spectrometric analysis. (Reproduced by permission from Cipolla and Shire, 1991.)

from batch to batch, although these batches were made from the same lots of raw materials. The RP-HPLC chromatogram of relaxin gel samples stored at 5°C for 6 months (Fig. 12) suggests that under these conditions the major degradation product is relaxin oxidized at the B-chain methionines. In addition to a small amount of des-Asp relaxin, there are five to six other minor degradation peaks which have not yet been definitively identified. Figure 13 illustrates the stability behavior of relaxin gel formulation stored for a year at 5°C. The ratio of the area under the intact relaxin peak over the total area under all the peaks was first plotted against time exhibiting about 10% loss in intact relaxin over a period of 1 year. However, when the intact relaxin peak area was normalized against a relaxin standard injected at the same time, the loss was more pronounced, indicating that there was a gradual loss in area under the relaxin peak without corresponding appearance of degradation products. This loss in area under the RP-HPLC chromatogram was also observed in metal-catalyzed oxida-

**Table VI. Major MH⁺ Ions of Tryptic Digest Fragments
of Light-Exposed Human Relaxin with 33-Amino-Acid B Chain[b]**

Tryptic fragment	Theoretical mass	Observed mass[a]			
		Sample A "Alt T_6"	Sample B "Alt T_5–T_9"	Sample C "Alt T_5–T_9"	Sample D "Alt T_6"
T_6	1137.3				
T_6 Met-sulfoxide	1153.3	1153.0			1152.4
T_6 kynurenine	1141.3				
T_6 N-formylkynurenine	1169.3				
T_1 (pyroglu)	990.2		990.3	991.0	
T_5–T_9	1662.9				
T_5–T_9 Met-sulfoxide	1678.9		1678.5	1678.5	
T_5–T_9 kynurenine	1666.9				
T_5–T_9 N-formylkinurenine	1694.9				
T_9	1395.6				
T_9 Met-sulfoxide	1411.6		1411.7	1411.8	

[a]Samples A–D as shown in Fig. 10.
[b]Reproduced by permission from Cipolla and Shire (1991).

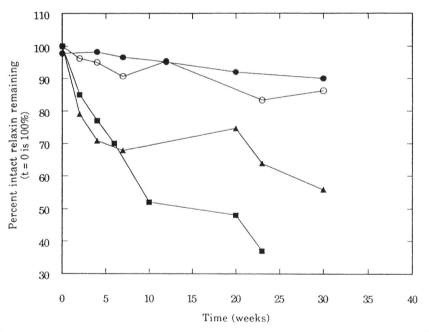

Figure 11. Stability of rhRlx at 5°C as measured by RP-HPLC. (●) aqueous solution pH 5.0; (▲) 3% methylcellulose, pH 5.0, lot 1; (■) 3% methyl cellulose pH 5.0, lot 2; (○) 3% methylcellulose pH 5.0 containing 20% (v/v) glycerol, and 1% (w/v) methionine.

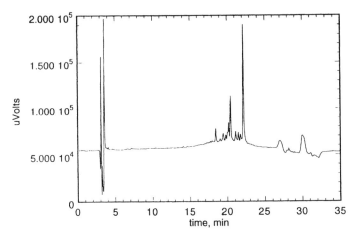

Figure 12. RP-HPLC chromatogram of rhRlx in 3% methylcellulose stored at 5°C for 6 months.

tion experiments described earlier (Li *et al.*, 1995). Thus, the data suggest that slow oxidation of histidine accompanied by protein precipitation may have also occurred in this gel formulation.

Storage of the gel at 5°C exposed to normal lighting conditions greatly accelerated the degradation of relaxin as shown in Fig. 14. The RP-HPLC chromatograms

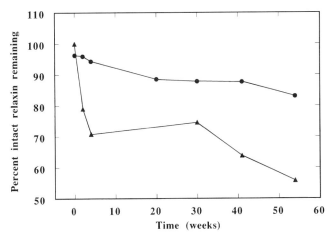

Figure 13. Stability of rhRlx in 3% methylcellulose gel stored at 5°C. (●) percent intact rhRlx remaining relative to total area of all peaks in the chromatogram; (▲) data normalized to standard rhRlx injected at the same time.

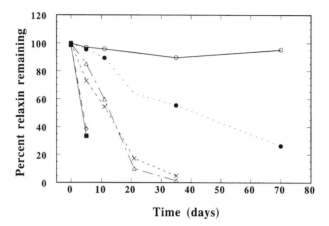

Figure 14. Effect of various storage conditions and formulation components on the stability of rhRlx in 3% methylcellulose gel. (○) stored at 5°C protected from light; (■) stored at 5°C exposed to fluorescent light; (◇) stored at 5°C, exposed to light, nitrogen headspace; (△) stored at 5°C, exposed to light, formulation containing 20% v/v ethanol; (×) stored at 5°C, exposed to light, formulation containing 0.5% ascorbic acid; (●) stored at 5°C, exposed to light, formulation containing 20% v/v glycerol.

obtained from these samples did not show any different peaks when compared to chromatograms of samples stored at 5°C in the absence of light. Thus, the types of degradation products, as detected by reversed-phase chromatography, were similar during storage either in the absence or presence of light at 5°C. These results suggest that accelerated stability studies of samples exposed to light at 5°C could be used to screen potential antioxidants and stabilizers. Figure 14 illustrates some of the attempts to stabilize the formulation by addition of various antioxidants or cosolvents. Inclusion of a nitrogen headspace or addition of thioglycerol (data not shown) did not offer any protection against oxidation. Addition of sodium *meta*-bisulfite resulted in total loss of protein in 1 week (data not shown). Ascorbic acid (0.5% w/v), ethyl alcohol (20% v/v), glycerol (20% v/v) offered some protection against light-induced oxidation. However, a gel formulation containing 1% methionine w/v and 20% v/v glycerol was found to be as stable as the liquid formulation (Fig. 11). Methionine added in large excess (500:1 molar ratio) probably acted as a scavenger of trace amounts of oxidant present in the formulation.

4. CONCLUSIONS

Relaxin was discovered more than 50 years ago. However, only with the advent of recombinant DNA technology have sufficient amounts of human relaxin been produced and made available for in-depth biochemical characterization and pharmacological studies. These investigations have characterized the solution and stability behavior of this hormone. In particular, degradation routes and conditions for formulation as a liquid for systemic administration or gel-based formulations for local application have been established. Pharmacological studies of human relaxin have identified the involvement of relaxin in many physiological processes, ranging from collagenolysis, inhibition of myometrial contraction, enhancement of sperm motility, to its effect of the cardiovascular system leading to lowering of blood pressure. However, the differences in relaxin activities among the different animal models have led to some contradictory observations. Thus, the full elucidation of the biology of this important human hormone lags behind the understanding of its biochemical and stability behavior. Human parturition involves a temporal sequence of events and interplay between different hormones and effector molecules (Porter, 1983; Sortino *et al.*, 1989). It is very likely that a successful clinical application of this protein will require additional knowledge of when in the parturition cycle rhRlx should be given, how often, and in what combination with other molecules that are normally produced during labor and delivery. Not until the biology of rhRlx in humans is thoroughly understood, will it be possible to design proper human clinical trials that will demonstrate the therapeutic value of this protein.

REFERENCES

Bagna, B., Schwabe, C., and Anderson, L. L., 1991, Effect of relaxin on facilitation of parturition in beef heifers, *J. Reprod. Fertil.* **91:**605–615.

Bell, R. J., Eddie, L. S., Lester, A. R., Wood, E. C., Johnston, P. D., and Niall, H. D., 1988, Antenatal serum levels of relaxin in patients having preterm labour, *Br. Obstet. Gynecol.* **95:**1264–1267.

Bell, R. J., Permezel, M., MacLennan, A., Hughes, C., Healy, D., and Brennecke, S., 1993, A randomized, double blind, placebo-controlled trial of the safety of vaginal recombinant human relaxin for cervical ripening, *Obstet. Gynecol.* **82:**328–333.

Bongers-Binder, S., Burgardt, A., Voelter, W., and Lippert, T. H., 1991, Distribution of immunoreactive relaxin in the genital tract and in the mammary gland of non-pregnant women, *Clin. Exp. Obstet. Gynecol.* **18:**161–164.

Bryant-Greenwood, G. D., 1982, Relaxin as a new hormone, *Endocrine Rev.* **3:**62–91.

Bryant-Greenwood, G. D., 1991a, The human relaxins: consensus and dissent, *Mol. and Cell. Endocrinol.* **79:**C125–C132.

Bryant-Greenwood, G. D., 1991b, Human decidual and placental relaxins, *Reprod. Fertil. Dev.* **3:**385–389.

Bryant-Greenwood, G. D., and Schwabe, C., 1994, Human relaxins: chemistry and biology, *Endocrine Rev.* **15:**5–26.

Canova-Davis, E., Baldonado, I. P., and Teshima, G. M., 1990a, Characterization of chemically synthesized human relaxin by high-performance liquid chromatography, *J. Chromatogr.* **508:**81–96.

Canova-Davis, E., Kessler, T. J., Lee, P.J., Fei, D. T. W., Griffin, P., Stults, J. T., Wade, J. D., and Rinderknecht, E., 1991, Use of recombinant DNA derived human relaxin to probe the structure of the native protein, *Biochemistry* **30:**6006–6013.

Canova-Davis, E., Tishima, G. M., Kessler, T. J., Lee, P. J., Kuzzetta, A.W., and Hancock, W.S., 1990b, Strategies for an analytical examination of biological pharmaceuticals, in: *Analytical Biotechnology: Capillary Electrophoresis and Chromatography* (C. Horvarth and J. G. Nikelly, eds.), American Chemical Society Symposium Series 434, Washington, D. C., pp. 90–112.

Chang, C. T., Wu, C. C., and Yang, J. T., 1978, Circular dichroic analysis of protein conformation: inclusion of the B-turns, *Anal. Biochem.* **91:**13–31.

Chen, S. A., Perlman, A. J., Spanski, N., Peterson, C. M., Sanders, S. W., Jaffe, R., Martin, M., Yalcin-kaya, T., Cefalo, R. C., Chescheir, N. C., Menard, M. K., and Mordenti, J., 1993, The pharmacokinetics of recombinant human relaxin in non-pregnant women after intravenous, intravaginal, and intracervical administration, *Pharm. Res.* **10:**834–838.

Chen, S. A., Reed, B., Tue, N., Gaylord, N., Fuller, G., and Mordenti, J., 1992, The pharmacokinetics and absorption of recombinant human relaxin in nonpregnant rabbits and Rhesus monkeys after intra-venous and intravaginal administration, *Pharm. Res.* **10:**223–227.

Cipolla, D. C., and Shire, S. J., 1991, Analysis of oxidized human relaxin by reverse phase HPLC, mass spectrometry and bioassays, in: *Techniques in Protein Chemistry II* (J. J. Villafranca, ed.), Academic Press, New York, pp. 543–555.

Cossum, P. A., Dwyer, K. A., Roth, M., Chen, S. A., Moffat, B., Vandlen, R., and Ferraiolo, B., 1992, The disposition of human relaxin (hRlx-2) in pregnant and non-pregnant rats, *Pharm. Res.* **9:**419–424.

Du, Y.-C., Minasian, E., Tregear, G. W., and Leach, S. J., 1982, Circular dichroism studies of relaxin and insulin peptide chains, *Int. J. Peptide Protein Res.* **20:**47–55.

Eichner, E., Herman, T., Kritzer, L., Platock, G. M., and Rubinstein, L., 1958, The effect of relaxin on term and premature labour, *Ann. N.Y. Acad. Sci.* **75:**1023.

Eigenbrot, C., Randal, M., Quan, C., Burnier, J., O'Connell, L., Rinderknecht, E., and Kossiakoff, A. A., 1991, X-ray structure of human relaxin at 1.5 Å, *J. Mol. Biol.* **221:**15–21.

Evans, M. I., Dougan, M.-B., Moawad, A. H., Evans, W. J., Bryant-Greenwood, G. D., and Greenwood, F. C., 1983, Ripening of the human cervix with porcine ovarian relaxin, *Am. J. Obstet. Gynecol.* **147:**410–414.

Fei, D. T. W., Gross, M. C., Lofgren, J. L., Mora-Worms, M., and Chen, A. B., 1990, Cyclic AMP response to recombinant human relaxin by cultured human endometrial cells—a specific and high throughput *in vitro* bioassay, *Biochem. Biophys. Res. Commun.* **170:**214–222.

Ferraiolo, B. L., Cronin, M., Bakhit, C. R., M., Chesnut, M., and Lyon, R., 1989, The pharmacokinetics and pharmacodynamics of a human relaxin in the mouse pubic symphysis bioassay, *Endocrinology* **125:**2922–2926.

Frieden, E. H., and Hisaw, F. L., 1953, *Recent Progress in Hormone Research*, Vol. 8 (G. Pincus, ed.), Academic Press, New York, p. 333.

Golub, M. S., Working, P. K., Cragun, J. R., Cannon, R. A., and Green, J. D., 1994, Short term infusion of recombinant human relaxin on blood pressure in the late-pregnant rhesus macaque, *Obstet. Gynecol.* **83:**85–88.

Han, X., Habuchi, Y., and Giles, W. R., 1994, Relaxin increases heart rate by modulating calcium current in cardiac pacemaker cells, *Circ. Res.* **74:**537–541.

Harris, M. A., Rees, J. M., Laughlin, E. A., Ford, W. C. L., Wardle, P. G., Hull, M. G. R., and Wathes, D. C., 1988, An evaluation of the role of relaxin in the penetration of cervical mucus by spermatozoa, *Hum. Reprod.* **3:**856–860.

Hisaw, F. L., 1926, Experimental relaxation of the pubic ligament of guinea pig, *Proc. Soc. Exper. Biol. Med.* **23:**661–663.

Hudson, P., Haley, J., John, M., Cronk, M., Crawford, R., Haralambidia, J., Tregear, G., Shine, J., and Niall, H., 1983, Structure of a genomic clone encoding biologically active human relaxin, *Nature* **301:**928–631.

Hudson, P., John, M., Crawford, R., Haralambidis, J., Scanlon, D., Gorman, J., Tregear, G., Shine, J., and Niall, H., 1984, Relaxin gene expression in human ovaries and the predicted structure of a human preprorelaxin by analysis of cDNA, *EMBO J.* **3:**2333–2339.

Hwang, J. J., Lee, A. B., Fields, P. A., Haab, L. M., Mojonier, L. E., and Sherwood, O. D., 1991, Monoclonal antibodies specific for rat relaxin V: Passive immunization with monoclonal antibodies throughout the second half of pregnancy disrupts development of the mammary apparatus and, hence, lactational performance in rats, *Endocrinology* **129:**3034–3042.

Kakouris, H., Eddie, L. W., and Summers, R., 1993, Relaxin: more than just a hormone of pregnancy, *T.I.P.S.* **181**:1306.

Kemp, B. E. and Niall, H. D., 1984, Relaxin, *Vitam. Horm.* **41**:79–115.

Kibblewhite, D., Larrabee Jr., W. F., and Sutton, D., 1992, The effect of relaxin on tissue expansion, *Arch. Otolaryngol. Head Neck Surg.* **118**:153–156.

Lessing, J. B., Brenner, S. H., Schoenfield, C., Goldsmith, L. T., Amelar, R. D., Dubin, L., and Weiss, G., 1985, The effect of relaxin on the motility of sperm in freshly thawed human semen, *Fertil. Steril.* **44**:406–409.

Li, S., Nguyen, T. H., Schoneich, C., and Borchardt, R. T., 1995, Aggregation and precipitation of human relaxin induced by metal-catalyzed oxidation, *Biochemistry* **34**:5762–5772.

MacLennan, A. H. and Grant, P., 1991, Human relaxin—in vitro response of human and pig myemetrium, *J. Reprod. Med.* **36**:630–634.

MacLennan, A. H., Grant, P., Ness, D., and Down, A., 1986a, Effect of porcine relaxin and progesterone on rat, pig and human myometrial activity *in vitro*, *J. Reprod. Med.* **31**:43–49.

MacLennan, A., Green, R. C., Bryant-Greenwood, G. D., Greenwood, F. C., and Seamark, R. F., 1981, Cervical ripening with combinations of vaginal prostaglandin F2a, estradiol and relaxin, *Obstet. Gynecol.* **58**:601–604.

MacLennan, A. H., Green, R. C., Grant, P., and Nicolson, R., 1986b, Ripening of the human cervix and induction of labor with intracervical purified porcine relaxin, *Obstet. Gynec.* **68**:598–601.

Musah, A. I., Schwabe, C., Wilham, R. L., and Anderson, L. L., 1986, Pelvic development as affected by relaxin in three genetically elected frame sizes of beef heifers, *Endocrinology* **34**:363–369.

Neuwinger, J., Jockenhovel, F., and Nieschlay, E., 1990, The influence of relaxin on motility of human sperm in vitro, *Andrologia* **22**:335–339.

Nguyen, T. H., Burnier, J., and Meng, W., 1993, The kinetics of relaxin oxidation by hydrogen peroxide, *Pharm. Res.* **10**:1563–1571.

Norstrom, A., Bryman, I., Wiquist, N., Sahni, S., and Lindblom, B., 1984, Inhibiting action of relaxin on human cervical smooth muscle, *J. Clin. Endocrinol. Metab.* **59**:379–382.

Osheroff, P. L., and Phillips, H. S., 1991, Autoradiographic localization of relaxin binding sites in rat brain, *Proc. Natl. Acad. Sci.* **88**:6413–6417.

Peterson, L. K., Skajaa, K., and Uldbjerg, N., 1992, Serum relaxin as a potential marker for preterm labour, *Br. J. Obstet. Gynecol.* **99**:292–295.

Porter, D. G., 1983, The possible involvement of relaxin in the regulation of uterine contraction, in: *Biology of Relaxin and Its Role in the Human* (M. Bigazzi, F. C. Greenwood, and F. Gasparri, eds.), Excerpta Medica, Princeton, NJ, pp. 114–124.

Provencher, S. W., and Glockner, J., 1981, Estimation of globular protein secondary structure from circular dichroism, *Biochemistry* **20**:33–37.

Rawitch, A. B., Moore, W. V., and Frieden, E. H., 1980, Relaxin-insulin homology: predictions of secondary structure and lack of competitive binding, *Int. J. Biochem.* **11**:357–362.

Schwabe, C., and Harmon, S. J., 1978, A comparative circular dichroism study of relaxin and insulin, *BBRC* **84**:374–380.

Sherwood, O. D., 1988, Relaxin, in: *The Physiology of Reproduction* (E. Knobil and J. Neill, eds.), Raven Press, New York, pp. 585–673.

Sherwood, O. D., 1993, Relaxin, in: *The Physiology of Reproduction* (E. Knobil and J. Neill, eds.), Raven Press, New York, pp. 861–1009.

Sherwood, O. D., Downing, S. J., Guico-Lamm, M. L., Hwang, J. J., O'Day-Bowman, M. B., and Fields, P. A., 1993, The phsiological effects of relaxin during pregnancy: studies in rats and pigs, *Oxford Rev. Reprod. Biol.* **15**:143–189.

Shire, S. J., Holladay, L. A., and Rinderknecht, E., 1991, Self-association of human and porcine relaxin as assessed by analytical ultracentrifugation and circular dichroism, *Biochemistry* **30**:7703–7711.

Sortino, M. A., Cronin, M. J., and Wise, P. M., 1989, Relaxin stimulates prolactin secretion from anterior pituitary cells, *Endocrinology* **124**:2013–2015.

Steinetz, B. G., Beach, V. L., and Kroc, R. L., 1969, Bioassay of relaxin, in: *Methods in Hormone Research*, 2nd ed. (R. I. Dorfman, ed.), Academic Press, New York, pp. 481–513.

Steinetz, B. G., O'Byrne, E. M., Butler, M. C., and Hickman, L. B., 1982, Hormonal regulation of the connective tissue of the symphysis pubis, in: *Biology of Relaxin and Its Role in the Human* (M. Bigazzi, F. C. Greenwood, and F. Gaspari, eds.), Excerpta Medica, Princeton, NJ, p. 71.

Stults, J. T., Bourell, J. H., Canova-Davis, E., Ling, V. T., Laramee, G. R., Winslow, J. W., Griffin, P. R., Rinderknecht, E., and Vandlen, R. L., 1990, Structural characterization by mass spectrometry of native and recombinant human relaxin, *Biomed. Environ. Mass Spectrom.* **19:**655–664.

Unemori, E. L., and Amento, E. P., 1990, Relaxin modulates synthesis and secretion of procollagenase and collagen by human dermal fibroblasts, *J. Biol. Chem.* **265:**337–342.

Unemori, E. L., Bauer, E. A., and Amento, E. P., 1992, Relaxin alone and in conjunction with interferon-gamma decreases collagen synthesis by cultured human scleroderma fibroblasts, *J. Invest. Dermatol.* **99:**337–342.

Unemori, E. N., Beck, S. L., Lee, W. P., Xu, Y., Siegel, M., Keller, G., Liggit, H. D., Bauer, E. A., and Amento, E. P., 1993, Human relaxin decreases collagen accumulation *in vivo* in two rodent models of fibrosis, *J. Invest. Dermatol.* **101:**280–285.

Ward, D. G., Thomas, G. R., and Cronin, M. J., 1992, Relaxin increases rat heart rate by a direct action on the cardiac atrium, *Biochem. Biophys. Res. Commun.* **186:**999–1005.

Weiss, G., 1989, Relaxin in the male, *Biol. Reprod.* **40:**197–200.

Winslow, J. W., Shih, A., Bourell, J. H., Weiss, G., Reed, B., Stults, J. T., and Goldsmith, L. T., 1992, Human seminal relaxin is the same product gene as human luteal relaxin, *Endocrinology* **130:**2660–2668.

Wood, S. P., Blundell, T. L., Lazarus, N. R, and Neville, W. J., 1975, The relation of conformation and association of insulin to receptor binding; x-ray and circular-dichroism studies on bovine and hystri-comorph insulins, *Eur. J. Biochem.* **55:**531–542.

6

Interferon-β-1b (Betaseron®): A Model for Hydrophobic Therapeutic Proteins

*Leo S. Lin, Michael G. Kunitani,
and Maninder S. Hora*

1. INTRODUCTION

Interferon-β-1b is a form of interferon-β (IFN-β) which has shown biological activity in a variety of *in vitro* and *in vivo* systems. IFN-β belongs to a class of proteins known as interferons (IFNs). Interferons were originally classified based on the cell type from which they were derived. Thus, the three major classes of IFNs were designated as leukocyte-, fibroblast-, and immune-interferon as these species were predominantly synthesized by leukocytes, fibroblasts, and T-lymphocytes, respectively (Pestka, 1983; Zoon, 1987). With our increasing knowledge of IFN structure and function, the nomenclature of IFN has also evolved. Today, the three major classes of IFN are referred to as IFN-α, IFN-β, and IFN-γ. Human IFN-α and -β, are approximately 30% similar at their primary amino acid sequence level, while IFN-γ is similar to neither. It is also believed that IFN-α and IFN-β bind to the same IFN receptor while there is a separate receptor for IFN-γ (Faltynek and Baglioni, 1984).

Natural human IFN-β is a glycoprotein with an approximate molecular weight of 23,000 Daltons. Correctly engineered recombinant, nonglycosylated, IFN-β species (molecular weight 18,500 Daltons) display the same biological effects as the native molecule. The IFN-β protein has been associated with a variety of antiviral

Leo S. Lin and Michael G. Kunitani • Department of Analytical Development, Chiron Corporation, Emeryville, California 94608.   *Maninder S. Hora* • Department of Formulation Development, Chiron Corporation, Emeryville, California 94608.

Formulation, Characterization, and Stability of Protein Drugs, Rodney Pearlman and Y. John Wang, eds., Plenum Press, New York, 1996.

(Kerr and Stark, 1992; Soike, 1987), antiproliferative (Arabje *et al.*, 1993), anti-infective (Kirchner, 1986), and immunomodulating (Reiter, 1993; Murray, 1992) activities. A brief history of the interferons, including IFN-β, has been discussed by Dianzani and Dolei (1984).

2. MOLECULAR BIOLOGY AND PROTEIN CHEMISTRY

The human IFN-β gene was cloned and expressed in a variety of host systems under the control of different promoter systems. A production strain of the bacterium *Escherichia coli* (*E. coli*) harboring a recombinant plasmid containing the human IFN-β gene and capable of expressing a part of its cellular proteins as recombinant IFN-β was introduced into well-controlled fermentation processes. Recombinant human IFN-β (rhIFN-β) was extracted from cells and purified by a series of column chromatographic and other steps (Mark *et al.*, 1984). The resulting product, purified to >95% purity as determined by sodium dodecyl sulfate polyacrylamide gel electrophoresis (SDS-PAGE), displayed a specific activity that was about 10-fold less than that of IFN-β produced from cultured human fibroblast cells. It was also found that most of the IFN-β protein existed in its covalent-linked dimeric and higher oligomeric forms in *E. coli*. Furthermore, the purified rhIFN-β exhibited loss of purity and potency over time (Mark *et al.*, 1984).

IFN-β has three cysteine residues, located at amino acid positions 17, 31, and 141. One or more of these cysteines could be involved in intermolecular disulfide bridging, resulting in the formation of inactive dimers and oligomers. Likewise, the three cysteines may also interact randomly within each molecule, resulting in three types of molecular species in the cell, each one with one of the three possible intramolecular disulfide bridges. It was postulated that only one of these forms may resemble the native conformation and retain biological activity. Both these possibilities could together result in the formation of inactive monomers and oligomers in the cell. If the sulfhydryls were responsible for the lower specific activity of the IFN-β protein, then removal of one of the cysteines would allow only one unique intramolecular disulfide bridge formation, leaving no free-sulfhydryl group to generate dimers or oligomers. Therefore, it was sought to eliminate one of the three cysteine residues by site-specific mutagenesis of the IFN-β gene, whereby one of the codons for cysteine is changed to that of serine. Serine was chosen as a replacement for cysteine because the two amino acids differ by only a single atom: the cysteine residue has a sulfur atom that is replaced by an oxygen atom in the serine residue. Cys-141 of the IFN-β molecule was known to be required for biological activity (Shepard *et al.*, 1981). By analogy with the IFN-α molecules in which a -S-S- bond is formed between Cys-29 and Cys-138 (Wetzel *et al.*, 1981), it was thought that the Cys-141 of IFN-β could be involved in a disulfide bridge with Cys-31, leaving a free and reactive thiol group on Cys-17. The Cys-17 residue was therefore chosen for replacement with serine. A schematic diagram showing the primary sequence of IFN-β_{ser17} is presented in Fig. 1.

The biological activities of IFN-β_{cys17} and IFN-β_{ser17} were compared in a virus yield reduction assay. The purified IFN-β_{cys17} had a specific antiviral activity of 3×10^7 units/mg. In contrast, the purified IFN-β_{ser17} exhibited a specific activity of 2×10^8 units/mg, comparable to that of purified native IFN-β (Derynick *et al.*, 1980). The biological activity of purified preparations of IFN-β_{cys17} and IFN-β_{ser17} were compared in a number of studies. Figure 2 illustrates the activity profile of the two IFN species stored at $-70°C$. The activity of IFN-β_{ser17} remained unchanged over a period of 150 days, while IFN-β_{cys17} lost a significant amount of its antiviral activity in 75 days. In addition, when these preparations were analyzed by nonreducing SDS-PAGE, a significant amount of dimers and oligomers could be detected in the IFN-β_{cys17} sample but not in the IFN-β_{ser17} preparation (Mark *et al.*, 1984). These data demonstrate that substitution of the cysteine residue at position 17 in the IFN-β with a serine residue prevents the formation of incorrect disulfide bonds resulting in a stable and bioactive rhIFN-β molecule. The IFN-β_{ser17} mutein was further developed as Betaseron® by Cetus Corporation, now Chiron Corporation in collaboration with Berlex Biosciences. The IFN-β_{ser17} molecule has been assigned an USAN name of IFN-β-1b.

Similar to the situation with human IFN-β, the Cys-31–141 disulfide bond is also important for biological activity of recombinant murine IFN-β synthesized in *E. coli* (Day *et al.*, 1992).

3. PRECLINICAL AND CLINICAL APPLICATIONS OF IFN-β

3.1. Preclinical Studies

The pharmacokinetics and antiviral activity of IFN-β_{ser17} (Betaseron®) were evaluated in an African green monkey model. This animal model has been successfully used for the evaluation of efficacy and pharmacokinetics of antiviral agents (Soike *et al.*, 1987, 1990). IFN-β_{ser17} was administered by the intravenous, intramuscular, and subcutaneous routes. Following i.v. administration, mean clearance, steady-state volume of distribution and terminal half-life values were 0.36 ± 0.08 liters/hr-kg, 0.65 ± 0.09 liters/kg, and 1.9 ± 0.43 hr, respectively. Bioavailability values for IFN-β_{ser17} delivered by the intramuscular and subcutaneous routes were determined to be 51% and 31%, respectively. Despite only 30–50% bioavailability by these non-i.v. routes, antiviral activity was comparable for i.v., i.m., and s.c. administration of 1×10^6 IU/kg of IFN-β_{ser17} twice daily (Chiang *et al.*, 1993). These studies also indicated that higher doses of the protein resulted in increases of the area under the serum concentration-time curve and of its antiviral efficacy. Finally, these studies demonstrated that significant accumulation of IFN-β_{ser17} in serum occurred with

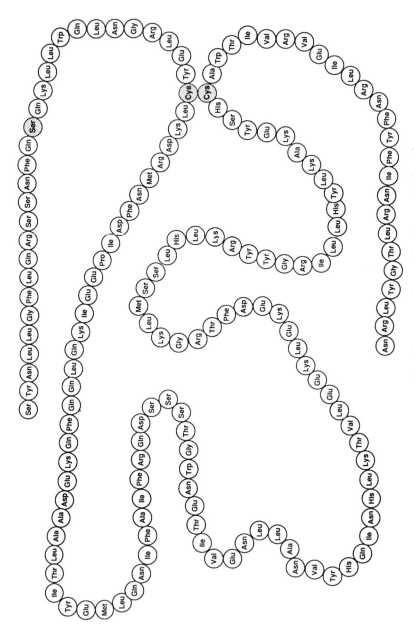

Figure 1. The primary amino acid sequence of recombinant human interferon-β_{ser17}.

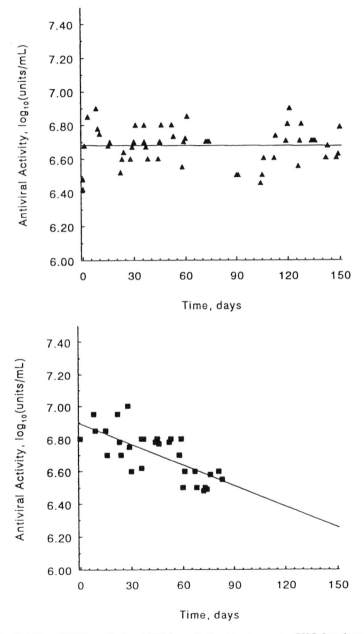

Figure 2. Stability of IFN-β$_{ser17}$ (top) and IFN-β$_{cys17}$ (bottom) to storage at $-70°C$. Interferon samples were thawed and the antiviral activities determined by a viral yield reduction bioassay at the indicated times. Each point represents the result of assays run in triplicate.

repeated twice-daily dosing and greatest antiviral efficacy of the molecule were observed under this dosing regimen.

3.2. Clinical Studies

Early clinical development of IFN-β, like other interferons, was directed toward its anticancer (Borden *et al.*, 1988, 1992; Quesada *et al.*, 1982; Reinhart, 1986) antiviral (Higgins *et al.*, 1986) and antiinfective indications (Schonfeld *et al.*, 1984). As for other indications, Jacobs *et al.* (1981) used natural IFN-β intrathecally in multiple sclerosis (MS) patients suspecting that the disease was caused by a viral infection. They reported a significant reduction in exacerbations experienced by the patients (Jacobs *et al.*, 1987). While the mechanism of action of IFN-β in MS is not fully understood, one or a combination of IFN-β activities, e.g., antiviral (Reder and Arnason, 1985), correction of deficient IFN secretion by immune cells (Neighbor and Bloom, 1979), reversal of the effects of IFN-γ (Fertsch *et al.*, 1987) and enhancement of suppressor T-cell function (Noronha *et al.*, 1990), have been implicated. A double-blind, dose-finding pilot study in subjects with relapsing-remitting MS showed that IFN-β_{ser17}, could be administered safely at a dose of 8 million IUs every other day, and demonstrated that treatment reduced the risk of exacerbations (Knobler *et al.*, 1993). A pivotal multicenter, randomized, double-blind, placebo-controlled trial of Betaseron® was conducted in 372 ambulatory patients with relapsing-remitting MS. The Betaseron® treatment caused significant reduction in exacerbation rates (compared to the placebo group), severity of exacerbations, and accumulation of magnetic resonance imaging abnormalities in the absence of serious side effects (IFNB Multiple Sclerosis Study Group, 1993; Patty *et al.*, 1993). Betaseron® (IFN-β_{ser17} or IFN-β-1b) is currently the only approved therapy in the United States for the treatment of relapsing-remitting multiple sclerosis.*

4. PHYSICOCHEMICAL CHARACTERISTICS OF IFN-β

4.1. Primary Structure

The primary structure of IFN-β_{ser17} was determined by amino acid composition, N-terminal amino acid sequencing, and peptide mapping.

---

*A second therapeutic, Interferon-β-1a (Avonex®, Biogen, Cambridge, MA) was approved by the FDA for the same indication in May 1996. Interferon-β-1a is a glycosylated version of the natural interferon-β.

Table I. Amino Acid Composition of Purified IFN-φ$_{ser-17}$

Residue	Hydrolysis time (hr) 24	48	72	Cumulative mean[a]	Predicted value from DNA sequence[b]
Asx	16.9	16.9	16.7	16.8 ± 0.5	17
Thr	7.2	7.1	6.8	7.0 ± 0.3	7
Ser	9.7	8.8	8.4	9.7 ± 0.3[c]	10
Glx	24.4	24.6	24.7	24.5 ± 0.7	24
Gly	6.3	6.4	6.4	6.3 ± 0.2	6
Ala	6.3	6.3	6.3	6.3 ± 0.2	6
Val	4.9	5.3	5.2	5.1 ± 0.2	5
Met	3.0	3.0	3.1	3.1 ± 0.2	3
Ile	10.2	10.7	10.7	10.7 ± 0.3[d]	11
Leu	24.6	24.6	24.6	24.6 ± 0.3	24
Tyr	9.9	9.8	9.9	9.9 ± 0.3	10
Phe	9.0	9.2	9.2	9.2 ± 0.4	9
Lys	10.6	10.7	11.1	10.8 ± 0.5	11
His	4.8	4.8	4.9	4.8 ± 0.2	5
Arg	11.1	10.9	11.1	11.0 ± 0.4	11
Trp	2.5	—	—	2.5 ± 0	3
Cys	2.0	—	—	2.0 ± 0.1[e]	2
Pro	1.0	—	—	1.0 ± 0.1	1

[a]The numbers representing the mean residues/molecule are averages from four separate hydrolysis series, each performed in duplicate. Cumulative mean values represent three hydrolysis times except where indicated. Uncertainties represent half the range of values averaged from cumulative mean.
[b]NH$_2$-terminal methionine omitted.
[c]24 hr values only.
[d]48 and 72 hr values only.
[e]Analyzed separately from the timed hydrolyses by performic acid oxidation.

4.1.1. AMINO ACID COMPOSITION

The primary amino acid sequence of IFN-β$_{ser17}$ consists of 165 amino acids. The amino acid composition was experimentally determined to be similar to that predicted from the DNA sequence. Table I presents these data.

4.1.2. N-TERMINAL AMINO ACID SEQUENCE

Purified IFN-β$_{ser17}$ was analyzed by N-terminal amino acid sequencing by subjecting it to automated Edman degradation in a Beckman Model 890M spinning-cup sequencer. The phenylthiohydantoin (PTH) amino acid derivatives formed in the instrument were identified using isocratic reversed-phase HPLC. These data, pre-

Table II. Partial Amino Acid Sequence of Purified IFN-β$_{ser-17}$

Residue number	Major residue	Yield (nmol)[a]	Minor residue	Yield (nmol)
1	Ser[b]	1.40		
2	Tyr	22.1		
3	Asn	13.9	Asp	0.91
4	Leu	17.0		
5	Leu	20.4		
6	Gly	14.8		
7	Phe	17.8		
8	Leu	15.4		
9	Gln	13.0	Glu	2.54
10	Arg	1.07		
11	Ser			
12	Ser			
13	Asn	6.46	Asp	0.51
14	Phe	9.05		
15	Gln	7.88	Glu	1.43
16	Ser			
17	Gln	6.94	Glu	1.72
18	Lys	2.31		
19	Leu	10.3		
20	Leu	10.2		
21	Trp	3.37		
22	Gln	4.54	Glu	2.11
23	Leu	9.93		
24	Asn	2.10	Asp	1.10
25	Gly	3.69		
26	Arg	1.94		
27	Leu	4.04		
28	Glu	4.37		
29	Tyr	4.17		
30	Cys[c]			

[a]A 35.7nmol sample of IFN-β$_{ser-17}$ was subjected to automated Edman degradation, and the PTH amino acids were analyzed by reverse-phase HPLC.
[b]Serine was recovered primarily as PTH-dehydroserine which could be detected at 313 nm.
[c]Cysteine was identified as PTH-cystine. Dehydroserine and cystine were not quantitated.

sented in Table II, indicate that the first 30 amino acids from the N-terminus yielded an amino acid sequence identical to the amino acid sequence (minus the methionine residue on the N-terminus) predicted by the DNA sequence of the IFN-β$_{ser17}$ gene. The N-terminal methionine of mature human IFN-β is used in *E. coli* as the initiation codon to direct the synthesis of the human protein. After initiation of translation, the N-terminal methionine is removed in *E. coli* by the enzyme methionine amino peptidase (MAP, Ben-Basset *et al.*, 1987). The removal of the N-terminal methionine from newly synthesized proteins by MAP is dependent on the identity of the penulti-mate residue and the biosynthetic rate of the recombinant protein. In the case of IFN-β$_{ser17}$ in the production strain used for manufacturing, the removal of amino

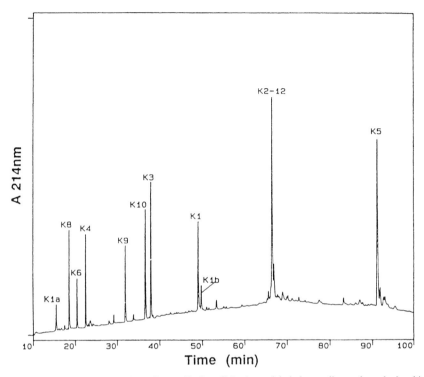

Figure 3.   Peptide map of IFN-β_{ser17} digested by Lys-C. Peaks are labeled according to the order in which the corresponding peptides occur in the IFN-β_{ser17} molecule (see Fig. 4). All expected peaks are displayed, with the exception of a tripeptide (K7) and a dipeptide (K11), which elute in the unretained peak from the RP-HPLC column. Two additional peaks, "K1a" and "K1b," resulting from cleavage of Arg_{11} and Ser_{12} bond, are seen as well.

terminal methionine is very efficient, resulting in IFN-β_{ser17} with a homogeneous amino terminal albeit one residue less than that predicted by the DNA sequence.

4.1.3. PEPTIDE MAPPING

The entire amino acid sequence of IFN-β_{ser17} was determined by peptide mapping using lysyl endopeptidase Lys-C. The Lys-C peptide map in conjunction with other protein fragmentation methods provided overlapping amino acid sequences for the entire IFN-β_{ser17} molecule. The results obtained provided the entire sequence of the IFN-β_{ser17} molecule and is identical to that predicted by the DNA sequence. Figure 3 shows a typical peptide map of this molecule.

Figure 4 displays the sequence of IFN-β_{ser17} showing the cleavage sites of Lys-C. Amino acid analysis, amino acid sequence analysis, and mass spectrometry of the peptides generated by Lys-C digestion confirmed that the generated peptide fragments were identical to those predicted.

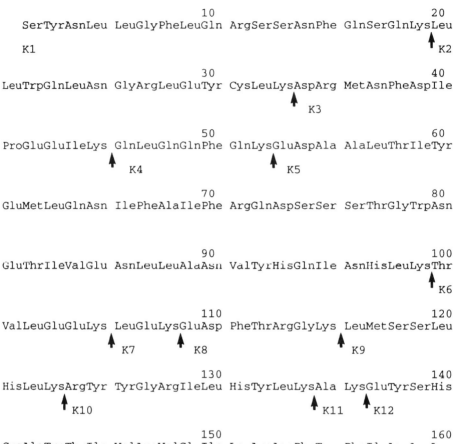

```
                        10                                      20
   SerTyrAsnLeu LeuGlyPheLeuGln ArgSerSerAsnPhe GlnSerGlnLysLeu
   K1                                                          ↑ K2

                        30                                      40
   LeuTrpGlnLeuAsn GlyArgLeuGluTyr CysLeuLysAspArg MetAsnPheAspIle
                                         ↑ K3

                        50                                      60
   ProGluGluIleLys GlnLeuGlnGlnPhe GlnLysGluAspAla AlaLeuThrIleTyr
                  ↑ K4           ↑ K5

                        70                                      80
   GluMetLeuGlnAsn IlePheAlaIlePhe ArgGlnAspSerSer SerThrGlyTrpAsn

                        90                                      100
   GluThrIleValGlu AsnLeuLeuAlaAsn ValTyrHisGlnIle AsnHisLeuLysThr
                                                              ↑ K6

                        110                                     120
   ValLeuGluGluLys LeuGluLysGluAsp PheThrArgGlyLys LeuMetSerSerLeu
                  ↑ K7           ↑ K8                 ↑ K9

                        130                                     140
   HisLeuLysArgTyr TyrGlyArgIleLeu HisTyrLeuLysAla LysGluTyrSerHis
               ↑ K10                               ↑ K11    ↑ K12

                        150                                     160
   CysAlaTrpThrIle ValArgValGluIle LeuArgAsnPheTyr PheIleAsnArgLeu
```

ThrGlyTyrLeuArg Asn

Figure 4.   Amino acid sequence of IFN-β_{ser17} showing sites of proteolysis by Lys-C. Residues are numbered as in native IFN-β. Lys-C cleavage sites are indicated by bold arrows. Names of the theoretical fragments generated by Lys-C proteolysis appear beneath the sequence near their N-terminal ends.

4.2. Secondary and Tertiary Structure

4.2.1. CD AND NMR SPECTROSCOPY

Utsumi *et al.* (1986) examined the conformation of fibroblast IFN-β (glycosy-lated) and *E. coli*–derived IFN-β (nonglycosylated) by circular dichroism (CD) and ^{1}H nuclear magnetic resonance spectroscopy. The two interferon preparations were studied by the CD and NMR methods in an acidic pH environment (pH 4.6 to

1.6) due to good solubility and stability of IFN under these conditions. The CD spectra indicated that both IFN-βs had approximately 70% α-helix content. The data indicated that fibroblast IFN-β and *E. coli*–derived IFN-β have very similar secondary structures, thus demonstrating that the lack of glycosylation of the recombinant molecule did not alter the secondary structure of the protein. Moreover, a slow conformational change was observed below pH 2.0 which was thought to induce the disruption of β-sheets. NMR analysis were used to study the folding of IFN-β and the two spectra showed that both fibroblast and recombinant IFN-β molecules possess characteristic features of globular proteins. The NMR data also confirmed the low-β-sheet content of IFN-β.

Boublik *et al.* (1990) recently examined the relationship between the conformation and antiviral activity of *E. coli*–derived rIFN-β. The extent of ordered secondary structure was determined by CD spectroscopy in various buffer conditions. In contrast to the work of Utsumi *et al.* described above, they reported α-helical content of 40% to 50% in the pH range 2.9 to 7.2. At pH 2.9, IFN-β exhibited maximum stability to heat denaturation and highest antiviral activity. It was found that both helicity and antiviral activity of the IFN-β decrease in parallel with denaturation by urea, heat, or repeated freeze-thaw cycles. These authors also displayed the primary structure of rIFN-β in the form of a two-dimensional helical surface. Using a computer program, the potential for helix formation was calculated based on the knowledge of the primary structure. Using this model, the α-helical content of hIFN-β was estimated to be approximately 35%.

Acharya *et al.* (1985) compared the conformations of IFN-β$_{cys17}$ and IFN-β$_{ser17}$ by CD spectroscopy to assess whether the single amino acid substitution induces significant secondary structure changes. The studies were performed in the presence of 0.1% sodium dodecyl sulfate (SDS) at neutral pH. SDS was added to render the proteins soluble under these conditions. Both recombinant variants of IFN-β exhibited essentially the same CD spectra, consisting of approximately 35% to 40% α-helical content. These data on α-helix content of IFN-β$_{ser17}$ and IFN-β$_{cys17}$ were in good agreement with that obtained by Boublik *et al.* (1990) for rIFN-β and the value estimated for native human IFN-β.

The far-ultraviolet CD spectrum of IFN-β$_{ser17}$ is presented in Fig. 5. This shows α-helical content of 45% with the rest being β-sheet.

4.2.2. FLUORESCENCE SPECTROSCOPY

Fluorescence spectroscopy has successfully been used to characterize conformational properties of IFN-α (Vincent *et al.*, 1992) and other proteins (Poklar *et al.*, 1994). The IFN-β molecule has three tryptophan residues which are located at positions 22, 79, and 143 in the sequence. The fluorescence emission maximum of IFN-β under physiological pH conditions occurs at 338 nm. In contrast, free tryptophan under identical conditions exhibits an emission maximum at 351 nm. These data indicate that the tryptophan residues within the IFN-β molecule resides in a highly hydrophobic environment (Borukhov and Strongin, 1990). Moreover, the emission

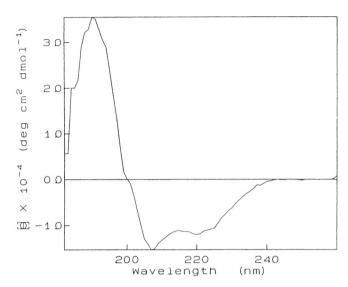

Figure 5. A representative far-ultraviolet circular dichroism spectrum of IFN-β_{ser17}.

maximum of IFN-β in its fully unfolded form (in 7 M guanidine hydrochloride) was seen at 352 nm. Further, the microenvironment of the tryptophan residues was studied in aqueous solutions at pH 2.0, 7.2, and 8.5 with KI, CsCl, and acrylamide as anionic, cationic, and neutral charge contact quenchers (Lehrer and Leavis, 1978). From these data, it was inferred that two of the three tryptophan residues of IFN-β were located near the surface of the protein. By analogy to IFN-α, tryptophan residues 22 and 143 would be expected to reside near the surface.

5. ANALYTICAL METHODS FOR EVALUATION OF PROTEIN PURITY

Besides structural information, the purity of the therapeutic protein under question is an important parameter before it is deemed suitable for use as a pharmaceutical product. The purity of the protein must also be assessed to evaluate its stability and for assignment of a shelf life to the product. Several analytical methods are used for this purpose; the primary among them being based on electrophoretic and chromatographic techniques.

5.1. SDS-PAGE

SDS-PAGE has widely been used for characterizing the purity of both native and recombinant forms of IFN-β. This method was first employed for detection of dimers, trimers, and higher oligomers of *E. coli*–derived IFN-β_{cys17} (Colby *et al.*, 1986; Lin *et al.*, 1986; Mark *et al.*, 1984). Visualization of gels was facilitated either by staining with Coomassie Brilliant Blue dye stain or Fast Green dyes or by an anti-IFN-β monoclonal antibody after transfer on a nitrocellulose paper (Western blots). The nonreduced SDS-PAGE is capable of showing dimers, trimers, and higher oligomers. In SDS-PAGE of IFN-β samples subjected to stress by placement at high temperatures, oligomers are observed. For example, a sample of IFN-β_{ser17} (1.2 mg/ml in 50 mM sodium acetate, 10 mg SDS, 2 mM EDTA, pH 5.5) formed approximately 30% oligomers after placement at 37°C for 3 months (Geigert *et al.*, 1988). Figure 6 shows a representative densitometric scan of SDS-PAGE analysis of a reduced sample. The reduced samples exhibit only dimers and some low-molecular-weight fragments. Since the dimers are present in reduced samples, it is likely that these dimers are not linked by disulfide bonds.

5.2. Isoelectric Focusing (IEF)

The IEF method is useful for separation and visualization of charge variants of IFN-β. Utsumi *et al.* (1987) compared the IEF profiles of fibroblast IFN-β and *E. coli* produced rIFN-β on silver stained gels. Whereas fibroblast IFN-β exhibited three distinct bands with pI of 8.9 ± 0.1, 8.6 ± 0.1, and 7.8 ± 0.1, the rIFN-β showed a single, trailing band at pI of 8.9 ± 0.1. The heterogeneity in the fibroblast preparation is ascribed to the presence of varying amounts of sialic acid on the carbohydrate moiety of the molecule. All three variants possessed antiviral activities. The trailing

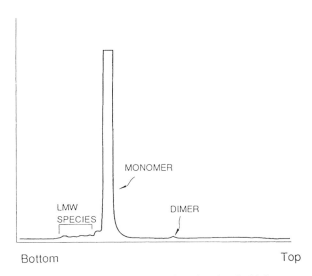

Figure 6. SDS-PAGE gel scan of reduced IFN-β_{ser17}. Sample reduced with 2-mercaptoethanol was run on a 12–15% linear gradient polyacrylamide gel, stained with Fast Green and scanned at 625 nm.

of the rhIFN-β band is presumably due to hydrophobic interaction between the protein and the acrylamide gel. IFN-β_{ser17} was electrofocused using the nonionic surfactant polyoxyethylene-12-lauryl ether (Laureth 12) to maintain the IFN-β_{ser17} solubility (Hershenson and Thomson, 1989). Because of the difficulties in calibrating IEF gels in the highly basic range (>pH 9), the pI for IFN-β_{ser17} was initially assigned by Hershenson as 9.6–9.7. Later, a more accurate calibration of the IEF gel was made, and a pI of 9.2 ± 0.1 was assigned.

5.3. RP-HPLC

Utsumi *et al.* (1987) reported the RP-HPLC profiles of fibroblast IFN-β and *E. coli*–derived IFN-β. They observed that the recombinant IFN-β was retained longer on the column than the fibroblast IFN-β, indicating that the former was more hydrophobic than the latter.

A representative RP-HPLC chromatogram of IFN-β_{ser17} is shown in Fig. 7. The second peak to elute (peak B) from the column represents the main IFN-β_{ser17} species. The first peak is known as peak A. Peak B can be converted to peak A under conditions specific for oxidation of methionines in proteins, suggesting that peak A is an IFN-β_{ser17} variant containing an oxidized methionine. Site-specific mutation was used to produce IFN-β_{ser17} analogues in which alanine was substituted for methio-

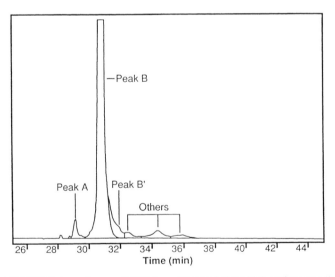

Figure 7. A RP-HPLC chromatogram of IFN-β_{ser17}. Reversed-phase high-performance liquid chromatography was conducted using a Vydac C_4 column. A gradient of 10% acetonitrile in 0.1% trifluoroacetic acid (TFA) to 100% acetonitrile in 0.1% TFA was used, and the elution was monitored by ultraviolet absorption at 214 nm.

nine at 36, 62, and 117 positions, respectively. Results of RP-HPLC analysis of the methionine analogues after chemical oxidation inferred that peak A contains an oxidized methionine at amino acid position 62. This was confirmed by peptide mapping of a Lys-C digest of isolated peak A.

The shoulder on the main peak, peak B′, was isolated by collecting fractions from the eluted column and thoroughly analyzed. The two isolated species had equivalent specific activities, IEF profiles, ELISA antibody responses, and peptide maps. These results indicated that peak B′ consists of a different conformational form(s) of IFN-β_{ser17} having a primary structure identical to that of peak B but resolvable by RP-HPLC.

The peaks eluting after peak B′ are mainly oligomeric forms of the IFN-β protein. These oligomers are primarily SDS-dissociable as they are not seen in the SDS-PAGE analysis (Geigert *et al.*, 1988).

6. *IN VITRO* BIOLOGICAL ACTIVITY OF IFN-β

The potency of IFN-β preparations are measured by *in vitro* biological activity assays. These assays are also important for assigning a shelf life for final commercial preparations and reference materials (Geigert *et al.*, 1988).

6.1. Antiviral Yield Reduction Assay

For measuring the antiviral activity of IFN-β, a virus yield reduction assay is employed. IFN-β containing samples are first added to GM2504 fibroblast cell for 24 hr at 37°C in a 7% CO_2 atmosphere. The cells are infected with 10^6 pfu of vesicular stomatitis virus (VSV) and incubated for 50 min. The cells are rinsed with Dulbecco's modified Eagle's medium to remove unadsorbed VSV and further incubated at 37°C for 24 hr in a 7% CO_2 atmosphere. The reduction in virus production as a result of the added IFN-β was measured in a plaquing assay by transferring the supernatant and adding to baby hamster kidney cells followed by incubation for 60 min. The number of plaques is inversely proportional to IFN-β activity. A standard curve is generated using a reference preparation of IFN-β from which the activity of an unknown IFN-β sample is determined. The potency of IFN-β_{ser17} in the yield reduction assay was found to be equivalent to that reported for native human IFN-β.

6.2. Cytopathic Effect Bioassay

A second assay that is used for measuring the potency of IFN-β preparations is based on the ability of IFN-β to inhibit viral cytopathic effects (Grossberg *et al.*,

1985). In this assay, IFN-β induced protection of A549 human lung carcinoma cells from infection with encaphlomyocarditis virus (ECV) is measured by a colorimetric method based on the ability of viable cells to reduce a dye 3-(4,5-dimethylthiazol-2-yl)-2,5-diphenyltetrazolium bromide (or MTT). Samples containing IFN-β are serially diluted and then A549 human lung carcinoma cells added. A dose-dependent antiviral state is induced in the cells by the interferon and the cells subsequently infected with ECV and IFN-β-induced cell protection measured by a spectrophotometric assay utilizing the MTT stain. The mitochondrial enzymes in viable cells reduce MTT to a dark blue formazan product which exhibits peak absorbance around 580 nm after solubilization with an alcohol/detergent solution (Mossman, 1983). Potency of IFN-β samples are determined relative to the National Institute of Health recombinant IFN-β reference material which is included on each assay plate. An interassay precision of approximately 15% has been recorded for this assay. Betaseron potency determined using the CPE assay is equivalent to potency obtained using the antiviral yield reduction assay.

7. FORMULATION STUDIES

7.1. Solubility Aspects

7.1.1. SOLUBILITY OF IFN-β_{ser17}

One major challenge with *E. coli*–derived IFN-β, partly due to it being unglycosylated, is its strongly hydrophobic character. This property of IFN-β is encountered time and again during its production and analyses. Lin *et al.*, (1986) report that IFN-β_{ser17} can be solubilized at neutral pH in the presence of surfactants such as 0.1% SDS or chaotropic agents such as 4 M guanidine hydrochloride at concentrations in the range 1–5 mg/ml. The ready solubility of IFN-β in SDS-containing solutions has been utilized throughout the purification procedure described by Lin and co-workers. Hershenson and Thomson (1989) reported the use of a nonionic surfactant (Laureth 12) for solubilizing IFN-β_{ser17} for the purpose of running an IEF gel on the protein. Utsumi *et al.* (1987) described the hydrophobicity of the *E. coli*–derived IFN-β based on longer retention of the recombinant molecule on the RP-HPLC column as compared to the retention of the fibroblast human IFN-β.

The rIFN-β_{ser17} protein is sparingly soluble (<0.05 mg/ml) at neutral pH on its own. The protein is fairly soluble (at approximately 1 mg/ml concentrations) at acidic pHs (pH 3 and below) or strongly alkaline pHs (pH 10 and above). The low solubility of this protein in the absence of stabilizers is most likely due to its hydrophobic nature. The protein tends to precipitate out due to protein–protein aggregate formation presumably through hydrophobic interactions at neutral or near-neutral pHs in the absence of solubilizing agents. These aggregates are "reversible" as they are rendered soluble again by readdition of a solubilizer such as 0.1% SDS (Fernandes and Taforo, 1991). These data are similar to the results obtained for human fibroblast IFN-β by Utsumi *et al.* (1989). These authors reported that IFN-β formed predominantly tetrameric aggregates through hydrophobic interaction which were dissociable by 1% SDS or 1% lithium dodecyl sulfate (LDS). These tetramers were seen by size-exclusion chromatography but migrated as monomers on SDS-PAGE. Moreover, tetramers retained only 10% of the biological activity displayed by the IFN-β monomeric form but retained full activity upon 1% SDS addition.

While solubility of IFN-β in other solvent systems has not been studied in a systematic manner, selected reports present such information in an indirect way. Thus, Utsumi *et al.* (1987) used a 100 μg/ml solution of *E. coli*–derived rIFN-β in a 10 mM sodium phosphate buffer (pH 6.8) containing 0.5 M NaCl and 40% ethylene glycol. In the same report, the authors describe the use of a 2 mg/mL rIFN-β solution in 10 mM sodium phosphate buffer prepared with deuterium oxide (pD 6.8) containing 0.5 M NaCl and 40% perdeuterated ethylene glycol for NMR studies. In agreement with these data, Boublik *et al.* (1990) used 0.5 mg/ml solutions of *E. coli*–derived IFN-β in 50% ethylene glycol, 1 M NaCl, and 50 mM sodium phosphate (pH 7.2) for their studies. Solutions of 50 μg/ml rIFN-β were also prepared in 50% ethylene glycol in a citric acid–sodium phosphate buffer (pH 2.9) and ammonium acetate–NaCl buffer (pH 5.1) for CD spectral studies. Boublik *et al.* also reported that ethylene glycol had strong cryoprotective and helix-promoting effects on IFN-β and that IFN-β was fully active in these systems. These studies demonstrate that rIFN-β has reasonable solubility in 40–50% ethylene glycol perhaps in the presence of 0.5 to 1 molar NaCl. No information regarding solubility of IFN-β in glycerol, propylene glycol, and polyethylene glycol exists currently.

7.1.2. SOLUBILITY-ENHANCING STRATEGIES USED FOR IFN-β$_{ser17}$

rIFN-β$_{ser17}$ is readily soluble under physiological pH conditions in the presence of the anionic surfactant SDS. Reference preparations of IFN-β$_{ser17}$ in 0.1% SDS are described by Geigert *et al.* (1988). The minimum concentration of SDS required for solubility of 1 mg of IFN-β$_{ser17}$ at pH 7.0 was found to be approximately 660 μg. The amount of SDS needed for IFN-β$_{ser17}$ solubility could be reduced to 175 μg/mg of the protein by addition of 1 mg of a nonionic surfactant polysorbate-80 (Durafax-80, Durkee Chemicals). These data indicate that SDS is a more effective solubilizer for IFN-β$_{ser17}$ than polysorbate-80. These results are in excellent agreement with data from Utsumi *et al.* (1989), who reported that SDS and LDS are effective solubilizers for rIFN-β.

A number of nonionic surfactants were evaluated for solubilization of this hydrophobic protein (Shaked *et al.*, 1993). The solubility of IFN-β$_{ser17}$ was evaluated using an ultracentrifugation assay. In this assay, recovery of the IFN-β$_{ser17}$ protein in the supernatant of a test solution at a given protein concentration (usually 250 to

500 μg/ml) after subjecting it to ultracentrifugation at 35,000 g for 1 hr at ambient temperature was measured. A recovery value of 80% protein in the supernatant was considered as an evidence of good solubility by this test. While this method does not provide the absolute maximum solubility of a protein in the test solution, it is useful for measuring solubility of the protein under rigorous conditions. In addition, it is a valuable tool for screening effective solubilizers for a given protein concentration and has often been used as such in the biochemical literature (Schein, 1990). A large number of nonionic surfactants were evaluated to aid solubilization of IFN-β_{ser17} (Hershenson *et al.*, 1989). Selected results from the ultracentrifugation screening are shown in Fig. 8.

Four formulations of IFN-β_{ser17}, containing surfactants such as Laureth 12 (trade name Trycol LAL12), an oxyalkylated alcohol (trade name Plurafac C-17), octoxynol-30 (trade name Triton X305), polyethylene glycol-8-oleate (trade name Nopalcol 4-O), or their mixtures were selected for further optimization studies (described next) based on the visual clarity, UV absorption, and ultracentrifugation data. A complete

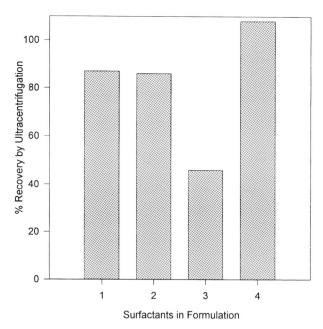

Figure 8.   Comparison of four surfactant systems for formulation of IFN-β_{ser17}. Formulations containing 0.25 mg/mL IFN-β_{ser17} in 10 mM sodium phosphate and one of the following surfactant(s): 0.15% laureth-12 (1), 0.10% oxyalkylated alcohol (Plurafac C-17), (2) a combination of 0.10% octoxynol-30 and 0.05% PEG-8-oleate (3) or a combination of 0.10% laureth-12 and 0.05% PEG-8-oleate (4) were evaluated by the ultracentrifugation assay. Individual bars show the recovery of IFN-β_{ser17} in the top half of the solution after centrifugation at 35,000 g for 1 hr by A_{280} measurements.

cross-reference of generic and trade names of these surfactants is available (Ash and Ash, 1993). A comparison of buffers indicated that for lyophilized IFN-β_{serl7} formulations, sodium phosphate was better for maintaining solubility of the protein upon reconstitution than sodium citrate and sodium maleate buffers. It was also surmised by Hershenson *et al.* (1989) that pH change caused by the well-known crystallization of the disodium phosphate component of the phosphate buffer during freezing may have helped in preserving the solubility of IFN-β_{serl7}.

For maintaining solubility of IFN-β_{serl7} after lyophilization, formulations with potential bulking agents were evaluated by the ultracentrifugation assay. The data, shown in Fig. 9, indicate that dextrose or a combination of dextrose and mannitol were suitable for this purpose while dextran, mannitol, or a dextrose/glycine mixture were unable to preserve solubility of IFN-β_{serl7} upon reconstitution (Hershenson *et al.*, 1989).

Finally, carrier proteins, such as human serum albumin (HSA) and plasma protein fraction (PPF), have also been found to be useful for rendering the IFN-β_{serl7}

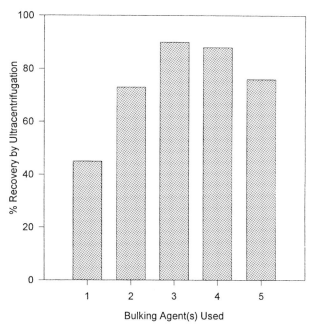

Figure 9. Effect of different bulking agents on the solubility of IFN-β_{serl7} upon reconstitution of the freeze-dried product. Formulations contained IFN-β_{serl7} (0.25 mg/ml) in 0.15% laureth-12 and 10 mM sodium phosphate buffer (pH 7) and one of the following bulking agents: 2.0% dextran (1), 2.0% mannitol (2), 2.0% dextrose (3), a combination of 0.1% dextrose and 2.0% mannitol (4) or a combination of 0.1% dextrose and 2.0% glycine (5). Individual bars show the recovery of IFN-β_{serl7} in the top half of the solution after ultracentrifugation at 35,000 g for 1 hr.

soluble under physiological pH conditions (Fernandes and Taforo, 1991). IFN-β_{ser17} could be solubilized by adding HSA to a 1:50 weight/weight (wt/wt) ratio. Formulations at 1 mg/ml IFN-β_{ser17} concentration were prepared using the 1:50 IFB-β_{ser17} ratio. PPF, which consists of 83% HSA and a maximum of 17% globulins (α- and β-), was also shown to solubilize IFN-β_{ser17} at similar wt/wt ratios. Solubilization of IFN-β_{ser17} in HSA and PPF solutions is thought to occur via interaction between the hydrophobic segments of IFN-β_{ser17} and HSA.

7.2. Parenteral Formulations of IFN-β_{ser17}

A recombinant form of IFN-β, interferon-β-1b or IFN-β_{ser17} (Betaseron®, a product of Chiron Corporation), is available commercially in the United States since 1993. Betaseron® is supplied as a lyophilized powder consisting of 0.25 mg of interferon-β-1b and contains 12.5 mg each of human serum albumin and dextrose. Appropriate amounts of sodium hydroxide and hydrochloric acid may have been used for adjustment of pH of the solution to 7.5. A diluent vial containing 0.54% sodium chloride is supplied along with Betaseron®. This concentration of sodium chloride yields an isotonic solution upon reconstitution of lyophilized Betaseron® as directed in the package insert. Each vial of Betaseron® is reconstituted with 1.2 ml of the supplied diluent and 1.0 ml of the reconstituted solution is injected subcutaneously by patients for the treatment of relapsing-remitting multiple sclerosis (Betaseron, Physician Desk Reference, 1995).

7.3. Long-Acting Formulations of IFN-β_{ser17}

Considerable research has been done to prolong the *in vivo* delivery of IFN-β_{ser17}. To enhance solubility and *in vivo* half-life of the recombinant molecule, it was modified by attachment of water-soluble polymers such as polyethylene glycol (PEG) and polyoxyethylene glycol (POG) (Katre and Knauf, 1990). Attachment with such polymers has successfully been used for altering the hydrodynamic radius of the resulting PEG–protein yielding a product with a desired *in vivo* half-life (Knauf *et al.*, 1988). The solubility of IFN-β_{ser17} could be greatly enhanced by PEG-attachment while maintaining the bioactivity of IFN-β. Similarly, the *in vivo* half-life of IFN-β_{ser17} was enhanced severalfold by the modification (Katre and Knauf, 1990).

Liposomal formulations of IFN-β have also been evaluated. Felgner and Epstein (1985) described a liposomal formulation of IFN-β_{ser17} made by hydrating a lyophilized mixture of multilamellar vesicles with an IFN-β_{ser17} solution. The encapsulated IFN-β retained full antiviral activity. The controlled release of IFN-β_{ser17} from this system was demonstrated in a mouse model after intramuscular injection. In control animals, free IFN-β_{ser17} disappeared from the injection site in 1 day while IFN-β_{ser17}

from liposomes was maintained at the injection site up to 9 days. In a subsequent study, this formulation was tested in a Simian *Varicella* virus infected African green monkey model (Eppstein *et al.*, 1989). It was observed that intramuscularly injected liposomal IFN-β_{ser17} resulted in a sustained release of the IFN-β from the injection site. Finally, the liposomal preparation exerted antiviral efficacy in the primate model superior to that obtained with the identical dosing regimen of free IFN-β_{ser17}.

The biodegradable polylactide-*co*-glycolide (PLG) polymer system has also been used for the controlled release of rIFN-β_{ser17} (Eppstein and Schryver, 1990). The protein was incorporated in the PLG matrix by a spray-casting technique. Prior to the encapsulation process, the IFN-β_{ser17} was spiked with a small amount of radiolabeled (^{125}I-IFN-β_{ser17}). No loss in the antiviral activity of IFN-β_{ser17} was seen by the process of encapsulation. Hollow cylindrical devices of PLG containing IFN-β_{ser17} films (300 μ thick, 5 mm long with ~0.5 mm external diameter) were sterilized by gamma irradiation and implanted subcutaneously in mice. No information on the effect of gamma irradiation on the integrity of encapsulated protein was provided in the report. The devices were removed surgically at periodic intervals and assayed for remaining radioactivity. Release of IFN-β_{ser17} was extended over a period of approximately 70 days.

8. STABILITY OF IFN-β

8.1. Stability-Indicating Assays

Several stability-indicating methodologies for IFN-β are available. The choice of the method depends upon the nature of the formulation. In formulations containing a carrier protein such as albumin, the normal methods used for the protein-purity analyses of IFN-β can be difficult because of interference from the carrier protein. In such cases, methods based on immunological detection of IFN-β are employed. Thus, enzyme-linked immunosorbent assays (ELISAs) based on monoclonal antibodies raised against the rhIFN-β molecule are used for quantification of IFN-β in the presence of a carrier protein. Similarly, the SDS-PAGE gels used for evaluation of oligomers and fragments of the IFN-β protein, are visualized by monoclonal antibodies after transfer to a nitrocellulose paper in the Western blot format. A common limitation of the immunological methods is that they can only detect only certain epitopes on the molecule.

In formulations utilizing no carrier protein, the regular SDS-PAGE method has been applied for detection and quantitation of oligomers and fragments of the IFN-β_{ser17} protein (Geigert *et al.*, 1988). Additionally, the RP-HPLC method has been used which is capable of tracking increases in the oxidized methionine form as well as oligomers of IFN-β. Based on RP-HPLC data of IFN-β_{ser17} formulated in the absence of a carrier protein, no increase in the oxidized methionine IFN-β_{ser17} peak was observed even after placement at 37°C for 3 months. By RP-HPLC, only oligomer formation was observed in the IFN-β_{ser17} product. These oligomers were not seen by the SDS-PAGE method, indicating that the oligomers were SDS-dissociable.

8.2. Stability of IFN-β_{ser17}

As expected, stability of IFN-β_{ser17} is a function of the formulation parameters. In the noncarrier protein solution formulation of IFN-β_{ser17} (per milliliter composition: 1.2 mg IFN-β_{ser17}, 10 mg SDS in 50 mM sodium acetate and 2 mM EDTA, pH 5.5) described by Geigert *et al.* (1988), an Arrhenius fit of the data was attempted. Based on the SDS-PAGE and RP-HPLC data, a t_{90} (i.e., time to reach 90% IFN purity) of 7 years was predicted at 5°C (2–8°C). An activation energy of 24 kcal/mole was reported for the rate of IFN-β degradation.

In IFN-β_{ser17} formulations containing human serum albumin as a solubilizing and stabilizing agent, the biological potency of IFN-β_{ser17} was reported during storage of the lyophilized product at 5°C (Geigert *et al.*, 1987). While no changes in the potency of the three subject formulations were observed at 5°C over 2 years, temperature-dependent decreases in this parameter were observed at elevated temperatures (25, 37, 55, 75, and 80°C). Based on the elevated temperature data, an activation energy of 25 kcal/mole was obtained.

Figure 10 presents data on the stability of the Betaseron® product as measured by its biological potency.

IFN-β_{ser17} formulations have also been evaluated by linear nonisothermal stability (LNS) studies (Geigert *et al.*, 1987; Jameson *et al.*, 1979). In this method, lyophilized IFN-β_{ser17} formulations were heated from 50°C to 80°C at a linear rate of 1.5°C/hr and samples were withdrawn at pre-determined set points and analyzed for biological potency. This method is best used for comparing different formulations within a short time frame. For example, Geigert *et al.* (1987) evaluated three slightly different IFN-β_{ser17} formulations based on HSA. The three formulations contained 0.06, 0.30, and 1.20 mg of IFN-β_{ser17} with 15, 15, and 60 mg of HSA, respectively; and each formulation used 15 mg dextrose as a bulking agent. All formulations contained ≤1% moisture by weight at the start of the study. Formulation containing the highest amount of HSA showed maximal stability by the real-time, multiple isothermal, and LNS studies demonstrating the usefulness of this technique for comparative purposes.

Lyophilized formulations of IFN-β_{ser17} based on the surfactant Laureth 12 were analyzed by the LNS method (Fig. 11). An HSA-based formulation was used as a control in this study as a relative relationship of stability indicated by the real-time and LNS studies had already been established for this formulation. IFN-β_{ser17} formu-

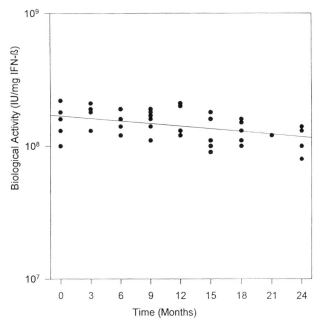

Figure 10. Potency stability of Betaseron® at 5°C. Stability of six different batches of IFN-β$_{ser17}$ formulated with human serum albumin as measured by the virus yield reduction biological activity assay as a function of the time of incubation under refrigeration conditions. The potency in international units per milligram of the IFN-β protein on a logarithmic scale on the *y*-axis and the time of incubation at 5°C on the *x*-axis are shown.

lations containing Laureth 12 with either dextrose or dextrose/mannitol appear to have potency stability characteristics similar to that of the HSA formulation of IFN-β$_{ser17}$.

9. CONCLUSIONS

In this chapter, we have attempted to provide a brief historical perspective on the development of human recombinant interferon beta, with a special emphasis on the research and development of Betaseron®, a recombinant human IFN-β, as a therapeutic protein drug. Brief summaries of the molecular biology and protein chemistry of IFN-β and its preclinical and clinical evaluations are presented to familiarize the reader with the complexity of the drug development process as it applies to therapeutic protein molecules.

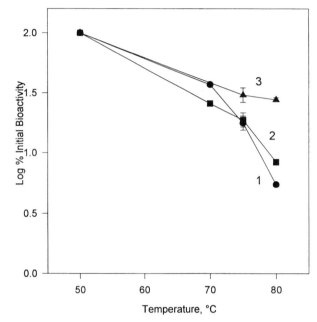

Figure 11. Stability comparison of three different formulations of IFN-β_{ser17} by linear nonisothermal studies. IFN-β_{ser17} formulations (0.25 mg/ml) containing 1.25% HSA and 1.25% dextrose (1), 0.15% laureth-12 and 5% dextrose (2), or 0.15% laureth-12 and 5% mannitol (3) are compared. The *x*-axis represents the temperature at which the IFN-β sample was withdrawn during linear nonisothermal heating and the *y*-axis shows the biological potency of the sample measured by the yield reduction bioassay and represented as the logarithmic of the initial value.

Betaseron® was one of the first few recombinant protein drugs to be tested in human clinical trials at the time when the recombinant DNA technology was at its infancy. We have described to the reader some of the difficulties that were encountered during its development, especially due to the strong hydrophobic nature of the molecule. We have presented the important physicochemical properties of this protein and a description of the analytical methods used for defining its purity. Finally, IFN-β formulations and their stability have been discussed.

ACKNOWLEDGMENTS. The authors would like to thank the many people from Chiron and Berlex who have worked on development of Betaseron® from its inception to the present time. This important therapy would not have been available to multiple sclerosis patients without their hard work and dedication.

REFERENCES

Acharya, A. S., Manjula, B. N., and Drummond, R. J., 1985, Conformational analysis of human fibroblast interferon cloned and expressed in *E. coli* poster presented at FASEB Meeting, Anaheim, CA.

Arabje, Y. M., Bittner, G., Yingling, J. M., Storer, B., and Schiller, J. H., 1993, Antiproliferative effects of interferons -α and -β in combination with 5-fluorouracil, cisplatin and *cis-* and *trans*-retinoic acid in three human lung carcinoma cell lines, *J. Interferon Res.* **13**:25–32.

Ash, M., and Ash, I. 1993, *Handbook of Industrial Surfactants*, Gower, Hants, UK.

Ben-Bassat, A., Bauer, K., Chang, S.-Y., Myabo, K., Boosman, A., and Chang, S., 1987, Processing of the initiation methionine from proteins: Properties of the *Escherichia coli* methionine aminopeptidase and its gene structure, *J. Bacteriol.* **169**:751–757.

Betaseron, 1995, *Physician Desk Reference*, pp. 622–626.

Borden, E. C., Hawkins, M. J., Sielaff, K. M., Storer, B. M., Schiesel, J. D., and Smalley, R. V., 1988, Clinical and biological effects of recombinant interferon-β administered intravenously daily in phase I trial, *J. Interferon Res.* **8**:357–366.

Borden, E. C., Kim, K., Ryan, L., Blum, R. H., Shiraki, M., Tormey, D. C., Comis, R. L., Hahn, R. G., and Parkinson, D. R., 1992, Phase II trials of interferons-α and -β in advanced sarcomas, *J. Interferon Res.* **12**:455–458.

Borukhov, S. I., and Strongin, A. Y., 1990, The intrinsic fluorescence of the recombinant human leukocyte interferon-αA and fibroblast-β1, *Biochem. Biophys. Res. Comm.* **169**:282–288.

Boublik, M., Moschera, J. A., Wei, C., and Kung, H., 1990, Conformation and activity of recombinant human fibroblast interferon-β, *J. Interferon Res.* **10**:213–219.

Chiang, J., Gloff, C. A., Soike, K. F., and Williams, G., 1993, Pharmacokinetics and antiviral activity of recombinant human IFN-β$_{ser17}$ in African green monkeys, *J. Interferon Res.* **13**:111–120.

Colby, C. B., Geigert, J. H., Ruzicka, F. J., Schiller, J. H., Willson, J. K. V., Chen, B. P., Sondel, P. M., and Borden, E. C., 1986, *In vitro* biological assessment of an interferon beta with a site specific amino acid substitution, in: *The Biology of the Interferon System* (W. E. Stewert II and H. Schellekens, eds.), Elsevier, pp. 273–278.

Day, C., Schwartz, B., Li, B.-L., and Pestka, S., 1992, Engineered disulfide bond greatly increases specific activity of recombinant murine interferon-β. *J. Interferon Res.* **12**:139–143.

Derynick, R., Remaut, E., Saman, E., Stranssens, P., De Clercq, E., Content, J., and Fiers, W., 1980, Expression of human fibroblast interferon gene in *Escherichia coli*, *Nature (London)* **287**:193–197.

Dianzani, F., and Dolei, A., 1984, From Isaacs to *Escherichia coli*, in: *Contributions to Oncology* (L. Borecky and V. Lackovic, eds.), Karger, Basel, pp. 1–14.

Eppstein, D. A., and Schryver, B. B., 1990, Controlled release of macromolecular polypeptides, U.S. Patent No. 4,962,091.

Eppstein, D. A., Van Der Pas, M. A., Gloff, C. A., and Soike, K. F., 1989, Liposomal interferon-β: sustained release treatment of simian varicella virus infection in monkeys, *J. Infect. Dis.* **159**: 616–620.

Faltynek, C. R., and Baglioni, C., 1984, Interferon is a polypeptide hormone, *Microbiol. Sci.* **1**:81–85.

Felgner, P. L., and Eppstein, D. A., 1985, Stable liposomes with aqueous-soluble medicaments and methods for their preparation. European Patent Publication No. 0172007A2.

Fernandes, P. M., and Taforo, T., 1991, Formulations for lipophilic IL-2 proteins, U.S. Patent, No. 4,992,271.

Fertsch, D., Schoenberg, D. R., German, R. N., Tou, J. Y. L., and Vogel, S. N., 1987, Induction of macrophage 1a antigen expression by rIFN-Γ and down-regulation by IFNα/β and dexamethasone are mediated by changes in steady-state levels of 1a mRNA, *J. Immunol.* **139**:244–249.

Geigert, J., Panschar, B. M., Fong, S., Huston, H., Wong, D. A., Wong, D. Y., Taforo, C., and Pemberton, M., 1988, The long-term stability of recombinant (serine-17) human interferon-β, *J. Interferon Res.* **8**:539–547.

Geigert, J., Ziegler, D. L., Panschar, B. M., Creasey, A. A., and Vitt, C. R., 1987, Potency stability of recombinant (serine-17) human interferon-β, *J. Interferon Res.* **7**:203–211.

Grossberg, S. E., Taylor, J. L., Seibenlist, R. E., and Jameson, P., 1985, Biological and immunological assays of human interferons, in: *Manual of Clinical Immunology* (N. R. Rose, H. Friedman, and J. L. Fahey, eds.), American Society of Microbiology, pp. 295–299.

Hershenson, S., Stewart, T., Carrol, C., and Shaked, Z., 1989, Formulation of recombinant interferon-β using laureth-12, a novel nonionic surfactant, in: *Therapeutic Peptides and Proteins: Formulation, Delivery and Targeting* (D. Marshak and D. Liu, eds.), Cold Spring Harbor, NY, pp. 31–36.

Hershenson, S., and Thomson, J., 1989, Isoelectric focusing of recombinant interferon-β, *Appl. Theor. Electrophor.* **1**:123–125.

Higgins, P. G., Al-Nakib, W., Willman, J., and Tyrell, D. A. J., 1986, Interferon-β$_{ser}$ as prophylaxis against experimental rhinovirus infection in volunteers, *J. Interferon Res.* **6**:153–159.

IFNβ Multiple Sclerosis Study Group, 1993, Interferon beta-1b is effective in relapsing-remitting multiple sclerosis. I. Clinical results of a multicenter, randomized, double-blind, placebo-controlled trial, *Neurology* **43**:655–661.

Jacobs, L., O'Malley, J., Freeman, A., and Ekes, R., 1981, Intrathecal interferon reduces exacerbations of multiple sclerosis, *Science* **214**:1026–1028.

Jacobs, L., Salazar, A. M., Herndon, R., *et al.*. 1987, Intrathecally administered natural human fibroblast interferon reduces exacerbations of multiple sclerosis: results of a multicenter, double-blinded study, *Arch. Neurol.* **44**:589–595.

Jameson, P., Grieff, D., and Grossberg, S. E., 1979, Thermal stability of freeze-dried mammalian interferons. Analysis of freeze-drying conditions and accelerated storage tests for murine interferon, *Cryobiology* **16**:301–314.

Katre, N., and Knauf, M. J., 1990, Solubilization of immunotoxins for pharmaceutical compositions using polymer conjugation, U.S. Patent No. 4,917,888.

Kerr, I. M., and Stark, G. R., 1992, The antiviral effects of the interferons and their inhibition, *J. Interferon Res.* **12**:237–240.

Kirchner, H., 1986, The interferon system as an integral part of the defense system against infections, *Antiviral Res.* **6**:1–17.

Knauf, M. J., Bell, D. P., Hirtzer, P., Luo, Z. P., Young, J. D., and Katre, N. V., 1988, Relationship of effective molecular size on systemic clearance in rats of recombinant interleukin-2 chemically modified with water soluble polymers, *J. Biol. Chem.* **263**:1564–1570.

Knobler, R. L., Greenstein, J. I., Johnson, K. P., *et al.*, 1993, Systemic recombinant human interferon-β treatment of relapsing-remitting multiple sclerosis: pilot study analysis and six-year follow-up, *J. Interferon Res.* **13**:333–340.

Lehrer, S. S., and Leavis, P. C., 1978, Solute quenching of protein fluorescence, in: *Methods in Enzymology*, Vol. 49, Academic, New York, pp. 222–254.

Lin, L. S., Yamamoto, R., and Drummond, R. J., 1986, Purification of recombinant human interferon-β expressed in *Escherichia coli*, in: *Methods in Enzymology*, Vol. 119, Academic, New York, pp. 183–192.

Mark, D. F., Lu, S. D., Creasey, A. A., Yamamoto, R., and Lin, L. S., 1984, Site-specific mutagenesis of the human fibroblast interferon gene, *Proc. Natl. Acad. Sci. USA* **81**:5662–5666.

Mossman, T., 1983, Rapid colorimetric assay for cellular growth and survival: application to proliferation and cytotoxic assays, *J. Immunol. Methods* **65**:55–63.

Murray, H. W., 1992. The interferons: macrophage activation, and host defence against nonviral pathogens, *J. Interferon Res.* **12**:319–322.

Neighbor, P. A., and Bloom, B. R., 1979, Absence of viral-induced lymphocyte suppression and interferon production in multiple sclerosis, *Proc. Natl. Acad. Sci. USA* **76**:476–480.

Noronha, A., Toscas, A., and Jensen, M. A., 1990, Interferon beta augments suppressor cell function in multiple sclerosis, *Ann. Neurol.* **27**:207–220.

Patty, D. W., Li, D. K. B., *et al.*, 1993, Interferon beta-1b is effective in relapsing-remitting multiple sclerosis. II. MRI analysis results of a multicenter, randomized, double-blind, placebo-controlled trial, *Neurology* **43**:662–667.

Pestka, S., 1983, The human interferons: from protein purification and sequence to cloning and expression in bacteria: before, between and beyond, *Arch. Biochem. Biophys.* **221:**1–37.

Poklar, N., Vesnaver, G., and Lapanje, S. 1994, Denaturation behavior of α-chymotrypsinogen A in urea and alkylurea solutions: fluorescence studies, *J. Protein Chem.* **13:**323–331.

Quesada, J. R., Gutterman, J. U., and Hersh, E. M., 1982, Clinical and immunological study of beta interferon by intramuscular route in patients with metastatic breast cancer, *J. Interferon Res.* **2:** 593–599.

Reder, A. T., and Arnason, B. G. W., 1985, Immunology of multiple sclerosis, in: *Handbook of Clinical Neurology. Demyelinating Diseases*, Vol. 3 (J. C. Koetsier, G. W. Vinken, G. W. Bruyn, and H. L. Klawans, eds.), Elsevier, Amsterdam, pp. 337–395.

Reinhart, J., Malspies, L., Young, D., and Neidhart, J., 1986, Phase I/II trial of human recombinant β-interferon serine in patients with renal cell carcinoma, *Cancer Res.* **46:**5364.

Reiter, Z., 1993. Interferon—a major regulator of natural killer cell-mediated cytotoxicity, *J. Interferon Res.* **13:**247–257.

Schein, C. H., 1990. Solubility as a function of protein structure and solvent components, *Bio/Technology* **8:**308–315.

Schonfeld, A., Nitke, S., Schatner, A., Wallach, D., Crespi, M., Hahn, T., Lavavi, H., Yarden, O., Shoham, J., Doerner, T., and Revel, M., 1984, Intramuscular human interferon-β injections in treatment of condylomata acuminata, *Lancet* 1038–1042.

Shaked, Z., Stewart, T., Hershenson, S., Thomson, J. W., and Thomson, J., 1993, Formulation processes for pharmaceutical compositions of recombinant beta-interferon, U.S. Patent No. 5,183,746.

Shepard, H. M., Leung, D., Stebbing, N., and Goddel, D. V., 1981, A single amino acid change in IFN-β₁ abolishes its antiviral activity, *Nature (London)* **294:**563–565.

Soike, K. F., Chou, T.-C., Fox, J. J., Watanabe, K. A., and Gloff, C. A., 1990, Inhibition of simian *Varicella* virus infection of monkeys by 1-(2-deoxy-2 fluoro-1-D-arabinofuranosyl)-5-ethyl uracil (FEAU) and synergistic effects of combination with human recombinant interferon-β, *Antiviral Res.* **13:**165.

Soike, K. F., Eppstein, D., Gloff, C. A., Cantrell, C., Chou, T.-C., and Gerone, P. J., 1987, Effect of 9-(1,3-dihydroxy-2-propoxymethyl)guanine and recombinant human interferon alone and in combination on Simian *Varicella* virus infection in monkeys, *J. Infect. Dis.* **156:**607–614.

Utsumi, J., Yamazaki, S., Hosoi, K., Kimura, S., Hanada, K., Shimazu, T., and Shimizu, T., 1987, Characterization of *E. coli*–derived recombinant human interferon-β as compared with fibroblast human interferon-β, *J. Biochem.* **101:**1199–1208.

Utsumi, J., Yamazaki, S., Kawagucki, K., Kimura, S., and Shimizu, H., 1989, Stability of human interferon-β1: oligomeric human interferon-β1 is inactive but is reactivated by monomerization, *Biochim. Biophys. Acta* **998:**167–172.

Utsumi, J., Yamazaki, S., Hosoi, K., Shimizu, H., Kawaguchi, K., and Inagaki, F., 1986, Conformations of fibroblast and *E. coli*–derived recombinant human interferon-βs as studied by nuclear magnetic resonance and circular dichroism, *J. Biochem.* **99:**1533–1535.

Vincent, M., Sierra, I. M., Berbaron-Santos, M. N., Diaz, A., Diaz, M., Padron, G., and Gallay, J. 1992, Time-resolved fluorescence study of human recombinant interferon α₂ association state of the protein, spatial proximity of the two tryptophan residues, *Eur. J. Biochem.* **210:**953–961.

Wetzel, R., Johnson, P. D., and Czarniecki, C. W., 1983, Roles of the disulphide bonds in a human alpha interferon, in: *The Biology of the Interferon System* (E. De Maeyer and H. Schellekens, eds.), Elsevier, Amsterdam, pp. 101–120.

Zoon, K., 1987, Human interferons: structure and function, in: *Interferon 9* (I. Gresser, ed.), Academic, New York, pp. 1–13.

7

Characterization, Formulation, and Stability of Neupogen® (Filgrastim), a Recombinant Human Granulocyte-Colony Stimulating Factor

Alan C. Herman, Thomas C. Boone, and Hsieng S. Lu

1. INTRODUCTION

1.1. Clinical Uses of Granulocyte-Colony Stimulating Factor

Neutropenia is a condition that occurs when neutrophil counts fall below the nominal range of approximately 1.5×10^9/L (Hutchinson and Boxer, 1991). One of the major applications of granulocyte-colony stimulating factor (G-CSF) therapy has been in ameliorating neutropenia. Neutropenia occurs in a wide variety of disease settings, including congenital defects, bone marrow suppression following pharmacological manipulation, and infection. This condition also occurs in cancer patients undergoing cytotoxic chemotherapy. The neutropenia can, in turn, lead to bacterial and secondary fungal infections often requiring hospitalization. G-CSF can decrease the period of neutropenia or prevent it altogether. The maximum tolerated dose and dosing schedule of some chemotherapeutic drugs are limited by myelosuppression. Treatment

Alan C. Herman • Analytical Research and Development, Amgen Inc., Thousand Oaks, California 91320   *Thomas C. Boone* • Process Science, Amgen Inc., Thousand Oaks, California 91320   *Hsieng S. Lu* • Protein Structure, Amgen Inc., Thousand Oaks, California 91320.

Formulation, Characterization, and Stability of Protein Drugs, Rodney Pearlman and Y. John Wang, eds., Plenum Press, New York, 1996.

with G-CSF can enable a higher-dose-intensity schedule which, in turn, may allow better antitumor effects (Morstyn and Dexter, 1994). In 1991, the United States Food and Drug Administration approved Neupogen® (Filgrastim, r-met-huG-CSF) for use by those suffering from neutropenia during or after chemotherapy. It has since been approved by many other countries worldwide.

Neupogen® has been approved worldwide for use in bone marrow transplantation and more recently in the United States for treatment of severe chronic congenital neutropenia. Neupogen® also has a potential application in mobilizing peripheral blood progenitor cells for transplantation. Other clinical uses such as treatment of AIDS patients and infectious diseases are still under investigation (Morstyn and Dexter, 1994).

1.2. Molecular and Biological Characterization

1.2.1. ISOLATION AND CLONING OF G-CSF

Murine G-CSF was initially identified and partially purified by Nicola *et al.* (1983) and its action on hematopoietic cells was established by Metcalf and Nicola (1983). Natural human G-CSF was first purified from a medium conditioned by the human bladder carcinoma cell line 5637 (Welte *et al.*, 1985) and later reported to be purified from the squamatous carcinoma cell line CHU-2 (Nomura *et al.*, 1986). Nagata *et al.* (1986a) calculated the molecular weight of recombinant G-CSF to be 18,987 Daltons based on the cDNA. However, Souza *et al.* (1986) measured the apparent molecular weight of the secreted recombinant form of the protein at 19,600 Daltons. Treatment of the mature protein with *O*-glycanase reduced the molecular weight of native G-CSF to 18,800 Daltons, suggesting that the secreted protein is *O*-glycosylated. Recombinant G-CSF has been expressed in both *Escherichia coli* and mammalian cells. Recombinant G-CSF differs from the natural product in at least two respects. First, recombinant preparations are comprised of a single amino acid sequence species, whereas preparations from natural sources contain two amino acid sequence species (discussed below). Second, glycosylation incident to recombinant protein expression is different from that found in nature, and thus the glycosylation of recombinant G-CSF expressed in Chinese hamster ovary cells differs from the natural protein (see Oheda *et al.*, 1988). *E. coli* expressed G-CSF differs from the natural material in its lack of glycosylation and its N-terminal methionyl residue incident to bacterial expression (Lu *et al.*, 1989a).

Two different genes encoding the amino acid sequence of human G-CSF were isolated independently from different tissue sources. Human G-CSF cDNA prepared from a bladder carcinoma cell line encodes a predicted amino acid sequence of 174 amino acids (Souza *et al.*, 1986). Two G-CSF cDNAs from a squamatous cell line code for polypeptides of 174 and 177 amino acids (Nagata *et al.*, 1986a,b). The differences in the two isolates are caused by an alternative mRNA splicing site. Three additional amino acids are not spliced out between residues 32 and 33 of the 174-amino-acid polypeptide to make the 177-amino-acid form which has greatly diminished biological activity. Analyses of genomic human DNA showed that human G-CSF is encoded by a single gene which is located on chromosome 17 q[11–22] (Le Beau *et al.*, 1987; Simmers *et al.*, 1987). The 2.5-kb human G-CSF chromosomal gene is composed of five exons and four introns (Nagata *et al.*, 1986b).

1.2.2. BIOLOGICAL ACTIVITY

The primary effects of G-CSF on normal hematopoietic cells are limited to cells of neutrophil lineage. *In vitro*, G-CSF selectively stimulates proliferation and differentiation of neutrophil colony-forming cells and alters several functions of mature neutrophils (Metcalf and Nicola, 1983; Metcalf, 1984, 1989; Souza *et al.*, 1986). G-CSF acts on a relatively mature progenitor cell population that is committed to neutrophilic differentiation (Ema *et al.*, 1990). G-CSF commonly exhibits synergistic hematopoietic activity with other cytokines *in vitro*, such as IL-3, IL-6, or GM-CSF (Demetri and Griffin, 1991). Strong synergistic activity of G-CSF was observed in combination with the cloned ligand (stem cell factor) for c-kit proto-oncogene (Martin *et al.*, 1990), which acts on an extremely early cell population within the hematopoietic hierarchy (Zsebo *et al.*, 1990).

When injected *in vivo*, recombinant G-CSF increases the number of mature neutrophils in the circulation of rats, mice, hamsters, dogs, primates, and humans (for reference see Morstyn and Dexter, 1994). Treatment of animals with G-CSF in preclinical studies revealed several important biological phenomena of G-CSF including elevation of neutrophil counts, accelerated recovery of neutrophils, redistribution of hematopoiesis, and mobilization of peripheral blood stem cells. The production of lymphocytes is largely unaffected. Exposure of animals to high doses of G-CSF for a protracted period does not appear to have deleterious effects.

1.2.3. IMMUNOASSAY AND BIOASSAY

Several immunoassay and bioassay procedures have been reported. Motojima *et al.* (1989) reported the use of an enzyme-linked immunosorbent assay (ELISA) using a polyclonal rabbit antiserum. Similarly, Tanaka and Kaneko (1992) found that both a competitive radioimmunoassay and an ELISA assay were useful for the measurement of G-CSF in rat serum. A rabbit polyclonal antibody was used in both cases and the assays were specific to G-CSF. Other colony-stimulating factors and interleukins were not recognized in the assays. Similarly, several bioassays for G-CSF have also been reported. Tohyama *et al.* (1989) reported the use of a murine hematopoietic cell line (NFS-60) that was dependent on G-CSF. Cell growth could be measured by a colorimetric tetrazolium assay. Shirafuji *et al.* (1989) described the use of a [3H]thymidine uptake assay to monitor the growth of NFS-60 cells in response to G-CSF.

1.3. Chemical–Physical Characterization

1.3.1. PRIMARY STRUCTURE

Neupogen® is composed of a polypeptide chain of 175 amino acids in length (Souza *et al.*, 1986; Lu *et al.*, 1989b). Direct expression of the protein in *E. coli* leads to the accumulation of large quantities of expressed product in inclusion bodies. Clinical grade, biologically active G-CSF is obtained through a series of manufacturing processes including solubilization of inclusion bodies, oxidation and folding, and ion-exchange chromatographic isolation. Neupogen® is a monomeric molecule in solution with a molecular weight of 18,799.94 based on sequence. N-terminal sequence analysis of purified G-CSF reveals that methionine is the only amino terminus, suggesting that the initiator of protein synthesis is not processed after translation. The two intramolecular disulfide bonds, Cys^{37}-Cys^{43} and Cys^{65}-Cys^{75}, form two small loop structures that maintain the biologically active conformation of G-CSF (Fig. 1). Reduction of any of the disulfide bonds causes reduction of activity. Neupogen® also contains a free cysteine at position 18 which is not required for activity (Lu *et al.*, 1989a).

1.3.2. THREE-DIMENSIONAL STRUCTURE

Circular dichroic analysis, which predicts 69% α-helix for Neupogen® (see below), and secondary structure analysis by Bazan (1990) and Parry (1988) suggested that G-CSF has a four-helical-bundle motif. Recently, the X-ray crystallographic atomic structure of Neupogen® was determined at high resolution (Hill *et al.*, 1993). The crystal structure confirmed the predicted topology and showed that Neupogen® has four antiparallel helices with cross angles of about 18°, which is close to that expected for an ideal left-handed helical bundle (see Fig. 2 for the depicted ribbon model). This four-helical structure, also called the cytokine fold, is similar to the helical topology of human growth hormone (DeVos *et al.*, 1992) and other cytokines such as GM-CSF (Diederichs *et al.*, 1991) and CSF-1 (Pandit *et al.*, 1992). The molecule contains four helices referred to as helices A, B, C, and D and three interconnecting loops, AB, BC, and CD. The AB loop (residues 39–72) and the CD loop (residues 123–143) are long overhand loops, while the BC loop (residues 91–100) is the more typical hairpin type. There is also a short helical section (the E helix or 3_{10} helix) within the AB loop. The topology is described as being "up-up-down-down." The crystal structure of Neupogen® indicates that the A helix is extended from the core helical bundle and is mobile since the first 10 N-terminal residues are not visible in the electron density map. The mobility of this region is consistent with the suggestion that the first 10 residues do not participate in the overall function or stability of the protein (Okabe *et al.*, 1990; Osslund and Boone, 1994). The long AB loop is also extended and structurally disordered.

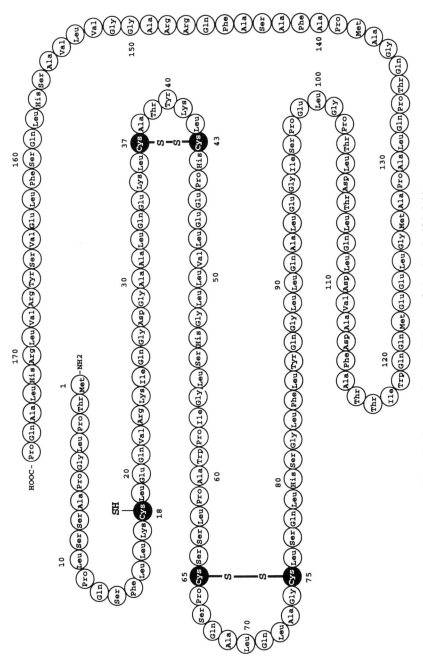

Figure 1. Sequence diagram of Neupogen® showing disulfide bridges.

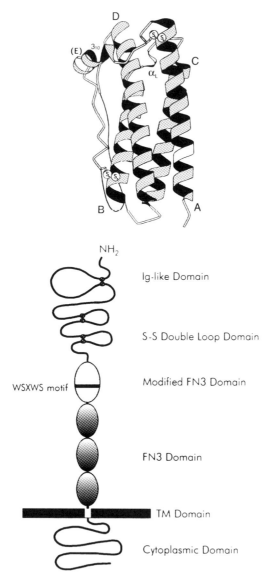

Figure 2. A ribbon model showing the four helical bundle structure of Neupogen® (top) and structural domains of G-CSF receptor (bottom).

1.3.3. DISULFIDE BOND FORMATION

The kinetics of the formation of the two disulfide bonds is dramatically different. The first disulfide bond (Cys^{37}-Cys^{43}) is between the first helix of the helical bundle and the short E helix. In contrast, the second disulfide bond (Cys^{65}-Cys^{75}) is positioned at the carboxyl terminal end of the E helix to helix B. Typically, G-CSF is oxidized in Sarkosyl at slightly alkaline pH with the addition of copper sulfate. In the process of folding and oxidation of Neupogen®, the protein rapidly undergoes formation of a partially oxidized intermediate containing a single Cys^{37}-Cys^{43} bond. Refolding and oxidation to form the Cys^{65}-Cys^{75} disulfide bond is the rate-limiting step in the formation of native Neupogen® (Lu *et al.*, 1992).

1.3.4. NEUPOGEN®–RECEPTOR INTERACTION

The mechanism by which Neupogen® stimulates the cell to produce its biological effects is poorly understood. It is clear that Neupogen® binds to a specific receptor causing subsequent transduction of signals and cellular response. cDNA clones encoding murine and human G-CSF receptors have been isolated (Fukunaga *et al.*, 1990a,b; Larson *et al.*, 1990). These receptors have a single transmembrane domain and consist of 813 and 812 amino acids, respectively. Within the extracellular domain, there are several unique domains which were identified to have statistically significant identity to other proteins. These are the disulfide-linked IgG-like domain, the cysteine-rich double-loop domain, three fibronectin type 3 (FN3) repeat units and the WSXWS motif which is typical of the cytokine receptor family (Fig. 2). In addition, these G-CSF receptors show significant sequence similarity to the signal transduction component (gp130) of the IL-6 receptor complex (Hibi *et al.*, 1990). Growth and differentiation signals stimulated by G-CSF are mediated by different regions in the cytoplasmic domain, which has limited similarity to other cytokine receptors (Mosely *et al.*, 1989). Although the downstream signal transduction pathway in response to Neupogen® receptor interaction is far from understood, recent data appear to indicate that many of the cytokine signal transductions including EPO, G-CSF, IL-3, GM-CSF, IL-6, and growth hormone are associated with the JAK family of protein tyrosine kinases (Wilks and Harpur, 1994; Kishimoto *et al.*, 1994).

Recent studies using epitope-mapping techniques revealed that the receptor-binding region of Neupogen® is restricted to a small region that includes residues 35 to 45. This small segment includes only the first disulfide loop (residues 36 to 42) and a portion of the first turn of 3_{10} helix. Several charged residues in this region, i.e., Lys^{41}, His^{44}, Glu^{46}, and Glu^{47}, may be contributing to the receptor binding. Other evidence also implicates the extended portion of the D helix (residues 165–175) as part of a receptor-binding domain (Osslund and Boone, 1994). Mutation of the carboxyl terminus of Neupogen® abolishes activity in a similar manner to the loss of activity in human growth hormone (Cunningham and Wells, 1989). Related cytokines, IL-6 and GM-CSF, predicted to have similar topology to G-CSF, also center their biological activity at the carboxyl terminus of the D helix (Bazan, 1990).

1.4. Glycosylated versus Nonglycosylated G-CSF

Since natural G-CSF has not been isolated in quantities sufficient for complete carbohydrate characterization, most of the carbohydrate analysis has been performed on recombinant G-CSF produced in Chinese hamster ovary cells.

1.4.1. CARBOHYDRATE STRUCTURE

Oheda *et al.* (1988) first analyzed the sugar composition of G-CSF and compared the recombinant to the natural product (Table I). The overall sugar composition of the two G-CSF sources was found to be different in sialic acid content. The recombinant product was analyzed in more detail by NMR spectroscopy following purification of the oligosaccharide alditols. Two sugar chains were observed with structures of NeuAcα2-3Galβ1-3GalNAcol and NeuAcα2-3Galβ1-3(NeuAcα2-6)GalNAcol. These two chains were found to be *O*-linked to a single site on the protein, Thr[134]. This structure was later confirmed by Clogston *et al.* (1993) by complementary methods.

1.4.2. PHYSICAL AND BIOLOGICAL DIFFERENCES OF GLYCOSYLATED AND NONGLYCOSYLATED G-CSF

Arakawa et. al (1993) have completed a detailed study of the apparent stability differences of glycosylated and nonglycosylated G-CSF by studying the accessibility of the free cysteinyl residue at position 18. Their work showed that the cysteine is partially solvent exposed in both glycosylated and nonglycosylated forms. At low pH, where the cysteine is protonated, both forms have greater stability. In the glycosylated form the carbohydrate appears to affect the reactivity of the sulfhydryl group either through steric hindrance or local conformational changes. Both forms show essentially identical conformation by circular dichroism, fluorescence, and infrared spectroscopy. Additionally, the kinetics of unfolding of the two forms is identical, indicating that any difference in stability of the two forms in not conforma-

**Table I. Sugar Compositions of Recombinant
Human G-CSF and Human G-CSF[a]**

	Galactose	Galactosamine	Sialic acid
rhG-CSF	0.97	0.82	1.54
hG-CSF	0.90	0.83	1.40

[a]Values are expressed as moles/mole of protein. (From Oheda *et al.*, 1988).

tional. Similarly, Wingfield *et al.* (1988) found that a Cys → Ser substitution at position 18 resulted in no measurable changes in physical or biological properties. Wild-type and mutant recombinant-derived, nonglycosylated proteins yielded bioassay results similar to those obtained with glycosylated, recombinant-derived human G-CSF produced in monkey cells. Although it has been proposed that the nonglycosylated G-CSF will aggregate and, subsequently, have diminished bioactivity (Oh-eda *et al.*, 1990), the presence of carbohydrate on G-CSF appears to have little effect on the ability of G-CSF to promote the proliferation and differentiation of the granulocyte progenitor lineages *in vitro* or *in vivo* (Zsebo *et al.*, 1986; Cohen *et al.*, 1987; Souza *et al.*, 1986).

2. STRUCTURAL ANALYSIS

The remainder of this chapter will deal exclusively with the nonglycosylated form of G-CSF produced in *E. coli*, specifically, Amgen's Filgrastim product, Neupogen®.

2.1. Sequence Analysis and Peptide Mapping

2.1.1. ELUCIDATION OF COMPLETE AMINO ACID SEQUENCE

Structural characterization was performed to define Neupogen®'s chemical composition (e.g., amino acid analysis, peptide mapping, amino acid sequence) (Lu *et al.*, 1989a). Peptide fragments were generated by digestion of *S*-carboxymethylated Neupogen® by endoproteinase Glu-C or by digestion of the intact protein by subtilisin. These fragments were then separated by reverse-phase HPLC. Figure 3 shows a typical peptide map obtained from endoproteinase Glu-C digestion of alkylated Neupogen® and this analysis is routinely used as a product identity test. The results of the amino acid sequence determination are summarized in Fig. 4. This figure also shows the amino acid sequence determined for each peptide fragment obtained from enzymatic digestion of Neupogen®. Overlapping peptide fragments were used in the sequence determination. The protein sequence analysis of Neupogen® indicates that the amino acid sequence of this recombinant protein conforms to that deduced from the sequence of the coding DNA.

2.1.2. CARBOXY-TERMINAL ANALYSIS

The Neupogen® gene sequence predicts a proline residue at the C-terminus (position 175) of the molecule. Carboxypeptidase P digestion as well as isolation and

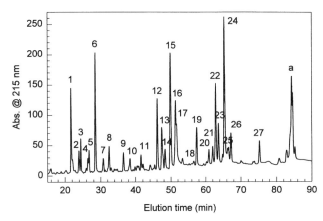

Figure 3. HPLC peptide map of reduced and carboxymethylated Neupogen® after endoproteinase Glu-C digestion.

characterization of the C-terminal peptide was performed to verify that the protein indeed ends with Pro[175]. The peptide CmS-8 (see Fig. 4), obtained from SV8 protease digestion of *S*-carboxymethylated derivative, was isolated by reverse-phase chromatography (RPC). Sequence analysis and amino acid composition determination of the peptide indicated that this is the C-terminal peptide. Electrospray mass spectrometric analysis of peptide CmS-8 is also consistent with data obtained from sequence and compositional analysis.

As confirmation, intact protein in 0.05% Brij-35, 10 mM NaAc, pH 4.0 was further treated with carboxypeptidase P (enzyme-to-substrate ratio = 1:400) at room temperature (Lu *et al.*, 1989b). The digest aliquots taken at different times were analyzed on an amino acid analyzer to determine the order of removed residues. The results indicated that … Leu-Ala-Gln-Pro-COOH is the C-terminal sequence of Neupogen® as predicted by the cDNA sequence. Confirmation of the C-terminal intactness can be assessed by electrospray mass spectrometric analysis. The measured mass of 18,799.77 is consistent with Neupogen® containing 175 amino acids (see Section 1.3.1).

2.1.3. AMINO ACID COMPOSITION

Amino acid composition analysis of Neupogen® was accomplished through acid hydrolysis of the protein at 110°C for 24 h *in vacuo*. Typical results of amino acid composition analysis are shown in Table II. The data indicate that the sample is a purified protein with an amino acid composition consistent with Neupogen®. Cysteine is quantified as the *S*-carboxymethylated derivative. Tryptophan is easily destroyed during normal acid hydrolysis and was recovered by an alternative hydrolysis

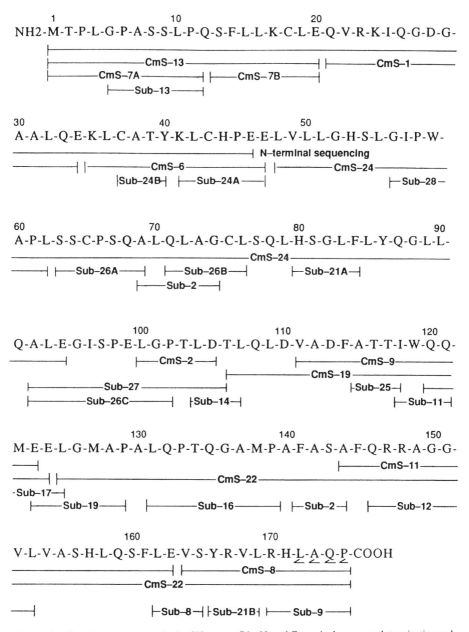

Figure 4. Complete sequence analysis of Neupogen® by N- and C-terminal sequence determination and characterization of isolated endoproteinase Glu-C and subtilisin-derived peptides (CmS- and Sub-, respectively).

Table II. Amino Acid Composition of Neupogen®

Amino acids	Method A[a]	Method B[b]	Method C[c]	Theoretical
Cysteic acid	—[d]	5.0	—	
Carboxymethyl cysteine	—	—	5.3	
Methionine sulfone	—	3.7	—	
Aspartic acid	4.2	4.2	4.1	4
Threonine	6.9	6.5	6.5	7
Serine	12.2	12.2	11.8	14
Glutamic acid	26.3	26.7	25.3	26
Proline	13.9	13.2	12.0	13
Glycine	14.8	14.5	14.0	14
Alanine	18.9	19.7	19.4	19
Half cystine	ND[e]	—	—	5
Valine	6.9	7.1	7.1	7
Methionine	3.6	—	3.0	4
Isoleucine	3.9	3.9	3.8	4
Leucine	33.4	33.8	33.1	33
Tyrosine	2.9	ND	2.7	3
Phenylalanine	6.0	5.6	5.9	6
Histidine	5.0	4.9	5.1	5
Lysine	4.3	4.3	3.7	4
Tryptophan	1.7	ND	ND	2
Arginine	4.6	5.2	5.0	5
Total	169.5	170.5	167.8	175

[a]Method A: hydrolysis of Neupogen® in 4 M methanesulfonic acid.
[b]Method B: hydrolysis of performic acid–oxidized Neupogen® in 6 N HCl.
[c]Method C: hydrolysis of carboxymethylated Neupogen® in 6 N HCl.
[d]—: Not present.
[e]ND: Not determined.

method using 4 M methane sulfonic acid containing 0.2% tryptamine. The results are consistent with the theoretical value of two tryptophans.

2.1.4. ASSIGNMENT OF DISULFIDE STRUCTURE

To elucidate the disulfide structure of Neupogen®, disulfide-containing peptides must be isolated. The protein was digested with subtilisin at pH 4 to minimize disulfide exchange, and the resulting peptide mixture was immediately separated by RP-HPLC. Peptides obtained from RP-HPLC were then subjected to amino acid composition, mass spectrometry, and sequence analyses to identify the disulfide-containing peptides. Some of the sequence assignments are shown in Fig. 4. In summary, peptides Sub-24 and Sub-26 are confirmed to be the disulfide-containing peptides and contain Cys[37]-Cys[43] and Cys[65]-Cys[75] bonds, respectively.

2.2. Biophysical Analysis

2.2.1. UV SPECTRUM

Analysis by ultraviolet spectroscopy of the purified protein showed an absorption maximum at 282 nm. In order to obtain a molar extinction coefficient, the protein concentration of the Neupogen® solution was determined by amino acid analysis. The absorbance at 280 nm as determined in buffer or 3 M GuHCl was nearly identical ($\pm 2.5\%$). The observed absorbance at 280 nm was divided by the measured protein concentration to yield an absorbance of 0.86 ± 0.015 for Neupogen® at 1.0 mg/ml.

2.2.2. CIRCULAR DICHROISM (CD) SPECTRA

The CD spectra of Neupogen® in 20 mM NaAc (pH 2.5 and 7.5) were obtained at room temperature over a spectral range of 188 to 320 nm (Lu *et al.*, 1989a; Narhi *et al.*, 1991). At the far-UV region, from 205 to 250 nm, the Neupogen® molecule exhibits strong CD patterns typical of globular proteins which are abundant in α-helical structure (Fig. 5). The double negative extrema at 222 nm and 209 nm, arising from the respective n-π^* and π-π^* (parallel) amide transitions, and a large positive maximum at 193–194 nm from π-π^* (perpendicular) amide transitions were observed. The estimated secondary structure of Neupogen® contains approximately 69% α-helix, 2.5% β-sheet, 4% β-turn, and the remaining unordered structure at pH 4.5.

Figure 5 shows the near-UV CD spectra of Neupogen®, representing distinct tertiary structural features of the molecule at both pH's. In particular, the Neupogen® molecule appears to exhibit a broad negative CD band around 270 nm, two positive CD extrema around 280 and 286 nm, and a shoulder at 290–295 nm, suggesting the contribution of tyrosine and tryptophan. pH and denaturant-induced conformational changes of the molecule have been visualized by far- and near-UV CD analyses (Narhi *et al.*, 1991).

2.2.3. FLUORESCENCE

Neupogen® contains two tryptophan and three tyrosine residues per molecule and hence is amenable to fluorescence studies (Narhi *et al.*, 1991). The fluorescence spectra of Neupogen® determined at pH 7.5 in 20 mM Tris, 100 mM NaCl, and at pH 2.5 in diluted HCl, are shown in Fig. 5. When the protein at pH 7.5 is excited at 280 nm, the spectrum appears to be symmetrical with a peak maximum at 344 nm, typical of tryptophan(s) being partially solvent exposed. Tyrosine fluorescence (around 300 nm) appears to be completely quenched by tryptophan, as is usually the case for globular proteins containing both tryptophan and tyrosine residues.

At pH 2.5, an entirely different fluorescence spectrum is observed after excita-

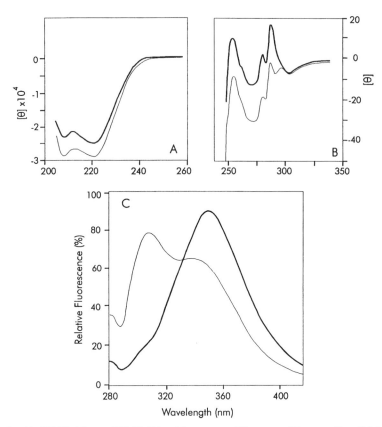

Figure 5. Far UV-CD (A), near UV-CD (B) and fluorescence (C) spectra of Neupogen® at pH 2.5 (heavy line) and pH 7.5 (light line). The overlaid spectra have been normalized for easier interpretation.

tion at 280 nm (Fig. 5). The spectrum is characterized by a peak at 308 nm and a shoulder at 344 nm, attributable to tyrosine fluorescence and the quenching of tryptophan fluorescence, respectively. The fluorescence intensity is considerably lower at pH 2.5 than at pH 7.5. These spectral changes suggest an altered conformation in acidic pH, relative to that at pH 7.5. This phenomenon may be related to the stability of various Neupogen® preparations (see Section 3).

2.3. Biochemical Analysis

2.3.1. POLYACRYLAMIDE GEL ELECTROPHORESIS

When Neupogen® is analyzed by polyacrylamide gel electrophoresis in sodium dodecyl sulfate (SDS-PAGE) under either reducing or nonreducing conditions (Laemmli, 1970), a single band with an apparent molecular weight of 18,800 Daltons

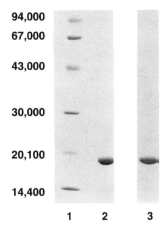

94,000
67,000

43,000

30,000

20,100

14,400

1   2   3

Figure 6. SDS-PAGE of Neupogen®. Neupogen® was separated on a 10–20% acrylamide gel under reducing and nonreducing conditions according to the method of Laemmli (1970). Proteins were visualized by staining with Coomasie Brilliant Blue R-250. Lane 1: Molecular weight standards. Lane 2: Reduced Neupogen®. Lane 3: Nonreduced Neupogen®.

is observed (Fig. 6). When Neupogen® is analyzed by isoelectric focusing (IEF), one major band at a pI of approximately 6.0 is observed which corresponds to methionyl G-CSF. The formylmethionine form of the molecule, if present, is well resolved from the major component (see Fig. 7).

2.3.2. ANALYTICAL HPLC

Over the past several years analytical high-pressure liquid chromatography (HPLC) has become quite useful as a tool for critically monitoring the purity and chemical stability of protein pharmaceuticals derived from recombinant technology. Proteins are subject to a variety of amino acid misincorporations and posttranslational modifications during fermentation, purification, formulation, and storage. Most of these changes are subtle and involve a limited amount of the protein. Typically, the goal of the analyst is to identify these modifications at levels of 1% or less of total protein. The variety of high-resolution HPLC techniques presently available has enabled the analyst to solve many of these problems. Since these modifications can affect a number of the properties of the protein (charge, hydrophobicity, size) a variety chromatographic methods have been successfully employed.

2.3.2a. Reverse-Phase Chromatography

Reverse-phase chromatography (RPC) is a highly discriminating type of HPLC that separates analytes on the basis of their relative hydrophobicity. One drawback of the technique is that proteins are usually denatured as they are adsorbed to the column

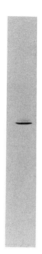

Figure 7. Isoelectric focusing of Neupogen®. Neupogen® was separated on an isoelectric focusing gel of 5% acrylamide and 6% urea. The pH gradient was 5–7. Proteins were visualized with Coomasie Brilliant Blue R-250. The f-metG-CSF band is barely visible some distance above the main band. The minor band just above the main G-CSF band is an artifact of the gel system.

matrix. Because of this, it is not usually possible to determine information about the protein other than chemical. Figure 8 shows a reverse-phase chromatogram of G-CSF. This is an atypical lot of G-CSF whose degradation has been artificially enhanced to illustrate various degradation pathways. Chromatographic conditions are detailed in the figure legend. Note that in order to achieve this level of resolution it is necessary to run the separation at relatively high temperatures (60°C). Because it is possible that artifacts may be generated at these temperatures, all of the peaks eluting from the column have been isolated and reinjected. In all cases, the reinjected peaks ran in the same position and did not generate additional peaks.

Several of the peaks in Fig. 8 have been identified. A commonly used method for identifying chemically modified species is by isolating the peak found on RPC, digesting it enzymatically, and comparing the peptide map to that obtained for the unmodified species. The peptide containing the modified amino acid will typically exhibit a retention time different from that of the control peptide. This modified peptide can then be further characterized by mass spectroscopy or N-terminal sequencing. This technique was used to characterize peaks 1 and 2 of Fig. 8 as containing an oxidized met[122] and met[127/138] respectively. Since both met[127] and met[138] reside on the same SV8 peptide, it is impossible to differentiate them by this method alone, and additional work is needed.

Peak 4 on the G-CSF reverse phase chromatogram is formylmethionine–G-CSF (f-metG-CSF). In a typical Neupogen® production lot this peak is below detectable levels (<1%). Similarly, the oxidized forms represent less than 2% of total Neu-

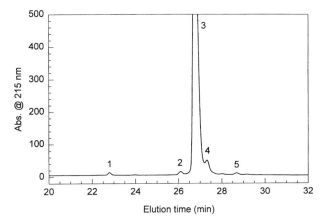

Figure 8. Reverse-phase chromatography of partially degraded G-CSF. The protein was chromatographed on a 4.6 × 150 mm C_4 column at 60°C using a linear gradient of 36% to 72% aceonitrile in 0.1% trifluoroacetic acid over 30 min. The flow rate was 0.8 ml/min. Peak 1: oxidized Met^{122} G-CSF. Peak 2: oxidized $Met^{127/136}$ G-CSF. Peak 3: unmodified G-CSF. Peak 4: f-met-G-CSF. Peak 5: partially reduced G-CSF. The chromatogram has been expanded along the X and Y axes for clarity. Absorbance is in milliabsorbance units (mAU).

pogen®. Finally, peak 5 represents a partially reduced G-CSF, a form typically present at less than 0.5%. This form of the protein has only the Cys^{37}-Cys^{43} disulfide bond (see Section 1.3.3).

2.3.2b. Ion-Exchange Chromatography

Ion-exchange chromatography (IEX) has been most useful for quantification of f-metG-CSF (Clogston *et al.*, 1992). Figure 9 shows an ion-exchange chromatogram of Neupogen®. IEF gels have, on occasion, shown several faint protein bands migrating between f-metG-CSF and G-CSF, suggesting deamidation of the protein. This has only been observed in samples that have been stored for extended periods at elevated temperatures. Although there is no asparagine in Neupogen®, the protein is rich in glutamine (see Table II). Similarly, IEX profiles will occasionally show a poorly resolved shoulder on the trailing edge of the f-metG-CSF peak or the leading edge of the G-CSF peak. Unfortunately, it has not been possible to obtain sufficient resolution of these IEX peaks for subsequent analysis.

2.3.2c. Size-Exclusion Chromatography

Glycosylated G-CSF is freely soluble in phosphate-buffered saline. When the carbohydrate is absent, however, the protein becomes quite hydrophobic and does not

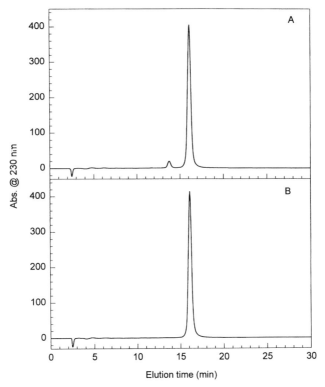

Figure 9.   Ion-exchange chromatography of Neupogen®. Neupogen® was applied to a 7.5 mm × 75 mm SP cation exchange column equilibrated in sodium acetate at pH 5.4. Protein was eluted with a linear gradient of 0–200 mM sodium chloride over 30 min at 1 ml/min. The peak eluting at 13.7 min is f-metG-CSF, the peak eluting at 16.3 min is met-G-CSF. Panel A: metG-CSF spiked with purified f-metG-CSF. Panel B: Typical released lot of Neupogen®. Absorbance is in mAU.

tolerate high salt concentrations or neutral pH. Because of this, it is necessary to run size-exclusion chromatography under acidic conditions (Watson and Kenney, 1988). At higher pH's monomer recovery is poor and any multimer is bound irreversibly to the column. Figure 10 shows a typical low pH SEC separation. Neupogen® characteristically shows a very small amount of high-molecular-weight aggregate (<0.2%) and will occasionally have a small amount of dimer present. The aggregate has been shown by laser light scattering to have a molecular weight of about 500,000 (Herman, unpublished observations). Interestingly, no intermediate multimers have been observed between the dimers and these large aggregates. It is possible that other forms are either bound irreversibly to the SEC column or are dissociated to monomer by the harsh acidic conditions.

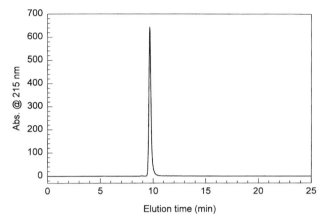

Figure 10. Acidic size-exclusion chromatography of Neupogen®. Neupogen® was applied to 7.8 mm × 300 mm TSK 3000 silica-based sizing column and chromatographed in pH 2.5 phosphoric acid. A small prepeak corresponding to dimer can be observed. Absorbance is in mAU.

2.3.2d. Identification of Translational Errors

The analytical methods described in the preceding paragraphs ensure that a product with an extremely high level of homogeneity is produced. Occasionally, these methods will reveal higher than expected levels of altered forms at certain stages of processing. When this occurs, steps are taken to characterize fully the altered material. In one such occurrence, three microheterogeneous forms were found by cation-exchange chromatography (Lu *et al.*, 1993). Each species was found to have a single histidine substituted by a glutamine. The substituted His positions were 53, 157, and 171. No differences in bioactivity were observed. The His → Gln substitution represents a single base change (CAU for His versus CAA/U for Gln), apparently due to mistranslation.

2.4. Analysis of the Free Cysteine Residue

There is a free cysteinyl residue in the Neupogen® molecule not accessible to carboxymethylation by a hydrophilic agent, iodoacetic acid, under native conformation. The SH group becomes fully reactive when Neupogen® is denatured. In other experiments, the free sulfhydryl has been shown to react very slowly with a hydrophobic modifying agent, dithiobis-nitrobenzoic acid (DTNB) under nondenaturing conditions (Arakawa *et al.*, 1993). It is postulated that the free cysteine may reside inside the hydrophobic environment of the molecule such that it is inaccessible to chemical modification by hydrophilic alkylating agents but is more accessible to hydrophobic agents. The free cysteinyl residue has been assigned to Cys[18] by identifying a ^{3}H-labeled peptide after SV-8 protease digestion and peptide mapping.

3. FORMULATION

The current market formulation for Neupogen® is a liquid stored at 2–8°C with a G-CSF concentration of 300 µg/ml. In this format the product is stable for more than 2 years.

3.1. Requirements for Nonglycosylated G-CSF

As can be seen in Table II, Neupogen® contains a high percentage of hydrophobic amino acid residues. Since the carbohydrate moiety of naturally occurring G-CSF masks some of this hydrophobicity, special considerations had to be made to obtain a long-term stable formulation for the *E. coli* product. Although natural G-CSF is quite stable under physiological conditions, at pH's above 5 Neupogen® was found to aggregate when tested at elevated temperatures. This was observed regardless of whether 5% mannitol or 150 mM sodium chloride was used as a tonicity modifier. However, Neupogen® was found to aggregate minimally at pH 4 with 5% mannitol. Additionally, chemical changes such as deamidation, oxidation, and proteolysis were minimized at this pH. Lower pH's resulted in increases in deamidation and proteolytic cleavage. Finally, 0.004% polysorbate-80 was added to the formulation to eliminate the formation of particulates that were occasionally observed at elevated temperatures. Currently, Neupogen® is formulated as a liquid in 10 mM sodium acetate, pH 4.0, 5% mannitol, and 0.004% polysorbate-80. With this formulation Neupogen® is stable for greater than 24 months at 2–8°C. No improvement in stability could be demonstrated by using a lyophilized formulation.

3.2. Sensitivity to Freezing—Packaging Solution

The primary drawback to the liquid-mannitol-containing formulation is that when Neupogen® is inadvertently frozen and thawed there is a tendency toward dimerization and aggregation. Since a significant percentage of Neupogen® is shipped to geographical areas subject to freezing temperatures for at least part of the year, there is a potential for a large amount of returned product. In order to solve this problem a special package was developed for Neupogen® called the SAFE-T-THERM®

tray. This is a tray filled with 100 ml of a gelled solution that is designed to freeze before the product itself freezes. The freezing of the gel prevents heat transfer out of the Neupogen®, which, in turn, prevents the product from freezing during extended exposure to subzero conditions. A temperature-indicating device is also part of the packaging. The indicator will turn red if the temperature goes below $-6° \pm 2°$. This is well above the actual freezing point of the product ($\sim -20°$). If the device turns red the pharmacist is instructed to return the product. Amgen was issued three U.S. patents on the freeze protection system (#5,181,394, #D332,397, and #D339,869).

3.3. Sensitivity to Freezing—Reformulation Solution

Although the SAFE-T-THERM® packaging system is an elegant solution to the freezing-sensitivity problem, prolonged exposure to subzero temperatures can still result in freezing of the product. New formulations were researched which would be tolerant of freezing. Other buffer systems capable of buffering at pH 4 ± 0.5 were investigated, but none of these completely eliminated the aggregation during freezing and thawing. Since mannitol crystallizes upon freezing, it was suspected that this crystallization may contribute to the aggregation of Neupogen®. Sorbitol is an optical isomer of mannitol but freezes in an amorphous form rather than a crystalline one. When mannitol was substituted with sorbitol in the existing formulation the freezing-sensitivity problem was eliminated. Presently, sorbitol is being substituted for mannitol in the formulation of Neupogen®.

4. STABILITY AND STABILITY-INDICATING ASSAYS

The current stability specifications for Neupogen® are the same as the release specifications. That is, product must remain within its initial specifications throughout its shelf life. Recombinant *E. coli* produced, nonglycosylated G-CSF is extremely stable when formulated as a liquid at pH 4 and has a typical shelf life of more than 2 years when stored at 2–8°C. Even so, current high-sensitivity analytical techniques have revealed several routes of degradation that occur at very low levels at 2–8°C and at faster rates during accelerated storage conditions.

4.1. Aggregation Analysis

Current specifications for Neupogen® allow for no more than 1% of the total protein to be aggregated. When stored as a liquid at controlled room temperature (29°C), Neupogen® begins to exhibit an accumulation of nondissociable aggregate detectable both by SDS-PAGE and acidic SEC. At 29°C, the the amount of aggregate present exceeds the specification in about 6–8 months. At 2–8°C, the product remains within specification for more than 36 months.

4.2. Oxidation and Detergent Effects

Freshly formulated Neupogen® typically has a baseline level of oxidized methionine of less than 1%. This level of oxidation is usually stable throughout the shelf life of the product. However, certain lots of Neupogen® have been shown to exhibit a slow but definite increase in the level of oxidized methionine. The polysorbate-80 used in the formulation (see section 3.1) has a tendency to produce peroxides, which, in turn, can lead to oxidation of the methionine residues. This peroxide contamination appears to have a greater effect on protein oxidation than the presence of atmospheric oxygen in the vial headspace or the effects of product foaming in the fill lines. There is a definite correlation between the peroxide level in the polysorbate-80 and the degree of oxidation. The methionine oxidation can be accelerated by formulating Neupogen® in very high polysorbate concentrations (0.05–0.10%). Under these conditions the oxidation is quite rapid (<1 day) and clearly dependent on the amount of peroxides in a particular lot of polysorbate-80 (see Fig. 11).

Polysorbate-20 appears to present much less of an oxidation problem than

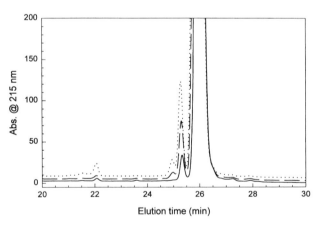

Figure 11. Oxidation of Neupogen® in polysorbate-80. Neupogen® was incubated at room temperatuure for 24 hr following the addition of 0.5% polysorbate-80 and then chromatographed as described in Fig. 8. Three lots of polysorbate-80 were used with 50 (solid line), 200 (dashed line), and 1000 (dotted line) ppm peroxides. All of the peaks except for the main peak eluting at 26 min represent oxidized forms of G-CSF. Absorbance is in mAU.

polysorbate-80. Comparative studies with polysorbate-80 and polysorbate-20 show that, even when the two detergents contain the same amount of peroxide, Neupogen® exposed to high concentrations of polysorbate-20 exhibits substantially less oxidation that when exposed to similar concentrations of polysorbate-80.

4.3. Glutamine Deamidation

The rate-limiting stability factor for Neupogen® is the formation of a series of acidic bands on IEF gels that migrate between G-CSF and f-metG-CSF. These bands are believed to represent deamidated forms of the protein. When Neupogen® is subjected to analytical chromatofocusing, it is possible to obtain a chromatogram that closely matches the pattern obtained on IEF gels. One of these minor components was subsequently analyzed by SV8 protease and a new peptide was found to be present. This new peptide had a mass consistent with an Gln → Glu substitution at position 68, indicating a possible deamidation at this position. Given the high glutamine content it is reasonable to assume that the other intermediate IEF bands observed also represent deamidation of the product. Both real-time and accelerated stability studies consistently show that deamidation occurs more rapidly than any of the other degradation routes.

4.4. Other Stability Issues

Several other forms of product degradation have been identified. These include proteolysis and disulfide rearrangement. However, these minor degradation routes occur much more slowly than the major ones described above. Because of this, efforts have been focused on understanding and controlling the more rapid degradation routes.

5. CONCLUSIONS

G-CSF is an extremely well-known and well-characterized molecule. Both the natural glycosylated form and the *E. coli*–produced nonglycosylated form are biologically active. A thorough understanding of the primary, secondary, and tertiary structures has enabled a rational approach to purification, folding, and formulation. Although the product can be considered mature, and testing and development of the second-generation formulation are complete, chemical and physical analysis of the product continue. It is this continued effort to understand the chemistry and stability of the product that ensure a safe and efficacious molecule.

REFERENCES

Arakawa, T., Prestrelski, S. J., Narhi, L. O., Boone, T. C., and Kenney, W. C., 1993, Cysteine 17 of recombinant human granulocyte-colony stimulating factor is partially solvent-exposed, *J. Protein Chem.* **112:**525–531.

Bazan, J. F., 1990, Haemopoietic receptors and helical cytokines, *Immunol. Today* **11:**350–354.

Clogston, C. L., Hsu, Y.-R., Boone, T. C., and Lu, H. S., 1992, Detection and quantitation of recombinant granulocyte colony stimulating factor charge isoforms: Comparative analysis by cationic exchange chromatography isoelectric focusing gel electrophoresis and peptide mapping, *Anal. Biochem.* **202:**375–383.

Clogston, C. L., Hu, S., Boone, T. C., and Lu, H. S., 1993, Glycosidase digestion, electrophoresis and chromatographic analysis of recombinant human granulocyte colony-stimulating factor glycoforms produced in Chinese hamster ovary cells, *J. Chromatogr.* **637:**55–62.

Cohen, A. M., Zsebo, K. M., Inoue, H., Hines, D., Boone, T. C., Chazin, V. R., Tsai, L., Ritch, T. and Souza, L. M., 1987, *In vivo* stimulation of granulopoiesis by recombinant human granulocyte colony-stimulating factor, *Proc. Natl. Acad. Sci. USA.* **84:**2484–8248.

Cunningham, B. C., and Wells, J. A., 1989, High-resolution epitope mapping of hGF-receptor interactions by alanine-scanning mutagenesis, *Science* **244:**1081–1084.

Demetri, G. D., and Griffin, J. D., 1991, Granulocyte colony-stimulating factor and its receptor, *Blood* **78:**2791–2808.

DeVos, A. M., Ultsch, M., and Kossiakoff, A. A., 1992, Human growth hormone and extracellular domain of its receptor: Crystal structure of the complex, *Science* **255:**306–312.

Diederichs, K., Boone, T., and Karplus, P. A., 1991, Novel fold and putative receptor binding site of granulocyte-macrophage colony-stimulating factor, *Science* **254:**1779–1782.

Ema, H., Suda, T., Miura, Y. and Nakauchi, H., 1990, Colony formation of clone-sorted human hemato-poietic progenitors, *Blood* **10:**1941–1946.

Fukunaga, R., Ishizaka-Ikeda, E., Seto, Y . and Nagata, S., 1990a, Expression cloning of a receptor for murine granulocyte colony stimulating factor, *Cell* **61:**341–350.

Fukunaga, R., Seto, Y., Mizushima, S. and Nagata, S., 1990b, Three different mRNAs encoding human granulocyte colony stimulating factor receptor, *Proc. Natl. Acad. Sci. USA* **87:**8702–8706.

Hibi, M., Murakami, M., Saito, M., Hirano, T., Taga, T., and Kishimoto, T., 1990, Molecular cloning and expression of an IL-6 signal transducer, gp130, *Cell* **63:**1149–1157.

Hill, C. P., Osslund, T. D., and Eisenberg, D. S., 1993, The structure of granulocyte colony-stimulating factor (r-huG-CSF) and its relationship to other growth factors, *Proc. Natl. Acad. Sci. USA* **90:**5167–5171.

Hutchinson, R. J., and Boxer, L. A., 1991, Disorders in granulocyte and monocyte production, in: *Hematology Basic Principles and Practice* (R. Hoffman, E. J. Benz, Jr., S. J. Shattil, B. Frurie, and H. J. Cohen, eds.), Churchill Livingstone, New York, pp. 193–204.

Kishimoto, T., Taga, T., and Akira, S., 1994, Cytokine signal transduction, *Cell* **76:**253–262.

Laemmli, U. K., 1970, Cleavage of structural proteins during the assembly of the head of bacteriophage T_4, *Nature* **227:**680–685.

Larson, A., David, T., Curtis, B. M. *et al.*, 1990, Expression cloning of a human granulocyte colony stimulating factor: A structural mosaic of hematopoietin receptor, immunoglobulin, and fibronectin domains, *J. Exp. Med.* **172:**1559–1570.

Le-Beau, M. M., Lemons, R. S., Carrino, J. J., Pettenati, M. J., Souza, L. M., Diaz, M. O., and Rowley, J. D., 1987, Chromosomal localization of the human G-CSF gene to 17q11 proximal to the breakpoint of the *t*(15;17) in acute promyelocytic leukemia, *Leukemia* **1:**795–799.

Lu, H. S., Boone, T. C., Souza, L. M., and Lai, P.-H., 1989a, Disulfide and secondary structure of recombinant human granulocyte colony stimulating factor, *Arch. Biochem. Biophys.* **268:**81–92.

Lu, H. S., Klein, M. L., and Lai, P. H., 1989b, Polypeptide C-terminal sequence analysis using carboxypep-tidase P and narrow bore HPLC of phenyl thiocarbamyl amino acids, *J. Chromatogr.* **454:**205–215.

Lu, H. S., Clogston, C. L., Narhi, L. O., Merewether, L. A., Pearl, W. R., and Boone, T. C., 1992, Folding and oxidation of recombinant human granulocyte colony stimulating factor produced in *E. coli* characterization of the disulfide-reduced intermediates and Cys Ala analogs, *J. Biol. Chem.* **267**:8770–8777.

Lu, H. S., Fausset, P. R., Sotos, L. S., Clogston, C. L., Rhode, M. F., Stoney, K. S., and Herman, A. C., 1993, Isolation and characterization of three recombinant human granulocyte colony stimulating factor his → gln isoforms produced in *Escherichia coli*, *Protein Expression Purification* **4**:465–472.

Martin, F. H., Suggs, S. V., Langley, K. E., Lu, H. S. *et al.*, 1990, Primary structure and functional expression of rat and human stem cell factor DNAs, *Cell* **63**:203–211.

Metcalf, D., 1989. Haemopoietic growth factors, *Lancet* April 15:825–827.

Metcalf, D., 1984, *The Haemopoietic Colony Stimulating Factors*, Elsevier, Amsterdam.

Metcalf, D., and Nicola, N. A., 1983, Proliferative effects of purified granulocyte colony stimulating factor (G-CSF) on normal mouse hemopoietic cells, *J. Cell Physiol.* **116**:198–206.

Morstyn, G., and Dexter, T. M., 1994, *Neupogen (r-metHuG-CSF) in Clinical Practice*, Marcel Dekker, New York.

Mosely, B., Beckmann, M. P., March, C. J. *et al.*, 1989, The murine interleukin-4 receptor: Molecular cloning and characterization of secreted and membrane bound forms, *Cell* **59**:335–348.

Motojima, H., Kobayashi, T., Shimane, M., Kamachi, S., and Fukushima, M., 1989, Quantitative enzyme immunoassay for human granulocyte colony stimulating factor (G-CSF), *J. Immunol. Methods* **118**:187–192.

Nagata, S., Tsuchiya, M., Asano, S., Kaziro, Y., Yamazaki, T., Yamamoto, O., Hirata, Y., Kubota, N., Oheda, M., Nomura, H. *et al.*, 1986a, Molecular cloning and expression of cDNA for human granulocyte colony-stimulating factor, *Nature* **319**:415–418.

Nagata, S., Tsuchiya, M., Asano, S. *et al.*, 1986b, The chromosomal gene structure and two mRNAs for human granulocyte colony-stimulating factor, *EMBO J.* **5**:575–581.

Narhi, L. O., Kenney, W. C., and Arakawa, T., 1991, Conformational changes of recombinant human granulocyte colony-stimulating factor induced by pH and guanidine HCl, *J. Protein Chem.* **10**:359–367.

Nicola, N. A., Metcalf, D., Matsumotu, M., and Johnson, G. R., 1983, Purification of a factor inducing differentiation in murine myelomonocytic leukemia cells: identification as granulocyte colony-stimulating factor, *J. Biol. Chem.* **258**:9017–9023.

Nomura, H., Imazeki, I., Oh-eda, M., Kubota, N., Tamura, M., Ono, M., Ueyama, Y., and Asano, S., 1986, Purification and characterization of human granulocyte colony-stimulating factor (G-CSF), *EMBO J.* **5**:871–876.

Oheda, M., Hase, S., Ono, M, and Ikenaka, T., 1988, Structures of the sugar chains of recombinant human granulocyte-colony-stimulating factor produced by Chinese hamster ovary cells, *J. Biochem.* **103**:544–546.

Oheda, M., Hasegawa, M, Hattori, K., Kuboniwa, H., Kojima, T., Orita, T., Tomonou, K., Yamazaki, T., and Ochi, M., 1990, *O*-linked sugar chain of human granulocyte colony stimulating factor protects it against polymerization and denaturation allowing it to retain its activity, *J. Biol. Chem.* **265**:11432–11435.

Okabe, M., Asano, M., Kuga, T. *et al.*, 1990, *In vitro* and *in vivo* hematopoietic effect of mutant human granulocyte colony stimulating factor, *Blood* **75**:1788–1793.

Osslund, T., and Boone, T. C., 1994, Biochemistry and structure of Neupogen® (r-metHuG-CSF), in: *Neupogen (r-metHuG-CSF) in Clinical Practice* (G. Morstyn and T. M. Dexter, eds.), Marcel Dekker, New York, pp. 23–31.

Pandit, J., Bohm, A., Jancarik, J., Halenbeck, R., Koths, K., and Kim, S.-H., 1992, Three-dimensional structure of dimeric human recombinant macrophage colony-stimulating factor, *Science* **258**:1358–1362.

Parry, D. A., Minasian, E., and Leach, S. J., 1988, Conformational homologies among cytokines: Interleukins and colony stimulating factors, *J. Mol. Recognition* **1**:107–110.

Shirafuji, N., Asano, S., Matsuda, S., Watari, K., Takaku, F., and Nagata, S., 1989, A new bioassay for human granulocyte colony-stimulating factor (hG-CSF) using murine myeloblastic NFS-60 cells as targets and estimation of its levels in sera from normal healthy persons and patients with infectious and hematological disorders, *Exp. Hematol.* **17:**116–119.

Simmers, R. N., Webber, L. M., Shannon, M. F., Garson, O. M., Wong, G., Vadas, M. A., and Sutherland, G. R., 1987 Localization of the G-CSF gene on chromosome 17 proximal to the breakpoint in the t(15;17) in acute promyelocytic leukemia, *Blood* **70:**330–332.

Souza, L. M., Boone, T. C., Gabrilove, J., Lai, P. H., Zsebo, K. M., Murdock, D. C., Chazin, V. R., Bruszewski, J., Lu, H., Chen, K. K., Barendt, J., Platzer, E., Moore, M. A. S., Mertelsmann, R., and Welte, K., 1986, Recombinant human granulocyte colony-stimulating factor: effects on normal and leukemic myeloid cells, *Science* **232:**61–65.

Tanaka, H., and Kaneko, T., 1992, Development of a competitive radioimmunoassay and a sandwich enzyme-linked immunosorbent assay for recombinant human granulocyte colony-stimulating factor. Application to a pharmacokinetic study in rats, *J. Pharmacobiodyn.* **15:**359–366.

Tohyama, K., Yoshida, Y., Kubo, A., Sudo, T., Moriyama, M., Sato, H., and Uchino, H., 1989, Detection of granulocyte colony-stimulating factor produced by a newly established human hepatoma cell line using a simple bioassay system, *Japanese J. Cancer Res.* **80:**335–340.

Watson, E., and Kenney, W. C., 1988, High-performance size-exclusion chromatography of recombinant derived proteins and aggregated species, *J. Chromatogr.* **436:**289–298.

Welte, K., Platzer, E., Lu, L., Gabrilove, J., Levi, E., Mertelsmann, R., and Moore, M., 1985, Purification and biological characterizaton of human pluripotent hematopoietic colony-stimulating factor, *Proc. Natl. Acad. Sci. USA* **82:**1526–1530.

Wilks, A. F., and Harpur, A. G., 1994, Cytokine signal transduction and JAK family of protein tyrosine kinases, *BioEssays* **16:**313–320.

Wingfield, P., Benedict, R., Turcatti, G., Allet, B., Mermod, J. J., DeLamarter, J., Simona, M. G., and Rose, K., 1988, Characterization of recombinant-derived granulocyte-colony stimulating factor (G-CSF), *Biochem. J.* **256:**213–218.

Zsebo, K. M., Cohen, A. M., Murdock, D. C., Boone, T. C., Inoue, H., Chazin, V. R., Hines, D., and Souza, L. M., 1986, Recombinant human granulocyte colony stimulating factor: molecular and biological characterization, *Immunobiology* **172:**175–184.

Zsebo, K., Wypych, J., McNiece, I., Lu, H. S. *et al.*, 1990, Identification, purification, and biological characterization of hematopoietic stem cell factor from Buffalo rat liver conditioned medium, *Cell* **63:**195–201.

8

Development and Shelf-Life Determination of Recombinant Human Granulocyte–Macrophage Colony-Stimulating Factor (LEUKINE®, GM-CSF)

John Geigert and Barbara F. D. Ghrist

1. THE HUMAN GM-CSF MOLECULE

Granulocyte–macrophage colony-stimulating factor (GM-CSF) belongs to a group of cytokine growth factors which promote white blood cell growth and function. GM-CSF induces partially committed progenitor cells to divide and differentiate in the granulocyte–macrophage pathways. GM-CSF also causes a response in granulocyte, monocyte, macrophage, and eosinophil mature end-stage cells.

The biological activity of GM-CSF occurs via interaction with cell-surface receptors (Park *et al.*, 1986). The GM-CSF receptor has been shown to exist in both low- and high-affinity states. The low-affinity GM-CSF specific receptor is an α-subunit (Gearing *et al.*, 1989). The high-affinity receptor is a heterodimer consisting of both the α-subunit and a β-subunit common to the receptors for GM-CSF, IL-3, and IL-5. The high-affinity receptor is formed only when both α- and β-subunits are bound to GM-CSF (Hercus *et al.*, 1994).

Recombinant human GM-CSF has found a medically useful role in bone marrow transplantation, for which one company, Immunex Corporation, has received marketed authorization from both the Food and Drug Administration (FDA) and the

John Geigert • Quality, IDEC Pharmaceuticals Corporation, San Diego, California 92121. *Barbara F. D. Ghrist* • Quality Control, Genentech Inc., South San Francisco, California 94080.

Formulation, Characterization, and Stability of Protein Drugs, Rodney Pearlman and Y. John Wang, eds., Plenum Press, New York, 1996.

European Committee for Proprietary Medicinal Products (CPMP). The product LEUKINE® (generic name Sargramostim), acting as a white blood cell stimulant, has been shown to reduce infection, antibiotic use, and hospital stays following autologous bone marrow transplantation in the treatment of certain cancers. Immunex has submitted supplemental filings with the FDA seeking approval for use of LEUKINE® following chemotherapy in patients with acute myeloid leukemia (AML), the most common form of acute leukemia in adults, and for use of LEUKINE® for allogeneic bone marrow transplantation.

The cloned gene for recombinant human GM-CSF has been expressed in bacteria, yeast, and mammalian cells. The recombinant preparation derived from bacterial cells is nonglycosylated, while the yeast- and mammalian-derived recombinant proteins are glycosylated, although to varying degrees and patterns. Glycosylation does not seem to be required for either *in vitro* or *in vivo* activity. However, the extent and pattern of glycosylation appear to influence pharmacokinetics and *in vivo* half-life (Donahue *et al.*, 1986; Moonen *et al.*, 1987).

Human GM-CSF is a glycoprotein of 127 amino acids. The primary amino acid sequence of Sargramostim, the recombinant human GM-CSF discussed in this chapter, is shown in Fig. 1. The amino acid sequence of Sargramostim differs from the natural human GM-CSF by a substitution of the amino acid leucine for arginine at position 23 to stabilize the protein within the expression system. Sargramostim, derived from yeast, contains both *N*-linked and *O*-linked oligosaccharides composed of mannose and *N*-acetylglucosamine.

H - Ala-	Pro-	Ala-	Arg-	Ser-	Pro-	Ser-	Pro-	Ser-	Thr-	Gln-	Pro-	Trp-	Glu-	His-
1	2	3	4	5	6	7	8	9	10	11	12	13	14	15
Val-	Asn-	Ala-	Ile-	Gln-	Glu-	Ala-	Leu-	Arg-	Leu-	Leu-	Asn-	Leu-	Ser-	Arg-
16	17	18	19	20	21	22	23	24	25	26	27	28	29	30
Asp-	Thr-	Ala-	Ala-	Glu-	Met-	Asn-	Glu-	Thr-	Val-	Glu-	Val-	Ile-	Ser-	Glu-
31	32	33	34	35	36	37	38	39	40	41	42	43	44	45
Met-	Phe-	Asp-	Leu-	Gln-	Glu-	Pro-	Thr-	Cys-	Leu-	Gln-	Thr-	Arg-	Leu-	Glu-
46	47	48	49	50	51	52	53	54	55	56	57	58	59	60
Leu-	Tyr-	Lys-	Gln-	Gly-	Leu-	Arg-	Gly-	Ser-	Leu-	Thr-	Lys-	Leu-	Lys-	Gly-
61	62	63	64	65	66	67	68	69	70	71	72	73	74	75
Pro-	Leu-	Thr-	Met-	Met-	Ala-	Ser-	His-	Tyr-	Lys-	Gln-	His-	Cys-	Pro-	Pro-
76	77	78	79	80	81	82	83	84	85	86	87	88	89	90
Thr-	Pro-	Glu-	Thr-	Ser-	Cys-	Ala-	Thr-	Gln-	Ile-	Ile-	Thr-	Phe-	Glu-	Ser-
91	92	93	94	95	96	97	98	99	100	101	102	103	104	105
Phe-	Lys-	Glu-	Asn-	Leu-	Lys-	Asp-	Phe-	Leu-	Leu-	Val-	Ile-	Pro-	Phe-	Asp-
106	107	108	109	110	111	112	113	114	115	116	117	118	119	120
Cys-	Trp-	Glu-	Pro-	Val-	Gln-	Glu-	OH							
121	122	123	124	125	126	127								

Figure 1. Primary amino acid sequence of Sargramostim (recombinant human GM-CSF).

2. THE LEUKINE® MANUFACTURING PROCESS

2.1. Fermentation and Purification

Sargramostim is produced in a yeast (*Saccharomyces cerevisiae*) expression system. Following fermentation, tangential flow filtration is used to separate the secreted, crude GM-CSF from the biomass and the filtrate is concentrated by ultra-filtration.

The concentrated crude GM-CSF filtrate is purified using successive reversed-phase high-performance liquid chromatography (RP-HPLC) columns. Purified GM-CSF is processed further by ion-exchange chromatography, and the protein is eluted and filtered to produce the bulk drug substance.

2.2. Formulation, Fill, and Finish

The bulk drug substance is transferred to a contract facility for compounding into the finished product. The compounded bulk is sterile filtered through a 0.2-micron filter, and aseptically filled, lyophilized (or filled as a liquid product), capped, labeled, and packaged.

LEUKINE® lyophilized formulation is a sterile, white, preservative-free, lyophilized solid. Each 5-cc glass vial with a 20-mm halobutyl isoprene blend rubber stopper contains either 0.25 or 0.50 mg Sargramostim, 40 mg mannitol, 10 mg sucrose, and 1.2 mg tromethamine (TRIS) at pH 7.4. LEUKINE® is reconstituted with 1 ml of either sterile water for injection, USP or bacteriostatic water for injection, USP (0.9% benzyl alcohol).

LEUKINE® liquid formulation is a sterile, clear, colorless liquid. Each 2-cc glass vial with a 13-mm halobutyl isoprene blend Purcoat rubber stopper contains either 0.50 mg or 1.00 mg Sargramostim, 40 mg mannitol, 10 mg sucrose, 1.2 mg tromethamine (TRIS), and 10 mg benzyl alcohol per mL at pH 7.4 in a 1-ml volume.

3. STRUCTURAL STUDIES OF GM-CSF

GM-CSF is an acidic glycoprotein belonging to the family of hematopoietic growth factors. Two review articles discuss structure–functional relationships of these proteins (Kaushansky, 1992; Kaushansky and Karplus, 1993). The three-dimensional X-ray crystal structure of nonglycosylated GM-CSF has been studied at both 6 Å resolution and at 2.8 Å resolution by using multiple isomorphous replacement techniques (Diederichs *et al.*, 1991b; Walter *et al.*, 1992). GM-CSF consists of a four-α-helix bundle arranged in a left-handed antiparallel array. When GM-CSF was studied at 2.4 Å resolution, a novel fold combining a two-stranded antiparallel β-sheet with the four α-helices was observed (Diederichs *et al.*, 1991a).

Proposed interactions of the hematopoietic cytokines with their receptors have been based on the accumulating structural information for many of these proteins. Two review articles compare and contrast the cytokines and their receptor complexes (Wlodawer *et al.*, 1993; Davies and Wlodawer, 1995). A number of papers have used a variety of techniques to study the interaction of GM-CSF with its receptor. Hercus *et al.* (1994) has reported a series of mutagenesis experiments which provide evidence implicating Asp[112] in the fourth helix to be pivotal in the binding of GM-CSF to the α-subunit of its receptor and Glu[21] in the first helix to the β-subunit. Demchuk *et al.*, (1994) performed electrostatic analyses of four-helix-bundle growth factors and produced evidence to support the binding of GM-CSF to a hetero-oligomeric receptor. Seelig *et al.* (1994) raised polyclonal antibodies to a synthetic peptide containing amino acids 110–127 present at the carboxy terminal of GM-CSF. They used these antibodies and their anti-idiotypic antibodies to probe the binding of GM-CSF to its receptor. Their data support the conclusion that the carboxy terminus of GM-CSF is critical for binding to the α-subunit of the receptor.

There are few reports regarding the solution stability of GM-CSF. Wingfield *et al.* (1988) compared the stability of glycosylated to nonglycosylated GM-CSF. They reported that the proteins are physically homogeneous and compact monomeric proteins, and that glycosylation did not affect conformational stability.

Tsarbopoulos *et al.* (1993) used mass spectrometry to confirm the existence of disulfide bonds between cysteine residues at positions 54 and 96 and between positions 88 and 121.

The accumulation of more data to further elucidate and confirm the sites of receptor binding in combination with other structural information should provide useful direction in the design of pharmaceutically beneficial GM-CSF analogues.

4. LEUKINE® STABILITY

4.1. LEUKINE® Stability Program

Manufactured lots of LEUKINE®, both lyophilized and liquid formulations, have been placed on the stability program.

The lyophilized formulations have CBER-approved expiry dating of 36 months from date of manufacture when stored at 2–8°C. The shelf life was determined from real-time storage with test data obtained throughout the 36-month time period.

The liquid formulations are currently under CBER review. To date, real time storage with test data obtained throughout an 18-month time period are available. At 2–8°C storage, the liquid product vials were placed in both the upright and inverted positions, with the assumption that the inverted position would be "worse case" due to maximizing for potential product–stopper interactions. Liquid product vials were also placed at both −20°C and 30°C in the inverted position to evaluate temperature stress conditions. The 2–8°C storage portion of this stability program is scheduled to continue through 36 months.

4.2. Potency by TF-1 Cell Proliferation Bioassay

The cell line-derived bioassay is based on the ability of recombinant human GM-CSF to induce proliferation of the TF-1 cells (an immature erythroleukemic human cell line) in a dose-dependent manner (Kitamura *et al.*, 1989). Proliferation is measured by quantifying radioactivity which is incorporated into viable cells when incubated with tritiated thymidine. The method is capable of detecting changes to the conformation or structure of the GM-CSF molecule which can alter its measured specific activity. The assay is calibrated using the First International Standard for GM-CSF and the results expressed as International Units (IU) per milligram GM-CSF (Mire-Sluis *et al.*, 1996). LEUKINE® has a nominal specific activity of 5.6×10^6 IU/mg GM-CSF.

Tables I and II provide examples of the potency results over time in storage. There was no statistically significant change in potency after 36 months at 2–8°C (lyophilized formulation), after 18 months at 2–8°C (liquid formulation, vial inverted), and even after 12 months at 30°C (liquid formulation, vial inverted).

Table I. Potency Stability of
LEUKINE® Lyophilized Product

Months in storage at 2–8°C	Measured potency (10^6 IU/mg)
0	8.1
3	7.5
6	5.6
9	7.1
12	4.5
18	5.9
24	6.5
30	6.6
36	5.6

Regression analysis of $\log_{10}$ transformed potency data versus months in storage:
Regression line slope: −0.002
p-value*: 0.36

*A *p*-value >0.05 documents that the null hypothesis for the slope being equal to zero cannot be rejected at the 5% level.

Table II. Potency Stability of LEUKINE® Liquid Product

Months in storage	Storage temp: 2–8°C Vial-inverted measured potency (10^6 IU/mg)	Storage temp: 30°C Vial-inverted measured potency (10^6 IU/mg)
0	5.1	5.1
3	5.0	5.0
6	6.9	6.8
9	5.0	4.8
12	5.0	5.3
18	5.3	—

Regression analysis of $\log_{10}$ transformed potency data versus months in storage:

Regression line slope:	−0.001	(2–8°C)	
	0.000	(30°C)	
p-value*:	0.87	(2–8°C)	
	1.00	(30°C)	

*A *p*-value >0.05 documents that the null hypothesis for the slope being equal to zero cannot be rejected at the 5% level.

4.3. Protein Integrity by SDS-PAGE Silver Stain

The protein integrity of GM-CSF is determined by sodium dodecyl sulfate–polyacrylamide gel electrophoresis (SDS-PAGE). The protein species are resolved by apparent molecular weight using a 10% to 20% linear gradient gel and then detected by staining with silver. Gels are run under reducing and nonreducing conditions. The method is capable of detecting fragmentation and oligomerization of the protein. By this method, recombinant human GM-CSF is resolved into three primary glycosylated components (referred to as bands 4, 3, and 2) of apparent molecular weight between 14 to 21 kDa, and a hyperglycosylated component (referred to as band 1) which generally appears as a broad band above 25 kDa.

Figure 2 provides an example of the SDS-PAGE results. There was no significant change in protein integrity after 36 months at 2–8°C (lyophilized formulation) and after 18 months at 2–8°C (liquid formulation). However, after 12 months at 30°C, under nonreducing conditions, band 4 in the liquid formulation product was becoming more diffuse, an indication of change taking place.

4.4. Protein Integrity by RP-HPLC

The protein integrity of GM-CSF is also determined by resolving the glycosylated protein species according to their hydrophobicity by RP-HPLC. Separation is performed on a C18 column using a linear gradient of 25% to 65% acetonitrile and 0.1% trifluoroacetic acid in water containing 1 M sodium chloride. Elution is mon-

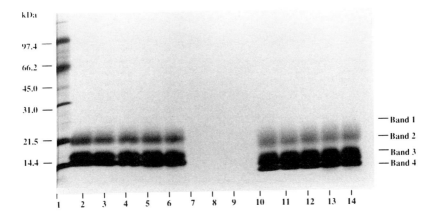

Figure 2.   Stability evaluation by SDS-PAGE of LEUKINE®. For each lane, the samples, amount loaded, and conditions are: 1, Low molecular weight makers; 2, LEUKINE®, lyophilized, 2–8°C, 24 months, 1 μg, reducing; 3, LEUKINES®, liquid, 2–8°C, 12 months, 1 μg, reducing; 4, LEUKINE®, liquid, 2–8°C, 12 months, 1 μg, reducing; 5, LEUKINE®, liquid, 30°C, 12 months, 1 μg, reducing; 6, LEUKINE®, liquid, 30°C, 12 months, 1 μg, reducing; 7–9, blank; 10, LEUKINE®, lyophilized, 2–8°C, 24 months, 1 μg, non-reducing; 11, LEUKINE®, liquid, 2–8°C, 12 months, 1 μg, non-reducing; 12, LEUKINE®, liquid, 2–8°C, 12 months, 1 μg, non-reducing; 13, LEUKINE®, liquid, 30°C, 12 months, 1 μg, non-reducing; 14, LEU-KINE®, liquid, 30°C; 12 months, 1 μg, non-reducing.

itored by absorbance at 220 nm. The method is capable of detecting changes in the protein. By this method, recombinant human GM-CSF is resolved into three primary glycosylated components (referred to as peaks 2, 3, and 4) and a hyperglycosylated component (referred to as peak 1). (Note, the 4 peaks observed by RP-HPLC correspond to the same number assigned to the four bands observed by SDS-PAGE.)

Figures 3 and 4 provide examples of the RP-HPLC results. There was no significant change in protein integrity after 36 months at 2–8°C (lyophilized formulation) and after 18 months at 2–8°C (liquid formulation). However, after 12 months at 30°C storage, the liquid formulation product showed significant denaturation. Note, changed GM-CSF co-elutes at the same retention time as the peak 1 component.

4.5. Protein Aggregation by SE-HPLC

The protein aggregation of GM-CSF is determined by resolving the monomeric protein species from the aggregated species according to their apparent molecular

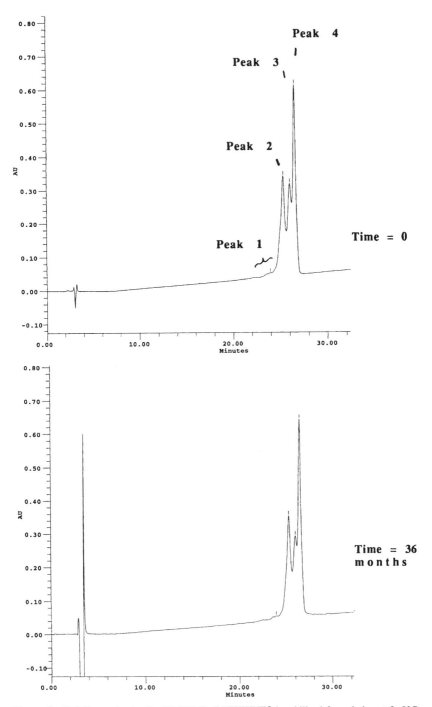

Figure 3.   Stability evaluation by RP-HPLC of LEUKINE® lyophilized formulation at 2–8°C.

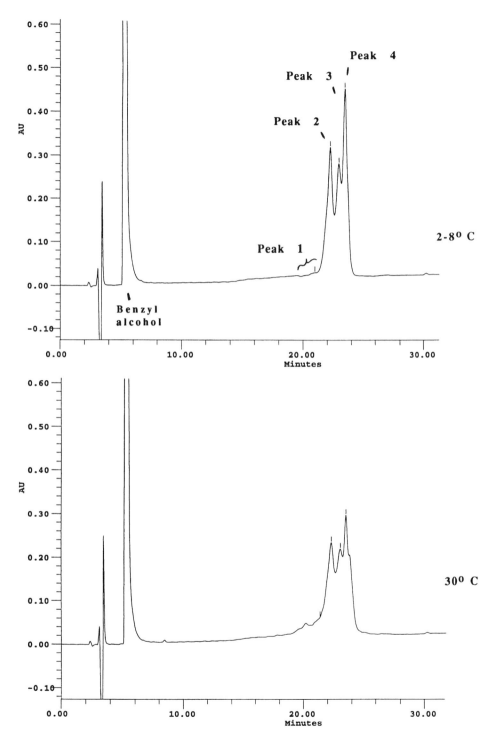

Figure 4. Stability evaluation by RP-HPLC of LEUKINE® liquid formulation after a 12-month time period at 2–8°C and 30°C.

size by size-exclusion high-performance liquid chromatography (SE-HPLC). Separation is performed on a Bio-Sil 125 column using an isocratic aqueous solvent of 100 mM sodium phosphate and 150 mM sodium chloride at pH 7.2. Elution is monitored by absorbance at 220 nm. By this method, recombinant human GM-CSF is resolved into a doublet monomeric component and an aggregated component.

Figures 5 and 6 provide examples of the SE-HPLC results. Aside from the minor amount of aggregation that is present at the time of preparation of the finished product, there was no significant change in protein aggregation after 36 months at 2–8°C (lyophilized formulation), after 18 months at 2–8°C (liquid formulation, inverted vial position), and even after 12 months at 30°C (liquid formulation, inverted vial position). However, the liquid formulation product, after being frozen at −20°C, showed some evidence of increased aggregation upon thawing.

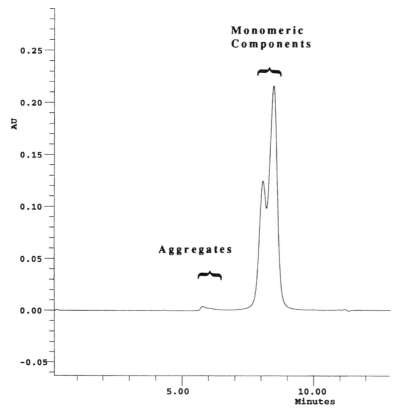

Figure 5. Stability evaluation by SE-HPLC of LEUKINE® lyophilized formulation after a 36-month time period at 2–8°C.

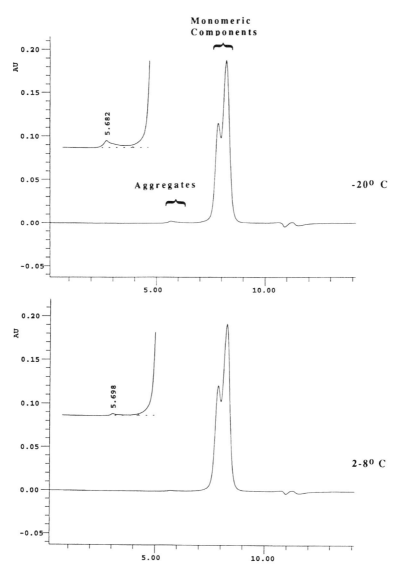

Figure 6. Stability evaluation by SE-HPLC of LEUKINE® liquid formulation after a 12-month time period at −20°C, 2–8°C and 30°C. Inserted in each chromatogram is an enhanced view of the aggregate region. (*Continued on next page*)

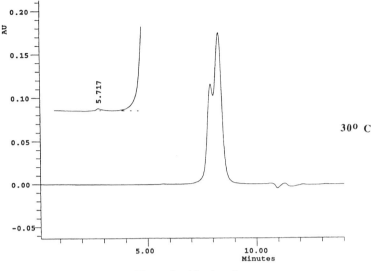

Figure 6. (*Continued*)

4.6. General Product Quality Parameters

The quality of the product (active protein ingredient plus excipients as well as integrity of the container-closure system) is assessed using several test methods: pH by pH meter; appearance (color and clarity) by visual inspection; sterility by USP Sterility Test; particulate matter by USP Particulate Test (HIAC); residual moisture by the Karl Fischer coulometric titration method (for the lyophilized formulation only); and antimicrobial preservative effectiveness by the USP Preservative Effectiveness Test (for the liquid formulation only).

For the appearance, sterility, residual moisture, and antimicrobial preservative effectiveness tests, there was no significant change in the product quality after 36 months at 2–8°C (lyophilized formulation) and after 18 months at 2–8°C (liquid formulation, inverted vial).

While the lyophilized formulation showed no significant change in measured pH after 36 months at 2–8°C, the liquid formulation showed a slight drop in measured pH (approximately 0.1 pH drop) after 18 months at 2–8°C. At 30°C storage, the drop in measured pH was accelerated (approximately a 0.3 pH drop after 18 months). For the liquid formulation, this change in pH was not totally unexpected, as TRIS buffer has a known weak buffering capacity for solutions at pH 7.4.

While the lyophilized formulation showed no significant change in number of particles per container after 36 months at 2–8°C, the liquid formulation showed a minor increase in measured particulates after 18 months at 2–8°C.

5. CONCLUSION

As these stability data demonstrate, LEUKINE® is a stable product, retaining biological potency, protein integrity and general quality parameters, when held at 2–8°C storage (36 months for lyophilized formulation and 18 months to date for liquid formulation). While the liquid formulation is more customer friendly (i.e., ready to use), it undergoes change more readily than the lyophilized formulation when exposed to warming to room temperature (i.e., protein denaturation, pH lowering) or to freezing (i.e., increased protein aggregation).

REFERENCES

Davies, D. R., and Wlodawer, A., 1995, Cytokines and their receptor complexes, *FASEB J.* **9**:50–56.

Demchuk, E., Mueller, T., Oschkinat, H., Sebald, W., and Wade, R.C., 1994, Receptor binding properties of four-helix-bundle growth factors deduced from electrostatic analysis, *Protein Sci.* **3**:920–935.

Diederichs, K., Boone, T., and Karplus, P. A. 1991a, Novel fold and putative receptor binding site of granulocyte-macrophage colony-stimulating factor, *Science* **254**:1779–1782.

Diederichs, K., Jacques, S., Boone, T., and Karplus, P. A., 1991b, Low-resolution structure of recombinant human granulocyte-macrophage colony stimulating factor, *J. Mol. Biol.* **221**:55–60.

Donahue, R. E., Wang, E. A., Kaufman, R. J., Foutch, L., Leary, A. C., Witek-Giannetti, J. S., Metzker, M., Hewick, R. M., Steinbrink, D. R., Shaw, G., Kamen, R., and Clark, S. C., 1986, Effects of N-linked carbohydrate on the *in vivo* properties of human GM-CSF, *Cold Spring Harbor Symp. Quant. Biol* **51**:685–692.

Gearing, D. P., King, J. A., Gough, N. M., and Nicola, N. A., 1989, Expression cloning of a receptor for human granulocyte-macrophage colony-stimulating factor, *EMBO J.* **8**:3667–3676.

Hercus, T. R., Cambareri, B., Dottore, M., Woodcock, J., Bagley, C. J., Vadas, M. A., Shannon, M. F., and Lopez, A. F., 1994, Identification of residues in the first and fourth helices of human granulocyte-macrophage colony-stimulating factor involved in biologic activity and in binding to the α- and β-chains of its receptor, *Blood* **83**:3500–3508.

Kaushansky, K., 1992, Structure-function relationships of the hematopoietic growth factors, *Proteins: Struct. Funct. Genet.* **12**:1–9.

Kaushansky, K., and Karplus, P. A., 1993, Hematopoietic growth factors: Understanding functional diversity in structural terms, *Blood* **82**:3229–3240.

Kitamura, T., Tange, T., Terasawa, T., Chiba, S., Kuwaki, T., Miyagawa, K., Piao, Y.-F., Miyazono, K., Urabe, A., and Takaku, F., 1989, Establishment and characterization of a unique human cell line that proliferates dependently on GM-CSF, IL-3 or Erythropoietin, *J. Cell. Physiol.* **140**:323–334.

Mire-Sluis, A. R., Das, R. G., and Thorpe, R., 1996, The International Standard for granulocyte-macrophage colony stimulating factor (GM-CSF): Evaluation of an international collaborative study, *J. Immunol. Methods*, in press.

Moonen, P., Mermod, J. J., Ernst, J. F., Hirschi, M., DeLamarter, J. F., 1987. Increased biological activity of deglycosylated recombinant human granulocyte macrophage colony-stimulating factor produced by yeast or animal cells, *Proc. Natl. Acad. Sci. USA* **84**:4428–4431.

Park, L. S., Friend, D., Gillis, S., and Urdal, D. L., 1986, Characterization of the cell surface receptor for human granulocyte macrophage colony-stimulating factor, *J. Exp. Med.* **164**:251–262.

Seelig, G. F., Prosise, W. W., and Scheffler, J. E., 1994, A role for the carboxy terminus of human granulocyte-macrophage colony-stimulating factor in the binding of ligand to the α-subunit of the high affinity receptor, *J. Biol. Chem.* **269**:5548–5553.

Tsarbopoulos, A., Pramanik, B. N., Labdon, J. E., Reichert, P., Gitlin, G., Patel, S., Sardana, V., Nagabhushan, T. L., and Trotta, P.P., 1993, Isolation and characterization of a resistant core peptide of recombinant human granulocyte-macrophage colony-stimulating factor (GM-CSF); confirmation of the GM-CSF amino acid sequence by mass spectrometry, *Protein Sci.* **2:**1948–1958.

Walter, M. R., Cook, W. J., Ealick, S. E., Nagabhushan, T. L., Trotta, P. P., and Bugg, C. E., 1992, Three-dimensional structure of recombinant human granulocyte-macrophage colony-stimulating factor, *J. Mol. Biol.* **224:**1075–1085.

Wingfield, P., Graber, P., Moonen, P., Craig, S., and Pain, R. H., 1988, The conformation and stability of recombinant-derived granulocyte-macrophage colony stimulating factors, *Eur. J. Biochem.* **173:** 65–72.

Wlodawer, A., Pavlovsky, A., and Gustchina, A., 1993, Hematopoietic cytokines: Similarities and differences in the structures, with implications for receptor binding, *Protein Sci.* **2:**1373–1382.

9

Formulation Development of an Antifibrin Monoclonal Antibody Radiopharmaceutical

Madhav S. Kamat, Glen L. Tolman, and John M. Brown

1. INTRODUCTION

Radiolabeled monoclonal antibodies (MAbs) and their fragments have been used in immunoscintigraphy in a variety of applications including detection of myocardial infarction (Khaw, 1987), deep venous thrombosis (Rosebrough, 1989; Knight, 1988), atherosclerosis (Fischman, 1989), detection of foci of bacterial infections (Rubin, 1989), detection and sizing of solid tumors (Pak, 1991; Goldenberg, 1993), and in monitoring the response to anticancer therapy (Pietersz, 1990).

In designing a formulation for an immunoscintigraphic agent, two components must be considered; the radionuclide and the MAb. The MAb is chosen on the basis of its specificity for an antigen associated with the target tissue. For efficient localization of this agent at the target site, with minimum nonspecific distribution, it is imperative that the specificity/avidity of the MAb toward the antigen be maintained throughout the shelf-life. Efforts to formulate an immunoscintigraphic agent for commercial use therefore must focus on preserving the chemical and physical integrity as well as the immunochemical properties of the MAb both during the shelf

Madhav S. Kamat, Glen L. Tolman, and John M. Brown • Pharmaceutical Development, Centocor Inc., Malvern, Pennsylvania 19355. *Present address of M.S.K.*: World Wide Pharmaceutical Technology, Bristol-Myers Squibb and Company, New Brunswick, New Jersey 08903.

Formulation, Characterization, and Stability of Protein Drugs, Rodney Pearlman and Y. John Wang, eds., Plenum Press, New York, 1996.

life of the product and then after labeling with the radionuclide in the clinic. The choice of radionuclide is based on a number of factors including its nuclear properties—energy and half-life, its availability and cost, and the labeling chemistry required to attach it to the MAb. The formulation of the radio-immunoscintigraphic agent must be compatible with the chemistry of radiolabeling to ensure that a pure and stable radiolabeled MAb is obtained in a quantitative and efficient manner.

The studies involved in the development of a formulation for an antifibrin murine MAb Fab′ fragment, radiolabeled with technetium-99m, are described in this chapter. Preformulation studies to identify critical factors with regard to the technetium-99m labeling chemistry and the physicochemical stability of the antifibrin Fab′ fragment are presented. Studies to establish the optimal composition of critical components in the formulation are also described. Finally, the results of the stability studies of the final formulation during long-term storage are summarized.

2. BACKGROUND ON MURINE Tc-99m–ANTIFIBRIN Fab′ FRAGMENT

2.1. The Antifibrin Murine MAb Fab′ Fragment

The murine antifibrin MAb T2G1s is an IgG1, κ light-chain antibody that binds to an epitope on the β chain in fibrin II and targets acute fibrin clots in deep venous thrombosis (DVT). The murine hybridoma cell line that produces T2G1s was prepared by fusing a murine myeloma cell line with murine splenocytes from a mouse immunized with the (T)N-DSK (thrombin-treated N-terminal disulfide knot) fragment (Kudryk, 1984). The immunogen (T)N-DSK is the highly soluble N-terminal fragment of fibrinogen called the "disulfide knot" and is obtained by treating cyanogen bromide-cleaved human fibrinogen (N-DSK) with thrombin (T) to remove fibrinopeptides A and B. The antigenic determinants exposed in the (T)N-DSK are identical to those exposed by thrombin cleavage of intact fibrinogen. These are the polymerization sites that are functional in the transition from fibrinogen to fibrin. The MAb T2G1s binds with high specificity and affinity ($K_d \sim 2.5 \times 10^{-9}$ M) to an epitope on the N-terminal end of the fibrin β-chain (Bβ 15–21). This epitope is cleaved by plasmin and, therefore, is not present on fibrin that has undergone fibrinolysis. Thus, because the T2G1s-reactive epitope is located at or in proximity to one of the polymerization sites, T2G1s binds to fibrin II but not to fibrinogen, fibrin I, or fibrin which has undergone fibrinolysis. Fibrin II is the transient intermediary between soluble fibrinogen and multiply cross-linked fibrin polymer and is only present in acute clots. The specificity of T2G1s therefore is uniquely suited to selectively target fibrin clots during active thrombosis before fibrinolysis and not the mature chronic thrombus characterized by tough fibrin weave produced after fibrin production, polymerization, and plasmin digestion (Kudryk, 1984).

The diagnostic performance of Tc-99m-antifibrin T2G1s Fab′ fragment was assessed in clinical studies enrolling patients with signs and/or symptoms of acute

DVT confirmed by ascending contrast venography. The Fab′ fragment of T2G1s, instead of complete T2G1s immunoglobulin (IgG) or papain-digested Fab fragment was chosen in these evaluations because it has several advantages over the intact IgG or the Fab: comparable immunoreactivity properties, availability of readily accessible sulfhydryl groups for chelation of radionuclide (Fab has none), favorable pharmacokinetics, and reduced immune response from the host. Each patient received 15–25 mCi of Tc-99m bound to 0.5 mg of T2G1s Fab′ and was imaged within 4–6 hr. The sensitivity (i.e., the number of positives out of patients with known clots) and specificity of Tc-99m–antifibrin T2G1s Fab′ for proximal (involving the knee and/or thigh), DVT were 79% and 91%, respectively. The clinical experience with Tc-99m–antifibrin T2G1s Fab′, specific for acute thrombi, indicates that it is a sensitive immunoscintigraphic agent for the rapid detection of DVT (Schaible, 1991).

2.2. Technetium-99m Labeling Chemistry

Technetium-99m has a half-life of 6 hr and emits a single 140-keV photon of gamma energy upon decay. These properties, and its availability in most hospitals from a commercially available Tc-99m/Mo-99 generator, make technetium-99m an ideal radionuclide for *in vivo* imaging applications. Several radiolabeling methods have been reported which describe the attachment of technetium-99m either through interaction with functional groups on the surface of the MAb or through interaction with a chelating group previously linked to the MAb (Hnatowich, 1991; Eckelman, 1989). To avoid the practical difficulties arising from the linking of a chelating agent to the antifibrin T2G1s, direct labeling of the endogenous sulfhydryl groups of the Fab′ fragment of antifibrin T2G1s with technetium-99m was chosen. Although the direct labeling of technetium-99m to Fab′ fragment theoretically requires less chemical manipulation, direct labeling methods have suffered from practical drawbacks, which include low purity of the Tc-99m-labeled final product, instability of the Tc-99m due to nonspecific binding to the Fab′, and loss of immunoreactivity of the Fab′ because of harsh radiolabeling conditions (Rhodes, 1991). These problems have been successfully addressed through the use of a mild reducing reagent and transfer ligand as described by Pak *et al.* (1992).

Technetium-99m is obtained in the form of aq. sodium [^{99m}Tc]pertechnetate from a commercially available Tc-99m/Mo-99 generator. In the pertechnetate ion ^{99m}TcO$_4^-$, the technetium, which is in the +7 oxidation state, is chemically unreactive and does not label any compound by direct addition. Reduction of ^{99m}TcO$_4^-$[Tc(VII)] to a lower oxidation state produces a highly reactive form that subsequently complexes strongly to many compounds, including free-sulfhydryl groups on proteins. Various reducing agents have been used for this purpose, including stannous chloride, stannous citrate, stannous tartrate, concentrated HCl, sodium borohydride, dithionite, and ferrous sulfate. Among these, stannous chloride has been proven to be the most effective due to its nearly optimal redox properties and lack of damage to immunoglobulins, and is the most often used reducing agent in the preparation of Tc-99m radiopharmaceuticals.

There are some drawbacks to this approach. In a typical preparation of a Tc-99m radiopharmaceutical, the presence of oxygen, particularly before the addition of the Tc-99m, can lead to the oxidation of stannous ion to stannic ion, thereby decreasing the amount of stannous ion available for the reduction of Tc(VII) and increasing free $^{99m}TcO_4^-$ in the radiopharmaceutical. Additionally, both reduced Tc-99m and Sn(II) can also undergo hydrolysis at physiologic pH to form insoluble technetium and tin oxides (colloidal species), which further complicate the use of Tc-99m-labeled MAbs for imaging purposes. To circumvent this problem, a weak chelating agent is generally added to the radiolabeling mixture that binds to the reduced Tc-99m and Sn(II) and prevents their subsequent hydrolysis.

The use of the weak chelating agent also addresses another major problem encountered in the labeling of MAbs with technetium, viz., the binding of the technetium to undesired low-affinity sites on the MAb. Paik *et al.* (1986) identified two sites on MAbs for technetium binding: high-affinity sites such as free-sulfhydryl groups, and low-affinity sites such as lysine groups (nonspecific binding sites). In the present studies, to achieve quantitative binding of Tc-99m to the high-affinity sites and minimize nonspecific binding, D-glucarate was used as a transfer ligand. Glucarate has an affinity for technetium which is intermediate between the high-affinity sulfhydryl groups and low-affinity nonspecific sites. In the presence of such transfer ligand and reducing agent the sequence of labeling reactions that occurs is postulated as follows:

$$^{99m}TcO_4^- + Sn(II) + \text{D-glucarate} \rightleftharpoons {}^{99m}Tc(V)\text{-D-glucarate} + Sn(IV) \qquad (1)$$

$$^{99m}Tc(V)\text{-D-glucarate} + \text{T2Gls-Fab}'\text{-SH} \rightleftharpoons {}^{99m}Tc\text{-S-T2Gls Fab}' \\ + \text{D-glucarate} \qquad (2)$$

In the first step, the stannous ion first reduces the [^{99m}Tc]pertechnetate to the proper oxidation state. In the presence of D-glucarate, 99m-Tc forms a transient complex consisting of reduced ^{99m}Tc-D-glucarate (Reaction 1). Upon exposure to free-sulfhydryl groups on T2Gls Fab' molecules in the surrounding solution, a transchelation reaction takes place, wherein Tc-99m from the ^{99m}Tc-D-glucarate complex is transferred to the higher-affinity sulfhydryl groups of the antifibrin T2Gls Fab', resulting in a stably labeled antifibrin T2Gls Fab'. Glucarate prevents transchelation to the lower-affinity nonspecific sites on the Fab'.

To achieve quantitative labeling of antifibrin Fab', and to keep the undesired side reactions to a minimum, the critical components in the labeling reaction mixture are the concentrations of the transfer ligand and stannous chloride and the maintenance of the free-sulfhydryl groups on the antifibrin Fab'. The experiments to evaluate factors which affect each of these components are described below. The studies involved in the preformulation development are described first. Based upon these observations, formulation studies were initiated, consisting of the selection of optimum buffer, pH, screening for the excipients, and evaluation of long-term stability.

3. ANTIFIBRIN Fab′ PRODUCTION, PURIFICATION, AND ANALYTICAL CHARACTERIZATION

3.1. Production and Purification of Antifibrin Fab′ (T2G1s)

Antifibrin T2G1s IgG1 was produced from the murine hybridoma in continuous perfusion cell culture and was purified by Protein A affinity chromatography (Bogard, 1989). The IgG was proteolytically cleaved with pepsin to yield the F(ab′)$_2$ fragment which was further purified by ion-exchange chromatography. The antifibrin F(ab′)$_2$ fragment was then mildly reduced with dithiothreitol (DTT) at room temperature to cleave H–H disulfides, yielding the Fab′ fragment (mol. wt. approx. 50 kDa). The reaction mixture was then exhaustively diafiltered to remove the DTT. The resulting product was sterile-filtered through a 0.22-μm filter and stored at 2–8°C under a blanket of argon gas until formulation.

3.2. Preparation of Antifibrin Fab′ Formulations

The bulk antifibrin Fab′ solutions were diafiltered into a buffer matrix which had been degassed to remove the dissolved oxygen. To this solution, other formulation components were added, and the pH and protein concentration of the solution were adjusted under anaerobic (nitrogen blanket) conditions. The final formulated bulk was filtered through a 0.22-μm filter and 1-ml solutions were filled into 10-ml borosilicate glass vials. For liquid formulation studies, the vials were blanketed with argon gas, stoppered with gray butyl rubber stoppers, and crimped with aluminum seals.

In the lyophilization studies, semistoppered filled vials were transferred to a freeze-dryer (model GT-20, Leybold). The shelf temperature was reduced to −40°C to freeze the solutions. After holding at this temperature for at least 6 hr, the primary drying was initially carried out with shelf temperature at 0°C for 8 hr and then at 15°C for up to 18 hr. The secondary drying phase was carried out at the shelf temperature of 25°C for up to an additional 18 hr. The drying was terminated after the product had reached the shelf temperature. It was held at this temperature for an additional 3 to 4 hr to ensure complete removal of moisture. The vials with less than 2% residual moisture were stoppered under a blanket of argon gas and crimped with aluminum seals.

3.3. Analytical Characterization

A number of analytical methods were employed to assess the radiochemical, biochemical, and physical properties of the Tc-99m–T2G1s Fab′. These were instant thin-layer chromatography (ITLC), high-performance size-exclusion liquid chromatography with UV and radiometric detection (HP-SEC), determination of free-sulfhydryl content, determination of stannous chloride, moisture determination, particle counting, and visual inspections. Radiolabeling was performed by mixing equal parts of T2G1s Fab′ formulation with eluate (0.9% saline) from a $^{99m}Tc/^{99}Mo$ generator. In the case of lyophilized formulations, the vials were reconstituted with 1 ml of eluate from the generator. The radiolabeled solutions were kept at room temperature for the analysis.

Potential radiochemical impurities in the final vialed product include both those common to stannous-reduced Tc-99m radiopharmaceuticals and those specific to the antifibrin Fab′ formulation. These impurities may include the following: (1) TcO_4^- due to incomplete reduction of starting TcO_4^-, as well as reoxidation of bound Tc-99m which then dissociates as free TcO_4^-; (2) Tc-glucarate, due to incomplete transfer of Tc-99m to the protein; (3) hydrolyzed reduced technetium (R-Tc), due to overreduction of TcO_4^- to Tc(IV) before tagging that can lead to insoluble R-Tc species such as technetium-99m dioxide and technetium-99m tin colloid; and (4) protein precipitate technetium (P-Tc), due to labeling of precipitated T2G1s Fab′. The radiochemical purity of the labeled T2G1s Fab′ was assessed using three types of assays specific for these different radiochemical species. The assays employed silica gel–impregnated ITLC (Gelman Sciences, ITLC-SG) as the stationary phase. The mobile phases used were 0.1 M sodium citrate, pH 5.0 (citrate), or a mixture of water: ethanol: concentrated ammonium hydroxide (75:25:2) (WEA) or methylethylketone (MEK).

When citrate buffer was used as the mobile phase, the Tc-99m-labeled T2G1s Fab′ remains at the origin while any free [^{99m}Tc] pertechnetate and other low-molecular-weight Tc-99m-labeled components such as ^{99m}Tc-D-glucarate or other labeled formulation excipients migrate with the solvent front. After spotting 20 µl of ^{99m}Tc–T2G1s Fab′ on the ITLC-SG strips, chromatograms were developed until the solvent front reached the top of the strip. The strip was immediately cut into halves, and the top and bottom halves were counted individually in a dose calibrator (Capintec). Technetium incorporation was reported as the activity in the bottom half (origin) divided by the total activity in both halves times 100%. In general, more than 90% of Tc-99m remains at the origin as radiolabeld T2G1s Fab′.

When the WEA mixture is used as the mobile phase, any hydrolyzed Tc-99m (insoluble colloids) present remains at the origin while ^{99m}Tc–T2G1s Fab′, ^{99m}Tc-D-glucarate, and other low-molecular-weight Tc-99m-labeled components move with the solvent front. The WEA-ITLC is run in the same manner as described for citrate ITLC. However, the technetium incorporation is reported as the activity in the top half of the strip (solvent front) divided by the total activity in both halves times 100%.

In general, less than 5% of technetium remains at the origin as insoluble Tc-99m colloids.

When MEK is used as the mobile phase, TcO_4^- migrates at the solvent front, while Tc-Fab$'$, R-Tc, P-Tc, and the majority of Tc-glucarate remain at the origin. The results are calculated as the percent of total counts remaining in the half containing the solvent front.

The radiochemical and chemical purity of Tc-99m-labeled antifibrin Fab$'$ samples were also analyzed by HP-SEC using either a Zorbax GF-250 or a Phenomenex SEP SEC-3000S size-exclusion column eluted with 0.2 M sodium phosphate buffer at pH 6.8. The eluate was monitored for UV absorbance at 214 nm and for 140-keV gamma emission of Tc-99m. To prevent both intermolecular disulfide bond and Fab$'$ dimer formation during chromatography, N-ethyl maleimide (NEM) was added to the T2G1s Fab$'$ samples before injection on the column to alkylate the free-sulfhydryl groups. The integrated peak area and the retention times from the UV and radiometric scans were compared to antifibrin Fab$'$ reference standard as criteria for purity and identity, respectively.

The immunoreactive fraction of the Tc-99m-labeled antifibrin Fab$'$ was measured by affinity column chromatography. The affinity column was prepared by covalent attachment to immobilized Sepharose 6B of a synthetic peptide corresponding to the first seven amino acids from the N-terminus of the β-chain of human fibrin and which contains the epitope for MAb binding. In this method, the radiolabeled sample was first diluted to 5 μg/ml with 1% bovine serum albumin (BSA) in phosphate-buffered saline (PBS). A 100-μl aliquot of this solution was applied to an affinity column (1 ml bed volume), which had been equilibrated with 1% BSA in PBS. The column was immediately eluted with a 10-ml portion of 1% BSA in PBS. This fraction contains activity associated with the nonbinding components of the sample (including the nonimmunoreactive or denatured antifibrin Fab$'$). The column was then eluted with a 10-ml portion of 0.1 M glycine, pH 2.5. Under this condition of low pH, the interactions between the antibody–antigen are broken up, resulting in the elution of the antibody. The eluted fraction then contains the activity which was immunoreactive and bound to the immobilized fibrin peptide. Aliquots (1 ml) of both the fractions were counted in a gamma scintillation counter. The percent immunoreactivity of Tc-99m-labeled antifibrin Fab$'$ was calculated as

$$\text{immunoreactive fraction} = \frac{\text{total counts eluted by glycine fraction} \times 100}{\text{total counts eluted by glycine and BSA fractions}}$$

This fraction was then corrected to exclude the contribution due to non-MAb–Tc-99m species by dividing by the fractional Tc-99m incorporation determined in the citrate–ITLC assay.

The sulfhydryl content of the Fab$'$ solutions was assessed spectrophotometrically at 412 nm after reacting with 5-5$'$-dithio-bis-(2-nitrobenzoic acid) (DTNB, Ellman's reagent) at pH 8.0 (Robyt, 1971). The bulk antifibrin Fab$'$ solutions were generally found to contain about 2–3 sulfhydryls per molecule of antibody fragment.

The Sn(II) content of the Fab' solutions was determined by titration with an iodine/iodide solution (standardized with arsenic oxide solution) to the starch/iodine endpoint, where the number of moles of iodine consumed is equal to the moles of Sn(II) present.

The moisture content of the lyophilized formulations was measured by Karl Fischer coulometry using a Mettler DL18 titrator. Five-milliliter portions of dry methanol were injected by a hypodermic needle into the vial through the rubber stopper to extract the residual moisture until no more water was detected (usually four times). The extracts were titrated with pyridine-free Karl Fischer reagent. The percent residual moisture was then calculated based upon the dry weight of the product. The sensitivity of the method was 0.3 mg of water and corresponded to about 0.5–1% moisture in the dry solids.

Following the reconstitution of lyophilized formulations in sterile 0.9% sodium chloride, each solution was visually inspected for the presence of insoluble particles, turbidity, and clarity against a black/white background using a 5× magnifying lens. The presence of subvisible particulate matter in the solution was evaluated using a particle counter (Climet, CI 2000) with a light obstruction detector (linear range of 4–250 μm). The results were expressed as the number of particles greater than 10 μm/ml in the sample.

4. PREFORMULATION STUDIES: DETERMINATION OF CRITICAL FACTORS

4.1. Antifibrin T2G1s Fab'

A dose of 15 to 25 mCi of Tc-99m–T2G1s Fab' is sufficient to produce a high-quality scintigraphic image at the site of the fibrin clot (Schaible, 1991). Therefore, the T2G1s Fab' must be radiolabeled with 25–30 mCi of Tc-99m to yield a patient dose equivalent to 15–25 mCi after losses due to radiolabeling efficiency, filtering, and after radioactive decay during storage for up to 2 hr. A 10-fold molar excess of T2G1s Fab' sulfhydryls over total technetium, i.e., approximately 0.5 mg of the 50-kDa MAb fragment, was chosen to achieve complete incorporation of the target dose of 25 mCi of Tc-99m (0.9×10^{-9} moles). The suitability of 0.5 mg of T2G1s Fab' was confirmed by measuring the Tc-99m incorporation in formulations in which the amounts of Tc-99m, stannous chloride, and glucarate were held constant, and the amount of Fab' was varied over 100-fold ranging from 0.01 to 1.0 mg. Incorporation of greater than 90% of the technetium presented was observed only when the amount of antifibrin Fab' was 0.5 or 1.0 mg (Table I). The Tc-99m incorporation was not optimal when the formulations contained lower than 0.5 mg of the T2G1s Fab'. Based upon these experiments, 0.5 mg of T2G1s Fab' was chosen as the final dose to ensure the incorporation of the desired dose of 25 mCi of Tc-99m.

**Table I. Effect of Amount of T2G1s
Fab′ on Incorporation of Tc99m[a,b]**

T2G1S Fab′ (mg/ml)	Tc-99m incorporation (%)
1.0	96.0
0.5	95.1
0.2	76.5
0.05	47.3
0.01	12.6

[a]Measured by citrate ITLC assay at 30 min.
[b]Radiolabeling was performed by mixing equal parts of
T2G1S Fab′ solution and eluate (0.9% saline, 25 mCi/ml)
from the generator.

In order to consistently incorporate 25 mCi of Tc-99m into antifibrin Fab′, the
sulfhydryl groups of the Fab′ must be in the reduced state and readily available for
chelation. The relationship between the available sulfhydryl groups on the T2G1s
Fab′ and the extent of Tc-99m incorporation as measured by the citrate ITLC test is
shown in Table II. The extent of Tc-99m incorporation into T2G1s Fab′ was shown to
be directly proportional to the level of free-sulfhydryl groups. When the sulfhydryl
groups were completely blocked after alkylation with N-ethylmaleimide, minimal
Tc-99m incorporation was observed. Based on these results, it was concluded that

**Table II. Relationship between
the Sulfhydryl Level and Tc-99m
Incorporation[a,b] into T2G1s Fab′**

Moles of −SH/ mole T2G1s Fab′[c]	Tc-99m incorporation (%)		
	15 min	30 min	60 min
0.0[d]	5.5	6.1	6.2
0.5	32.1	54.5	79.1
0.9	66.3	79.1	84.2
1.4	87.2	93.5	93.9
2.3	89.2	95.6	97.4
3.2	90.0	94.6	93.9

[a]Measured by citrate ITLC assay.
[b]Radiolabeling was performed by mixing equal parts of
T2G1S Fab′ solution with eluate (0.9% saline, 25mCi/mL)
from the generator.
[c]Measured by Ellman's reagent
[d]Treated with N-ethylmaleimide (NEM) to alkylate all −SH
groups.

≥1.4 mole of sulfhydryls per mole of T2Gls Fab′ was necessary for greater than 90% incorporation of Tc-99m at 30 min.

In aq. solutions, free-sulfhydryl groups are quite reactive and can oxidize to form inter- and intramolecular disulfide bonds, thereby making them unavailable for chelating the radionuclide. In Fab′ solutions, the result of such oxidation can lead to the formation of dimers of Fab′ wherein two molecules of Fab′ can covalently combine to produce a dimer with an approximate molecular weight of 100,000 Da (also referred as F(ab′)$_2$]. The loss of the sulfhydryl groups of T2Gls Fab′ and the formation of T2Gls Fab′ dimers as seen on HP-SEC is shown in Table III. During the course of eight weeks at 4°C and at pH of 6.8, a 40% decrease in sulfhydryl content was noted. This observation and the increase in the T2Gls F(ab′)$_2$ content, although small, indicated that in aq. solutions oxidation of the free sulfhydryls had occurred.

In general, the rate of oxidation of free-sulfhydryl groups is dependent upon the pH of the solution (the pK_a of most −SH is approximately 8) and the presence of catalysts such as divalent metal ions. Hence to minimize oxidation, the pH of the formulation of T2Gls Fab′ solutions must be adjusted to less than pH 8.0. The stability of the free-sulfhydryl groups was studied as a function of metal chelation, the concentration of Fab′, and the pH of the solutions. To do this, a number of solutions at different pH's were prepared with or without a chelating agent (EDTA) and stored in sealed borosilicate glass vials at 22°C. The extent of dimerization of T2Gls Fab′ was measured by HP-SEC, and the results are presented in Tables IV and V. Lowering the pH of the solution to 5.8 retarded the conversion of T2Gls Fab′ to dimer (Table IV). The presence of EDTA (1 mM) in the solution further reduced the extent of oxidation, presumably by chelating the metal ions present which catalyze sulfhydryl oxidation. The concentration of the T2Gls Fab′ in the solutions correlated inversely with the extent of dimerization; i.e., dilute solutions exhibited greater dimerization than the concentrated solutions over the period of time of the study (Table V). As expected, the addition of *N*-ethyl maleimide (NEM), which alkylates

**Table III. Stability of Sulfhydryl Groups
of T2Gls Fab′ (0.5 mg/ml)
at 4°C in aq. Solution (pH 6.8)**

Time (weeks)	SH/Fab′[a]	Fab′ monomer[b] (%)	F(ab′)2[b] (%)
0	3.0	100	0
1	3.5	100	0
2	3.1	100	0
4	3.0	100	0
5	2.9	97.5	2.5
8	2.4	97.1	2.9

[a] Measured by Ellman's reagent
[b] Measured by HP-SEC.

**Table IV. Stability of T2G1s Fab′
in Aqueous Solutions Stored at 22°C.
Effect of Various pH's on Percent Dimer Formation**[a]

pH	EDTA (mM)	10 min	24 hr	2 weeks	13 weeks
5.8	1	1.5	1.3	1.3	2.4
	0	1.5	1.9	3.1	6.7
7.2	1	1.4	1.4	3.2	11.0
	0	1.4	13.0	27.8	—
8.6	1	1.2	11.0	40.9	48.3
	0	1.3	33.0	42.1	—
9.5	1	1.3	32.0	54.0	71.2
	0	1.3	46.9	71.0	—

[a]Measured by HP-SEC.

the free-sulfhydryl groups, prevented the dimerization completely in the 0.5-mg/ml sample, confirming that the dimerization is mediated through the free-sulfhydryl groups only. It was also found that the monomer could be regenerated through reduction of the dimer with reducing agents such as dithiothreitol or β-mercaptoethanol (data not shown).

4.2. Stannous Ion [Sn(II)]

Stannous ion is required for the reduction of pertechnetate in the Tc-99m labeling of T2G1s Fab′, and therefore good stability of SnCl$_2$ in aq. solution was

**Table V. Stability of T2G1s Fab′
as a Function of Concentration at pH 7.2.
Percent Dimer Formation of T2G1s Fab′ at 22°C**[a]

Fab′ conc. (mg/ml)	10 min	24 hr	2 weeks	13 weeks
Control[b]	1.4	1.5	1.7	1.5
0.05	1.2	23.0	45.0	73.2
0.1	1.3	11.7	22.3	54.9
0.5	1.3	13.0	26.4	34.5
5.0	1.4	3.5	19.6	22.9

[a]Measured by HP-SEC.
[b]This sample at 0.5 mg/ml was treated with N-ethylmaleimide (NEM) to alkylate all −SH groups.

critical. Aqueous solutions of stannous chloride were studied with and without the protection of a blanket of inert gas. Stannous chloride (125 μg) was added to solutions containing D-glucaric acid (6 mg/mL) in 10 mM phosphate buffer at pH 8.0. The solutions were vigorously purged with argon gas for 60 min before the addition of $SnCl_2$, and the vessel holding the formulation was sealed to prevent further entry of oxygen. The results of the recovery of Sn(II) in this solution stored at 2–8°C are presented in Table VI. The recovery of stannous ion decreased rapidly in aq. solution when not protected by a blanket of argon gas; i.e., more than 50% of the SN(II) oxidized within 2 hr under ambient air conditions. Although the presence of an argon gas blanket retarded the oxidation of Sn(II), the recovery was still less than 20% in 24 hr. These studies indicated that Sn(II) is unstable in aq. solutions, suggesting that lyophilization of solutions containing $SnCl_2$ is essential. As seen from the results in Table VI, stannous chloride was found to be stable for more than 2 years at 2–8°C when stored in lyophilized solid form (although $SnCl_2$ oxidizes readily in solution at ambient conditions, during lyophilization, where low temperatures and vacuum prevail, its oxidation is minimal).

These results suggested that the T2G1s Fab′ slowly oxidizes in aq. formulations and that an optimum stability was achieved only in neutral-to-acidic conditions with EDTA present to preserve the free-sulfhydryl groups for the chelation of Tc-99m. Moreover, lyophilization of the final formulation was necessary to maintain the stability of Sn(II) throughout long-term storage.

4.3. Effect of Moisture

In order to establish the tolerance limits for residual moisture in lyophilized T2G1s Fab′ formulations containing Sn(II), the effect of residual moisture on lyophilized T2G1s Fab′ was assessed. Formulations containing T2G1s Fab′, Sn(II), and glucarate with a range of residual moisture content were prepared by placing

**Table VI. Percent Sn(II)Cl₂ Remaining in Aq. Solution[a]
and Lyophilized Solid[b] (2–8°C)**

Time	Solution with ambient air	Solution with argon	Lyophilized solid
0	79.0	74.7	—
15 min	68.8	75.5	—
2 hr	43.4	81.4	—
24 hr	0.0	19.2	91.0
6 months	0.0	0.0	87.5
2.1 yr	—	—	74.5

[a]10 mM phosphate with D-glucaric acid (6 mg/ml), pH 8.0.
[b]10 mM phosphate with D-glucaric acid (6 mg/ml), 3% potassium chloride, pH 8.0.

Table VII. Effect of Residual Moisture on T2G1s Fab′ Integrity in Lyophilized Samples Stored at 2–8°C for over 1 Month

Moisture (%)	Fab′ monomer[a] (%)	F(ab′)$_2$[a] (%)	Higher agg.[a] (%)	Tc-99m incorp.[b] (%)
1.5	97.8	1.4	0.8	96
2.1	96.9	2.2	0.7	96
3.2	94.2	4.6	1.2	94
4.0	92.9	4.7	2.4	93
6.7	71.3	17.4	11.3	83
9.1	69.2	17.3	12.5	69
12.3	54.9	31.0	14.1	42

[a]Measured by HP-SEC.
[b]Measured by citrate ITLC assay at 30 min.

semistoppered vials containing extensively dried T2G1s Fab′ in constant humidity chambers (at 25% and 75% RH at 2–8°C). The vials were removed periodically over 2 weeks after exposure to the humid environments and sealed. The samples were stored at 2–8°C for one additional month and were then analyzed by HP-SEC and by citrate ITLC after labeling. The extent of formation of dimer and higher-molecular-weight aggregates detected by HP-SEC and the Tc-99m incorporation of these samples are summarized in Table VII. These data demonstrated that as the moisture content of the lyophilized produce increased from 1.5% to 12.3%, the level of cross-linked Fab′ dimer and higher aggregates increased, accompanied by a significant decrease in Tc-99m incorporation. Based upon these data, a moisture content of <4% was considered essential to ensure >90% of T2G1s Fab′ in the lyophilized product remains as monomer with Tc-99m incorporation >90%.

5. FORMULATION STUDIES

Based upon the above preformulation studies the development phase for final formulation was initiated. The studies had already indicated that the essential components of the formulations were a lyophilized product containing T2G1s Fab′ at 0.5 mg/ml, SnCl$_2$ as reducing agent, D-glucaric acid as transfer agent, and appropriate buffer. Bulking agents were also considered essential for successful lyophilization to further improve the physical and chemical stability of the oxidation-prone components of the product. The criteria for acceptable performance of potential candidate formulations were based upon the interim specifications as described in Table VIII. The selection of the final formulation was based upon the comparative performance of the formulations in these stability-indicating tests.

**Table VIII. List of Analytical Tests and Acceptance Criteria
Used during Selection of the Optimum Formulation for T2G1s Fab′**

Test	Acceptance criterion
Purity by HP-SEC	>90% Fab′ monomer
Tc-99m incorporation by citrate ITLC	>90% in protein in 15 min
Tc-99m incorporation by radiometric HP-SEC	>90% in the Fab′ monomer
Visual examination	Clear solution; free of particles
Immunoreactive fraction by peptide-affinity column	>90%

5.1. Excipient Screening

5.1.1. EFFECT OF CONCENTRATION OF TRANSFER LIGAND

The potassium salt of D-glucaric acid (saccharic acid) was chosen as the transfer ligand for these formulations and the effect of its concentration on incorporation of Tc-99m into T2G1s Fab′ was studied. The first series of measurements examined the transfer of Tc-99m in solution to glucarate. The buffer solutions for the reaction included a fixed level of phosphate (50 mM) and stannous chloride (100 μg) and varied in their glucarate concentrations. The incorporation of Tc-99m in the glucarate complex was measured by citrate ITLC at 15 min and 3 hr after the addition of Tc-99m. The results, summarized in Table IX, showed that the transfer of Tc-99m to

**Table IX. Effect of D-Glucarate Concentrate
on Tc-99m Incorporation into Glucarate
(using glucarate alone) and into Fab′
(using glucarate with T2G1s Fab′)**

D-Glucarate (mM)	% Tc-99m Incorporation[a]			
	D-Glucarate alone[b]		D-Glucarate with Fab′	
	15 min	3 hr	15 min	3 hr
10	61.2	29.3	98.1	98.1
20	67.6	48.6	98.3	98.1
30	76.4	52.2	98.3	98.4
40	83.0	61.6	98.4	97.3
60	85.1	71.1	98.5	98.1

[a]Measured by citrate ITLC assay.
[b]To distinguish between 99mTcO$_4^-$ and 99mTc-glucarate, the ITLC strips were developed in methylethylketone (MEK).

the glucarate complex was not quantitative and was unstable with time at any concentration when the glucarate was used alone. However, when T2G1s Fab′ was included in the reaction mixture, a complete transchelation of Tc-99m from the glucarate complex to the free-sulfhydryl groups of the T2G1s Fab′ occurred, resulting in the formation of stable ^{99m}Tc–T2G1s Fab′. The citrate ITLC results also indicated that, in the presence of T2G1s Fab′, the concentration of glucarate in the buffer matrix was not critical. Based on these studies, a glucarate concentration in the middle of the test range, 6 mg/ml (24 mM), was chosen for further studies. At this concentration, the transfer ligand allowed quantitative incorporation of Tc-99m into Fab′, while limiting the amount of excipient present in the product.

5.1.2. EFFECT OF CONCENTRATION OF THE REDUCING AGENT

In order to minimize the presence of hydrolysis products of stannous chloride in the product, the amount of stannous chloride should be kept to a minimum. However, an excess quantity of Sn(II) must be present in the formulation to last throughout the shelf life of the product, since some Sn(II) is expected to be lost through oxidation over time. The effect of the concentration of stannous chloride on Tc-99m incorporation was examined, and the results, as summarized in Table X, show that Tc-99m incorporation was the greatest when the concentration of stannous chloride was between 10 and 100 μg/mL, and it decreased when the concentration was increased to 500 μg/mL. At the latter concentration, Tc-99m–colloid formation also increased. In order to ensure sufficient stannous chloride in the product through the shelf life, an initial concentration of 125 μg/ml was chosen (or 150 μg/ml of the dihydrate salt) for optimum recovery of stannous chloride. This initial concentration was found to achieve acceptable incorporation of Tc-99m into Fab′ ($>90\%$ in 15 min) even up to 2.5 years of storage.

**Table X. Effect of SnCl₂ Concentrate
on Tc-99m Incorporation into T2G1s Fab′**

SnCl₂ (μg/ml)	ITLC		HP-SEC (radiometric)		
	Tc-99m incorp.[a] (%)	Tc-99m colloids[b] (%)	T2G1s Fab′ monomer (%)	Low-MW species (%)	High-MW aggregates (%)
0	1.2	1.1	6.2	92.8	0.0
10	90.3	1.5	98.8	1.1	0.1
100	90.9	0.6	97.1	2.8	0.2
500	72.1	17.9	78.2	10.2	10.6

[a]As measured by citrate ITLC.
[b]As measured by WEA ITLC.

5.1.3. EFFECT OF BUFFER AND pH

Different buffer systems were tested for their ability to support incorporation of Tc-99m into T2G1s Fab'. All the reaction mixtures contained the same concentration of glucarate (24 mM), sodium chloride (0.3 M), stannous chloride (125 μg), and T2G1s Fab' (0.5 mg/ml). In these experiments, it was found that phosphate was the best buffer for efficient Tc-99m incorporation and hence was chosen for further use in the product formulation (Table XI). Using phosphate buffer at the concentration of 50 mM, the effect of pH was also examined as shown in Table XI. The lowest pH studied, 5.8, gave acceptable labeling, and solutions above pH 7.0 began to show a trend toward inhibition of Tc-99m incorporation. Based on these observations and other data from the solution stability of antifibrin Fab', a solution pH between 6.0 and 7.0 was considered appropriate for further use in the product formulation of T2G1s Fab'.

5.1.4. EFFECT OF BULKING AGENTS

Bulking agents facilitate lyophilization by providing a support structure and promoting removal of residual moisture during drying. A variety of agents were evaluated for their ability to produce an acceptable dried cake upon lyophilization and also yield clear, particle- and haze-free solutions upon reconstitution. Moreover, these agents must be chosen such that they do not participate in the radiolabeling

Table XI. Effect of Buffer and pH of Solutions on Tc-99m Incorporation into T2G1s Fab'

Buffer	Conc. (mM)	pH	% Tc-99m incorporation[a] 15 min	60 min
Barbiturate	50	7.5	62	61
Carbonate	200	8.0	70	84
Glycylglycine	50	7.9	66	94
Imidazole	50	5.8	51	81
Succinate	50	6.0	89	91
Tris	50	8.1	75	82
Phosphate	50	5.8	91	93
Phosphate	50	6.3	91	93
Phosphate	50	6.8	91	93
Phosphate	50	7.0	89	93
Phosphate	50	7.3	89	90
Phosphate	50	7.8	86	88

[a]As measured by citrate ITLC.

chemistry, adversely affecting Tc-99m incorporation into T2G1s Fab'. The use of 50 mM phosphate buffer at pH 6.8, a T2G1s Fab' concentration of 0.5 mg/ml, and D-glucaric acid at 6 mg/ml were kept constant in all of the test mixtures and the amounts of bulking agents were varied between 3% and 5% w/w. The physical characteristics of these formulations are summarized in Table XII. The inclusion of carbohydrates, in general, produced acceptable lyophilized products with good physical characteristics except in the products which contained glucose and sorbitol. These unacceptable products had a collapsed cake, turbidity on reconstitution, and higher moisture content. The dried samples containing salts exhibited good cake characteristics but also showed increased particulate matter, presumably as a result of adverse effects of high ionic strengths due to cryo concentration during the freezing and primary drying phases of lyophilization. The presence of amino acids such as arginine, glycine, and glutamine resulted in good cake characteristics and also

**Table XII. Effect of Bulking Agents
on the Physical Properties of Lyophilized T2G1s Fab'[a]**

Excipient	Cake	Solution[b]	Particles/ml ($>10\mu$m)	Moisture[c] (%)
Carbohydrate (5% w/w)				
Maltose	+	+	165	2.1
Lactose	+	+	190	1.8
Sucrose	+	+	120	2.3
Glucose	−	−	350	5.8
Sorbitol	−	+	210	5.2
Mannitol	+	+	290	1.5
Salts (3% w/w)				
Sodium chloride	+	−	1600	1.2
Sodium chloride and 0.1% Tween 80	+	−	465	1.8
Potassium chloride	+	+	2625	1.3
Amino acids (5%)				
Arginine	+	+	175	1.6
Glycine	+	+	210	1.6
Glutamate	+	+	190	1.4
Lysine	+	−	290	1.4
Others (3% w/w)				
Clyclodextrin	+	+	195	1.5
PVP	+	+	3515	1.8
Tween 80	+	+	110	1.9
Ficoll	+	−	260	1.8

+ = acceptable (e.g., good cake, clear solution).

− = unacceptable (e.g., collapsed cake, cloudy solution).

[a]in 50 mM potassium phosphate, 6 mg/ml D-glucaric acid, pH 6.8.

[b]Reconstituted with sterile water for injection.

[c]By Karl Fischer titration.

produced clear reconstituted solutions except when lysine was included. The inclusion of hydroxypropyl β-cyclodextrin, polyvinyl pyrolidone (PVP), Tween 80 (0.01%), or Ficoll produced good cakes. The PVP, however, showed increased particles in the reconstituted solutions, and the Ficoll-containing product required an excessively long time for complete reconstitution and produced a turbid solution.

The above lyophilized products were also tested for their radiochemical and immunochemical properties. The results of some representative formulations are shown in Table XIII. The samples containing carbohydrates (lactose and maltose) showed excellent Tc-99m incorporation and maintained high immunoreactivity toward fibrin peptide. The percent Tc-99m incorporation in the samples containing arginine, glutamic acid, cyclodextrin, and Tween 80 was quite low, with concomitant elevated levels of labeled low-molecular-weight species as seen on the radiometric HP-SEC, suggesting that these species competed with T2G1s Fab′ for the available Tc-99m. Figures 1A and 1B show representative HP-SEC profiles (with UV and radiometric signals) for samples containing maltose and arginine as bulking agents respectively. The UV scan for both these formulations indicated a predominant monomeric T2G1s Fab′ peak at a retention time of approximately 9 min. The large UV signal at a retention time of 14 min is due to the NEM which was used to prevent cross-linking of sulfhydryls during chromatography. However, the radiometric scans show radioactivity associated with the T2G1s Fab′ peak alone only in the case of maltose formulation (Fig. 1A), whereas in the case of arginine formulation almost 53% of the total radioactivity was associated with the low-molecular-weight peak, presumably radiolabeled arginine (Fig. 1B).

Thus, although many of the excipients used as bulking agents assisted in yielding optimally lyophilized products with good physical properties (Table XII) and good chemical stability of T2G1s Fab′ (Table XIII), some of these adversely

**Table XIII. Effect of Bulking Agents on the Radiochemical
and Immunochemical Properties of Lyophilized T2G1s Fab′**

Excipient	Fab′ monomer[a]	Tc-99m incorp.[b]	Tc-99m–Fab′ monomer[c]	Low-MW species[c]	Immuno fraction[d]
Lactose	100	94	100	0	95
Maltose	100	93	100	0	95
NaCl	100	90	100	0	91
Arginine	95	43	41	59	92
Gluta. acid	95	57	47	53	89
Cyclodextrin	98	35	40	60	89
Tween 80	76	27	22	78	79

[a]By HP-SEC (UV).
[b]By citrate ITLC.
[c]By HP-SEC (radiometric).
[d]By affinity column chromatography.

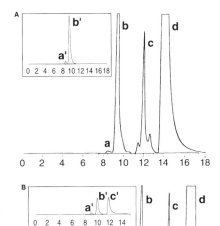

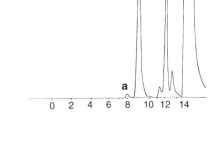

Figure 1. (A) UV and radiometric (inset) HP-SEC profiles of lyophilized samples containing maltose as bulking agent: a = dimer of T2G1s Fab'; b = T2G1s Fab' monomer; c = maltose; d = NEM (used to prevent chromatography artifact); a' = dimer of ^{99m}Tc-T2G1s-Fab'; b' = monomer of ^{99m}Tc-T2G1s-Fab'. (B) UV and radiometric (inset) HP-SEC profiles of lyophilized samples containing arginine as bulking agent: a = dimer of T2G1s Fab'; b = T2G1s Fab' monomer; c = arginine; d = NEM (used to prevent chromatography artifact); a' = dimer of ^{99m}Tc-T2G1s-Fab'; b' = monomer of ^{99m}Tc-T2G1s-Fab'; c' = ^{99m}Tc-arginine.

participated in the radiolabeling reaction and hence were incompatible with the product.

5.2. Stability Studies and Shelf-Life Determination

In order to study long-term stability to determine shelf-life, selected lyophilized formulations were stored at 4, 22, and 37°C and were tested over a period of 2 years. The results of 2-year-old samples are summarized in Table XIV. The products containing either sodium chloride or potassium chloride as excipients were stable for 2 years at 4°C. However, after 2 years at 22°C, these formulations showed decrease in monomeric Fab' content, Tc-99m incorporation, immunoreactivity, and increased levels of particulates. In contrast, the lyophilized products containing carbohydrates as excipients, such as with maltose and sucrose, exhibited excellent stability (Table XIV and Figs. 2A and 2B) over this time, maintaining physical, chemical, radiochemical, and immunochemical properties well above the acceptance criteria even after 2 years when stored at the elevated temperature of 37°C.

Table XIV. Two-Year Stability of Various Formulations of Lyophilized T2G1s[a]

Excipient	Moisture (%)	Particulate matter	Tc-99m incorp.[b]	% Fab' monomer UV	Radio.	Immun. fraction (%)
Maltose (5%)						
4°C	1.7	−	93	96	97	94
22°C	2.3	−	91	94	97	94
37°C	2.1	+	88	91	89	91
NaCl (3%)						
4°C	2.1	+	91	91	88	88
22°C	2.8	+ +	88	58	71	81
KCl (3%)						
4°C	3.3	+ +	94	95	89	87
22°C	6.0	+ + +	89	38	23	75
Sucrose (5%)						
4°C	2.1	−	87	90	85	90
22°C	4.1	−	89	91	87	91
Sucrose (5%) + EDTA (0.5mM)						
4°C	1.8	−	96	94	94	91
22°C	3.3	−	95	91	92	93
37°C	3.4	−	93	93	91	92

[a]All formulations contained T2G1s Fab' (0.5 mg/ml) in 50 mM potassium phosphate, 6 mg/ml D-glucaric acid, and 150 μg/ml of $SnCl_2 \cdot 2H_2O$.
[b]By citrate ITLC.
− = clear, no particles.
+ = <10 visible particles.
+ + = >10 visible particles.
+ + + = >100 visible particles.

6. SUMMARY

These studies have shown that formulation development of a monoclonal anti-body radio-immunoscintigraphy agent is a challenging task involving a number of issues related to the radiochemistry of labeling as well as the stability of the antibody. Through a systematic approach, as described in this study, a stable and efficacious product of high quality can be developed in a rational and efficient manner. In developing an optimized formulation of Tc-99m–antifibrin Fab' for use in immuno-scintigraphy of DVT, a number of critical components were examined in regard to technetium-labeling chemistry and the ability of the formulation to support the long-term stability of the product. It was found that the addition of glucarate as a transfer ligand, $SnCl_2$ as a reducing agent, and neutral-to-acidic pH of the solution were essential for optimum radiolabeling of 0.5 mg of antifibrin Fab' to a desired activity of 25 mCi of Tc-99m. The lyophilization of the final product was also required to further stabilize both the antifibrin Fab' fragment and the reducing agent. The addition of carbohydrate as bulking agent and lyoprotectant and inclusion of EDTA

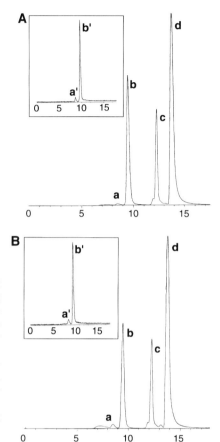

Figure 2. (A) UV and radiometric (inset) HP-SEC profiles of lyophilized stability samples containing maltose as bulking agent stored at 4°C for 2 years: a = dimer of T2Gls Fab′; b = T2Gls Fab′ monomer; c = maltose; d = NEM (used to prevent chromatography artifact); a′ = dimer of ^{99m}Tc-T2Gls-Fab′; b′ = monomer of ^{99m}Tc-T2Gls-Fab′. (B) UV and radiometric (inset) HP-SEC profiles of lyophilized stability samples containing maltose as bulking agent stored at 37°C for 2 years: a = dimer of T2Gls Fab′; b = T2Gls Fab′ monomer; c = maltose; d = NEM (used to prevent chromatography artifact); a′ = dimer of ^{99m}Tc-T2Gls-Fab′; b′ = monomer of ^{99m}Tc-T2Gls-Fab′.

as a chelating agent further improved the performance of the formulations, resulting in products with long shelf-life.

Many of the principles described in this study are not only useful in developing a technetium-based immunoscintigraphic agent but are also applicable to other immunopharmaceuticals, including products involving delivery of radionuclides, drugs, and toxins for immunotherapy of cancer and other diseases.

REFERENCES

Bogard, W., Dean, R., Deo, Y., Fuchs, R., Mattis, J., McLean, A., and Berger, H., 1989, Practical considerations in the production, purification, and formulation of monoclonal antibodies for immunoscintigraphy and immunotherapy, *Semin. Nucl. Med.* **19**:202–220.

Eckelman, W. C., Paik, C. H., and Steigman, J., 1989, Three approaches to radiolabeling antibodies with 99mTc, *Nucl. Med. Biol.* **16:**171–176.

Fischman, A., Rubin, R., Khaw, B. A., Krammer, P. N., Wilkinson, R., Ahamad, M., Nedelman, M., Locke, E., Nossiff, N. D., and Strauss, W. H., 1989, Radionuclide imaging of experimental atherosclerosis with non-specific polyclonal immunoglobulin G, *J. Nucl. Med.* **30:**1095–1100.

Goldenberg, D., Wlodkowski, T., Sharkey, R., Silberstein, E., Serafini, A., Garty, I., Van Heertum, R. L., Higginbotham-ford, E., Kotler, J., Balasubramaniam, N., Swayne, L., Hansen, H., and Pinsky, C., 1993, Colorectal cancer imaging with iodine-123-labeled CEA monoclonal antibody fragments, *J. Nucl. Med.* **34:**61–70.

Hnatowich, D. J., 1991, Recent developments in the radiolabeling of antibodies with iodine, indium, and technetium, *Semin. Nucl. Med.* **20:**80–91.

Khaw, B. A., Strauss, W. A., Moore, R., Fallon, J., Yasuda, T., Gold, H., and Haber, E., 1987, Myocardial damage delineated by indium-111 antimyosin Fab and technetium-99m pyrophosphate, *J. Nucl. Med.* **28:**76–82.

Knight, L., Maurer, A., Ammar, I., Shealy, D., and Mattis, J., 1988, Evaluation of indium-111-labeled anti-fibrin antibody for imaging vascular thrombi, *J. Nucl. Med.* **29:**494–502.

Kudryk, B., Rohoza, A., and Ahadi, M., 1983, A monoclonal antibody with ability to distinguish between NH_2-terminal fragments derived from fibrinogen and fibrin, *Mol. Immunol.* **20:**1191–1200.

Kudryk, B., Rohoza, A., and Ahadi, M., 1984, Specificity of a monoclonal antibody for the NH-2 terminal region of fibrin, *Mol. Immunol.* **21:**89–94.

Paik, C. H., Eckelman, W., and Reba, R., 1986, Transchelation of 99mTc from low affinity sites to high affinity sites of antibody, *Nucl. Med. Biol.* **13:**369–362.

Pak, K. Y., Nedelman, M. A., Fogler, W. E., Tam, S. H., Wilson, E., Van Haarlem, L. J. M., Colognola, R., Warnaar, S. A., and Daddona, P. E., 1991, Evaluation of the 323/A3 monoclonal antibody and the use of technetium-labeled 323/A3 Fab′ for the detection of Pan adenocarcinoma, *Nucl. Med. Biol.* **18:**483–497.

Pak, K. Y., Nedelman, M., Kanke, M., Khaw, B. A., Mattis, J. A., Strauss, W. H., Dean, R., and Berger, H. J., 1992, An instant kit method for labeling antimyosin Fab′ with technetium-99m: Evaluation in an experimental myocardial infarct model, *J. Nucl. Med.* **33:**144–150.

Pietersz, G. A., 1990, The linkage of cytotoxic drugs to monoclonal antibodies for the treatment of cancer, *Bioconj. Chem.* **1:**89–95.

Rhodes, B., 1991, Direct labeling of proteins with 99m-Tc, *Nucl. Med. Biol.* **18:** 667–676.

Robyt, J. F., Ackerman, R. J., and Chitrenden, C. G., 1971, Reaction of protein disulfide groups with Ellman's reagent: a case study of the number of sulfhydryl and disulfide groups in asporgillus oryzaed-amylase, papaine, and lysozyme, *Arch. Biochem. Biophys.* **147:**262–269.

Rosebrough, S., McAfee, J., Grossman, Z., and Schemancik, L., 1989, Immunoreactivity of 111-In and 131-I fibrin specific monoclonal antibody used for thrombus imaging, *J. Immunol. Methods* **116:**123–129.

Rubin, R., Fischman, A. J., Callahan, R., Khaw, B. A., Keech, F., Ahamad, M., Wilkinson, R., and Strauss, W. H., 1989, 111In-labeled nonspecific immunoglobulin scanning in the detection of focal infection, *N. Engl. J. Med.* **321:**935–940.

Schaible, T., and Alavi, A., 1991, Antifibrin scintigraphy in the diagnostic evaluation of acute deep venous thrombosis, *Semin. Nucl. Med.* **21:**313–324.

10

Biophysical Characterization and Formulation of TP40:

A Chimeric Protein That Requires a pH-Dependent Conformational Change for Its Biological Activity

Gautam Sanyal, Dorothy Marquis-Omer, and C. Russell Middaugh

1. INTRODUCTION

1.1. Rationale behind Designing a Recombinant Chimeric Protein Containing Transforming Growth Factor-α and a Fragment of *Pseudomonas* Exotoxin (PE)

TGF-α-PE40 is a genetically engineered chimeric protein composed of transforming growth factor-α (TGF-α), a 5-kDa peptide (Massagué, 1990), fused to 40-kDa segment (PE40) of *Pseudomonas* exotoxin (PE). In its unaltered form PE contains three distinct domains: (a) a cell binding portion that presumably binds to an α-2 macroglobulin/low density lipoprotein receptor which is present on most eukaryotic cell surfaces (Kounnas *et al.*, 1992), (b) a translocation domain which is responsible

Gautam Sanyal, Dorothy Marquis-Omer, and C. Russell Middaugh • Department of Vaccine Pharmaceutical Research, Merck Research Laboratories, West Point, Pennsylvania 19486.

Formulation, Characterization, and Stability of Protein Drugs, Rodney Pearlman and Y. John Wang, eds., Plenum Press, New York, 1996.

for transfer of PE across endosomal membranes into the cell cytoplasm, and (c) an enzymatic region which catalyzes ADP-ribosylation of elongation factor-2 (EF-2) which, in turn, inhibits protein synthesis. In TGF-α-PE40, the cell binding domain of PE is replaced with TGF-α, while domains (b) and (c) are retained (Pastan and FitzGerald, 1989). The rationale behind this design was to exploit the high affinity of TGF-α for EGF receptors (EGFr), thereby specifically targeting the toxic activity of PE40 toward certain tumor cells which express high concentrations of EGFr on their surface while minimizing the normally indiscriminate cytotoxicity of PE.

1.2. *In Vitro* Cytotoxic Activity of TGF-α-PE40 against Carcinoma Cell Lines Rich in Epidermal Growth Factor Receptors (EGFr)

In vitro experiments performed with a variety of cell lines clearly demonstrate the EGFr specificity of TGF-α-PE40 (Table I) (Edwards *et al.*, 1989). Cells containing little or no EGFr are not significantly affected by TGF-α-PE40 while virtually all of the cell lines tested are sensitive to PE itself. In contrast, TGF-α-PE40 manifests cell-killing activity against all cell lines containing EGFr, although quantitative differences in potencies exist that do not necessarily directly correlate with EGFr content. The PE40 segment of PE by itself manifests little or no cytotoxicity against any cell line examined.

Table I. Approximate Concentrations (nM) of PE and PE-Derived Toxins Required for Half-Maximal Cytotoxic Activity against Various EGFr-Rich and EGFr-Lacking Cells

Cell lines	EGFr × 10^{-4}/cell	Concentration (nM) required for half-maximal activity			
		TP40	TGF-α-PE40	PE	PE40
CHO	ND[a]	>300	100	0.96	>300
NR-6	ND[a]	>300		0.05	
U373MG	1.7	200		0.08	
HT29	4.4	0.67		1.2	>300
SCC-25	10	0.07		0.06	186
BT-20	12	0.09		0.22	35
SCC-4	17	0.45		0.15	43
HeLa	33	3.90	1.0	1.70	124
MDA-MB-468	160	0.25		2.00	68
A431	250	0.11	0.02	0.02	31

[a]Absent or not present at a detectable level.

1.3. Development of TP40, a Mutant Form of TGF-α-PE40, as a Potential Chemotherapeutic Agent

Within TGF-α-PE40, the TGF-α portion contains three disulfide bonds while PE40 contains two. The disulfides of TGF-α are essential for EGFr binding (Edwards *et al.*, 1989). To avoid scrambling between the TGF-α and PE40 disulfides during folding of the recombinant protein, all four cysteines in PE40 were mutated to alanines. This resulted in better process consistency during large-scale purification. This "Δ-cys mutant" of TGF-α-PE40 will be henceforth referred to as TP40. TP40 retains a very high cytotoxic activity against various EGFr-rich carcinoma cell lines, although its *in vitro* activity against A431 cells is approximately fivefold less than that of TGF-α-PE40 (Table I). The EGFr binding activity of TP40 is approximately 15-fold higher than that of TGF-α-PE40, while their ADP-ribosylation activities are of comparable magnitude (Edwards *et al.*, 1989). Since cell-killing activity is the end result of the sequential combination of EGFr binding, translocation and ADP-ribosylation activities of the conjugate proteins, one might assume that the translocation activity (for which there is no direct assay) must be somewhat compromised upon (cys to ala) mutation of TGF-α-PE40. The higher EGFr binding activity of TP40, however, suggests the potential for reduced nonspecific cell binding and, consequently, a wider therapeutic window for the mutated protein. Cell lines containing little or no EGFr are not significantly affected by either TP40 or TGF-α-PE40, further reinforcing the EGFr specificity of these chimeric proteins (Table I). Furthermore, when the three disulfide bonds in the TGF-α portion of TP40 are reduced and the resulting sulfhydryls carboxymethylated, the protein loses its EGFr binding activity (Edwards *et al.*, 1989). This observation provides confirmation that, as expected, binding of TP40 to the EGFr is mediated through the TGF-α domain. PE40 by itself is relatively non-toxic to most cells since it does not contain a region to mediate cell surface binding.

As desired, TP40 manifests marked antitumor activity against xenographic implants in nude mice (Heimbrook *et al.*, 1990) and against primary human tumors grown in soft agar (Von Hoff *et al.*, 1992). More recently, a phase I clinical study has been completed for human bladder cancer in which TP40 was found to be remarkably nontoxic. In addition, it displayed clinically significant activity against carcinoma *in situ* (CIS) (Goldberg *et al.*, 1995).

1.4. Expression and Purification of TP40

TP40 was produced from a bacterial expression system employing the plasmid vector pTAC-TGF57-PE40, as described by Heimbrook *et al.* (1990). This system was adopted from Linemeyer *et al.* (1987). This vector expresses a synthetic gene encoding TGF-α fused to a modified PE40 containing alanine codons instead of the four cysteine codons normally found in the PE40 segment of the PE gene. The pTAC-TGF57-PE40 plasmid was introduced into a strain of *E. coli* and induced with isopropyl-β-thiogalactopyranoside. TP40 was purified from these cultures using multiple chromatographic steps (George *et al.*, 1992; Yamazaki *et al.*, submitted). The resulting protein was identified by amino acid sequencing and found to be of 99% or greater purity by standard analytical criteria, e.g., SDS–polyacrylamide gel electrophoresis (SDS-PAGE), reverse-phase HPLC (RP-HPLC), HPLC size-exclusion chromatography (HPSEC), and hydrophobic interaction chromatography (HIC).

2. STRUCTURE–FUNCTION CORRELATION

2.1. Structural Characterization of TP40 Employing Biophysical Techniques

2.1.1. CIRCULAR DICHROISM (CD) SPECTROSCOPY

The three major domains of PE are evident in its three-dimensional structure as determined by X-ray crystallography (Allured *et al.*, 1986). The 40kDa PE40 segment contains the translocation and ADP-ribosylation domains II and III. Domain II is composed predominantly of (six) α-helical segments. Domain III contains primarily β-sheet secondary structure and a few stretches of α-helix. PE40Δcys constitutes approximately 89% of the mass of TP40, which contains a total of 421 amino acid residues. Therefore, it is not surprising that the CD spectra of TP40 and PE40Δcys are very similar, suggesting that PE40Δcys dominates the secondary structure of TP40 (Fig. 1). The secondary structure contents of the two proteins have been estimated by variable selection analysis (Manavalan and Johnson, 1987) of these CD spectra and found to be nearly identical (Sanyal *et al.*, 1993). In each case, α-helices and β-sheets make about equal contributions to the overall secondary structure (23–28% and 21–31%, respectively), the rest of which is composed of turns and unordered regions. These results are consistent with the crystal structure data of PE (Allured *et al.*, 1986). No NMR study of TP40, PE, or PE40 has yet been reported. The structure of TGF-α has been studied by NMR and FTIR spectroscopy (Kline *et al.*, 1990; Prestrelski *et al.*, 1992). It is composed primarily of disordered structures and turns. This structure could be altered, however, upon binding to EGF receptors.

2.1.2. FTIR SPECTROSCOPY

The amide I′ FTIR spectra of TP40 and PE40Δcys have also been measured in D_2O solutions buffered with 5 mM sodium phosphate at a pD of 7.2. The resulting

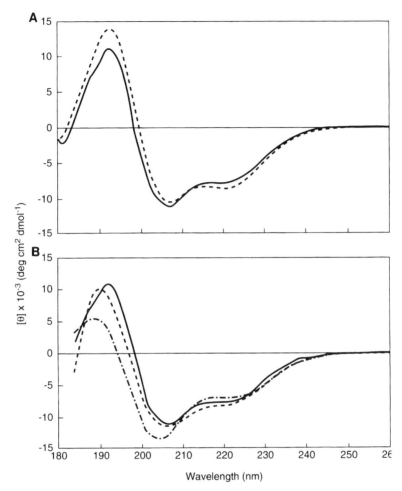

Figure 1. (A) Far-UV CD spectra of TP40 (-) and PE40Δcys (---) taken in 100 mM sodium phosphate buffer, pH 7.2 at 25°C. (B) CD spectra of TP40 at pH 2.5 (---), 7.2 (—), and 11.4 (-----) in 100 mM sodium phosphate buffer, at 25°C.

Fourier self-deconvolved spectra and underlying component bands, resolved by curve fitting, are shown in Fig. 2. Once again, there is a marked similarity between the spectra of TP40 and PE40Δcys, reinforcing the CD results which suggest that the secondary structure of the former is similar to that of the latter. The secondary structure assignments (Susi and Byler, 1986) of the individual bands for both proteins are indicated in Table II and are in general agreement with those estimated from CD spectra.

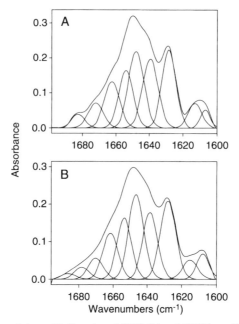

Figure 2.   FTIR spectra of the amide I′ region of TP40 (A) and PE40Δcys (B). The partially deconvoluted spectrum and the fully deconvoluted bands are shown. Peak frequencies, bandwidths, and areas
under the bands are listed in Table II.

2.1.3. FLUORESCENCE SPECTROSCOPY

TP40 contains four tryptophan residues all of which occur in the PE40Δcys
segment. Although the presence of multiple tryptophan residues prohibits detailed
interpretation of the protein's fluorescence spectrum, the overall tryptophan fluorescence signal has been conveniently utilized to study unfolding and folding of TP40
under various conditions (Sanyal *et al.*, 1993; Gress *et al.*, 1994). The (uncorrected)
wavelength of maximum emission is located between 329 and 336 nm depending on
the instrument used. The location of the emission maximum is independent of
excitation wavelength between 280 and 295 nm, suggesting that tyrosine residues
do not make a major contribution to the native protein's intrinsic fluorescence. Not
surprisingly, the tryptophan fluorescence emission spectra of TP40 and PE40Δcys
are very similar and respond to conformational perturbations in a similar manner. The
average tryptophan fluorescence lifetimes of both proteins are also similar and
sensitive to unfolding perturbations as described in detail elsewhere (Gress *et al.*,
1994).

**Table II. FTIR Amide I′ (1620–1700 cm⁻¹)
Spectral Characteristics of TP40 and PE40Δcys[a]**

Protein	Peak frequency (cm⁻¹)	Band[b] half-width (cm⁻¹)	Relative peak area	Assignment[c]
TP40	1628	4.8	0.20	β-strand
	1639	5.4	0.20	β-strand
	1648	5.3	0.22	Unordered
	1654	5.0	0.15	α-helix
	1662	5.3	0.13	Turn
	1672	5.3	0.07	Turn or β-strand
	1683	4.6	0.03	Turn
PE40Δcys	1628	5.3	0.21	β-strand
	1638	5.0	0.17	β-strand
	1646	5.2	0.23	Unordered
	1653	5.0	0.16	α-helix
	1662	5.2	0.12	Turn
	1670	5.1	0.06	Turn
	1678	5.0	0.03	β-strand
	1686	5.1	0.02	Turn

[a]Measurements were made at ambient temperature using approximately 5 mg/ml TP40 and 6 mg/ml PE40Δcys at pD = 7.2.

[b]Half-width at half-peak height.

[c]Based on the assignments of Susi and Byler (1986). Because of overlap between a pair of adjacent bands, assignment to individual secondary structure contents in the 1640–1660 cm⁻¹ region should be considered tentative. For example, the bands centered at 1648 and 1654 cm⁻¹ (TP40) may both contain contributions from α-helix and unordered structures. Also, the 1639 cm⁻¹ band may contain contributions from both β-sheet and unordered structure.

2.2. pH-Dependent Structural Changes of TP40

2.2.1. CD AND FLUORESCENCE SPECTRAL CHANGES IN SOLUTION

The secondary structure of TP40 is virtually invariant over a pH range of 5.0 to 9.0, as judged by CD spectra. At pH values above 10 unfolding is observed, as indicated by the relative increase in ellipticity at 200 nm relative to that at 220 nm (Fig. 3A). At acidic pH values, alterations in secondary structure are more subtle, and most of the ordered structure is retained. It should be emphasized that pH effects on the CD spectrum of TP40 are primarily determined by the PE40Δcys portion, and that no pH dependence is observed of the weak TGF-α spectrum (not illustrated; see Sanyal et al., 1993).

The pH-dependence of the fluorescence λ_{max} of TP40 is shown in Fig. 3B. Like

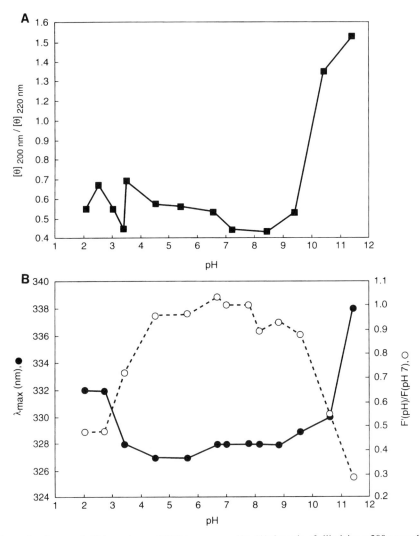

Figure 3. Structural pH dependence of TP40 as measured by (A) the ratio of ellipticity at 200 nm to that at 220 nm and (B) wavelength of maximum fluorescence (●) and fluorescence intensity (○) as a function of pH. Measurements were made at 25°C with 280-nm exciting light.

its CD spectrum, the tryptophan fluorescence emission spectrum of TP40 is independent of pH between pH 5 and 8, but a gradual red-shifting of the fluorescence spectrum is observed as the pH is lowered below pH 5. This suggests exposure of one or more hydrophobic regions at pH <5, while the overall secondary structure of the peptide backbone remains unchanged. At pH >8, on the other hand, a progressive red-shift of the fluorescence spectrum with increasing pH coupled with CD spectral changes suggests a more global unfolding of the protein's secondary as well as tertiary structure.

The above inference is further reinforced by the marked increase in the fluorescence intensity, as a function of decreasing pH, of the hydrophobic fluorescence probes 2-*p*-toluidinylnaphthalene-6-sulfonate (TNS) (Fig. 4). This effect is especially pronounced below pH 4, although a smaller but progressive increase in dye fluorescence with decreasing pH is observed between pH 7 and 5.

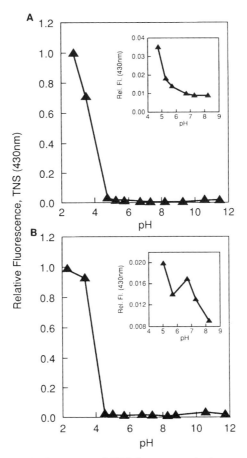

Figure 4. Low-pH-induced enhancement of TNS fluorescence in the presence of TP40 (A) and PE40Δcys (B). Excitation was at 315 nm at room temperature. Emission was monitored at the maximum, 430 nm, and emission intensities were normalized to the highest intensity observed at the lowest pH. The insets magnify the data between pH 4 and pH 9.

2.2.2. pH-DEPENDENT INTERACTION OF TP40 WITH LIPOSOMES

At low pH TP40 was also found to interact with anionic liposomes, as detected by a blue-shift of the protein's tryptophan fluorescence (Fig. 5A). These liposomes were prepared as reverse evaporation vesicles (REVs) employing distearoylphosphatidylcholine (DSPC) and dioleoylphosphatidylglycerol (DOPG) and TP40 was titrated with HCl in their presence. The observed blue-shift of tryptophan fluorescence

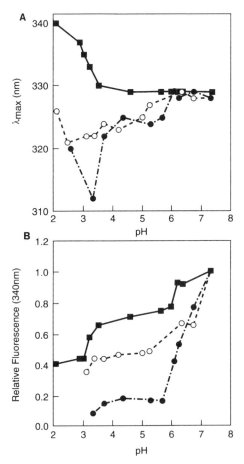

Figure 5. (A) Intrinsic tryptophan fluorescence emission maximum versus pH of TP40 (■), TP40 in the presence of 1:1 DSPC:DOPG REVs (○) and TP40 in the presence of 1:1 brominated DSPC:DOPG REVs (●). Samples in 10 mM sodium phosphate buffer (pH 7.4) were titrated in the cuvette with HCl. The wavelength of excitation was 280 nm. (B) Relative intrinsic tryptophan fluorescence intensity monitored at 340 nm versus pH of TP40 (■), TP40 in the presence of 1:1 DSPC:DOPG REVs (○) and TP40 in the presence of 1:1 brominated DSPC:DOPG REVs (●). Conditions were as in (A).

below pH 6 is in contrast to the fluorescence red-shift that is observed when TP40 is titrated with HCl in the absence of liposomes. Thus, at least one and possibly more of the protein's four tryptophan residues appear to be in a hydrophobic region which, at an acidic pH, becomes exposed and available to interact with anionic lipid bilayers. The presence of liposomes provides a hydrophobic surface for the exposed tryptophan(s) which, in turn, results in the observed blue-shift in tryptophan fluorescence. Neutral liposomes do not induce any change in the tryptophan fluorescence of TP40 at low pH, suggesting that interaction of this protein with membranes involves an electrostatic as well as a hydrophobic component. Thus, in addition to exposing one or more hydrophobic surfaces on the protein, acidic pH presumably also confers a net positive charge on the protein which enhances interaction with anionic membranes. Interestingly, the approximate midpoint of the anionic liposome-induced, pH-dependent, tryptophan fluorescence blue-shift of TP40 is ~5, which is near the presumed pH of endosomal membrane surfaces (Draper and Simon, 1980). On the other hand, half-maximal TNS binding to the free protein in solution occurs at approximately pH 3 in the absence of liposomes (Fig. 4). It appears that the negative charge on the membrane surface might lower the effective pH in the immediate environment of TP40, thereby inducing the observed structural transition at an apparently higher solution pH.

The evidence for interaction of TP40 with anionic liposomes was reinforced by the observed quenching of TP40's tryptophan fluorescence by brominated DSPC: DOPG vesicles (Fig. 5B). The rationale was to take advantage of the quenching effect of bromide on tryptophan fluorescence provided that these two moieties were within interacting distance so that static quenching was possible. This quenching is also pH-dependent and is pronounced at acidic pH values. Since the bromide concentration in the liposomes is much lower than that typically needed for dynamic tryptophan fluorescence quenching, the assumption that the mechanism of quenching is static and not collisional appears reasonable. Consequently, we conclude that one or more of the protein's tryptophan residues physically interacts with the liposomes.

2.2.3. LOW pH-INDUCED AGGREGATION OF TP40 IN SOLUTION

At low pH the protein in solution also self-associates to form large, soluble aggregates. This has been demonstrated by both equilibrium sedimentation and quasielastic light-scattering (QLS) measurements (Sanyal *et al.*, 1993). The molecular weight of TP40 estimated from such measurements is consistent with that of a monomer between pH 5.3 and 7.0. At pH 2.5, a molecular weight approximately 10 times that of monomer is observed by equilibrium sedimentation (Table III). This is consistent with QLS measurements which yield a z-average mean hydrodynamic diameter (D_h) of approximately 17 nm at pH values of 2.0 and 3.0 (Table IV). The relatively low polydispersity at these pH values suggests a fairly homogeneous solution containing a well-defined oligomeric species. Velocity sedimentation mea-

Table III. Estimates of Molecular Weights (MW) and Sedimentation Coefficients (*S*) of TP40 as a Function of pH as Determined by Equilibrium Sedimentation and Velocity Sedimentation Measurements

pH	Best-fit model[a]	MW[a]	$S_{20°C}$[b]
2.52	Single species[c]	443 090	2.42, 10.00
3.93[d]		Not determined (insoluble material)	Not determined
5.25	Single species	46 307	2.55
5.44	Single species	42 004	2.53
5.65	Single species	41 158	2.46
7.04	Single species	45 085	2.51

[a]Equilibrium measurements were performed with 1 mg/ml TP40 solutions at approximately 25 °C. Data from both 10,000 and 15,000 rpm centrifugations were used in the Nonlin analysis to generate the best-fit model and the MW.

[b]Velocity measurements were made on 1 mg/ml TP40 solutions at 20°C at a rotor speed of 40,000 rpm. Results are expressed in Svedberg units (S).

[c]Although the best fit was obtained assuming a single species of approximately 10 times the MW of a monomer, almost equally good fits resulted assuming equilibrium between multimers of different sizes. Measurements at 4°C yielded a monomer–hexamer equilibrium as the best fit for TP40 solutions (0.25 mg/ml) at pH 2.5 and 3.2. Velocity sedimentation data could also be fit to two components with widely different *S* values.

[d]Precipitation of TP40 from solution occurred during centrifugation. At 4°C, using 0.25 mg/ml TP40, a single species with a MW of 47,945 was obtained as the best fit.

surements at pH 2.5, however, were best described by a two-component fit with sedimentation coefficients of 2.5 S and 10.0 S. At pH values between 5.3 and 7.2, the sedimentation coefficient remained nearly invariant at 2.5 ± 0.05, reinforcing the evidence for the presence of a monomeric species (Table III). The theoretically calculated D_h for a spherical TP40 molecule is 8.4 nm. This calculation assumes a

Table IV. *Z*-Average Mean Hydrodynamic Diameter (D_h) of TP40 as a Function of pH[a]

pH	D_h (nm)	Polydispersity index	pH	D_h (nm)	Polydispersity index
2.00	17.6	0.183	7.20	8.2	0.282
2.96	16.7	0.163	7.78	9.7	0.330
3.59	24.8	0.120	8.66	9.1	0.290
4.36	>100	0.128	9.93	8.7	0.279
5.51	9.5[b]	0.604[b]	10.9	10.3	0.266
6.34	8.7	0.292			

[a]Measurements were made at 25°C on TP40 solutions at a concentration of approximately 1 mg/ml. Samples at different pH values were prepared by dialyzing a 1-mg/ml solution at pH 7 against 100 mM phosphate buffer of the desired pH.

[b]A small amount (~3%) of a larger material (D_h range of 35–48 nm) was detected, which accounts for the relatively high polydispersity index.

partial specific volume of 0.728 cm³/g (calculated from amino acid composition of TP40) and a hydration volume of 0.35 cm³/cm³ of the protein. For pH values from 5.5 to 9.9, QLS measurements yield nearly constant D_h values of 8.2–9.7 nm (Table IV), in agreement with equilibrium and velocity sedimentation results that indicate the presence of a monomeric species (Table III). pH's between 4 and 5 are impossible to study because of isoelectric precipitation of the protein. The most probable reason for aggregation at acidic pH is again the exposure of one or more hydrophobic surfaces, as evidenced by the red-shifted tryptophan fluorescence and TNS binding. Interpretation of the large enhancement of TNS binding at pH values below 4 is, however, complicated by aggregation, although one can speculate that these two observations are simply different expressions of the same phenomenon. The possibility that TNS is trapped by protein aggregates cannot be excluded. It should be noted, however, that TNS binding to TP40 is enhanced as pH is decreased from 7 to 5 while the protein apparently remains monomeric (as detected by QLS), although not as markedly as at pH values <4.

2.2.4. pH-DEPENDENCE OF *IN VITRO* BIOACTIVITY OF TP40

This has been determined in cell-killing experiments employing human epidermal carcinoma (A431) cells. TP40 was incubated at pH values between 3.4 and 11.5 and examined for cytotoxicity. No discernible difference in activity (beyond the ca. 27% standard deviation inherent in these experiments) is detected over a pH range of 3.4–8.2 (Table V). Because the pH of the cell medium was 7.4, the normal bioactivity observed for the samples incubated at different pH values suggests that any pH-induced change (between pH 3.4 and 8.2) is reversible. On the other hand, a TP40 sample incubated at pH 11.5 manifests an irreversible loss of activity. This is consis-

Table V. *In Vitro* Cell-kill Bioactivity of TP40 Samples Incubated at Different pH Values[a]

Incubation pH	Relative potency[b]	95% confidence interval
3.4	0.99	0.92–1.08
5.5	0.83	0.81–0.85
7.2	0.95	0.91–0.99
8.2	0.87	0.81–0.93
11.5	0.20	0.18–0.24

[a]Samples incubated at 5°C in 100 mM sodium phosphate buffers at the indicated pH were transferred and diluted into the assay medium at 37°C, pH 7.4.
[b]Relative potency represents the ratio of EC_{50} of the assay standard to that of the sample, where EC_{50} is the concentration of TP40 at which 50% cell survival is observed. Typical EC_{50} values were 35–50 pM under these assay conditions. The assay standard was structually well characterized, stored at −70°C, and fully bioactive.

tent with the loss of the protein's secondary structure at this high pH as detected by CD spectroscopy.

2.3. Speculations on the TP40 Translocation Mechanism

The data discussed above strongly suggest that at acidic pH values TP40 (and PE40Δcys) undergoes a conformational change in which its secondary structure remains intact but hydrophobic surfaces become partially exposed. This may be the key property of this protein which is required for its translocation across the endosomal membrane surface where the pH is thought to be approximately 5. The reversibility of such a change is important because the pH in the cytoplasm, where TP40 must ADP-ribosylate elongation factor-2 to exert its cytotoxic function, is approximately 7.4. Interestingly, a similar low-pH-induced conformational change has been implicated in the cytotoxic activity of *Pseudomonas* exotoxin (PE) (Zalman and Wisnieski, 1985; Sandvig and Moskaug, 1987; Farahbakhsh and Wisnieski, 1989; Jiang and London, 1990). The binding of hydrophobic fluorescence probes (ANS and TNS), changes in intrinsic tryptophan fluorescence, and susceptibility to proteolysis have all been utilized to investigate effects of reducing the pH on the structure and membrane interaction of PE. At pH values between 3.7 and 5.4, a largely folded conformation with a slightly blue-shifted tryptophan fluorescence compared to pH 7.0 is observed. When the pH is reduced below 3.7, unfolding of tertiary structure becomes more pronounced. The possibility of involvement of a "molten globule" (MG) structure has been suggested based on these observations (Jiang and London, 1990) but not systematically investigated. MG states of proteins are characterized by a substantial loss of tertiary structure compared to native states while extensive secondary structure and compact form are retained. In recent years, a large body of evidence has been gathered which suggests that MG states are early intermediates in the folding pathway of many proteins (Kuwajima, 1989; Baldwin, 1991; Christensen and Pain, 1991; Dobson, 1992; Mach *et al.*, 1993). Such states can often be induced in proteins by low pH and high anion concentrations as well as by relatively low denaturant concentrations insufficient to cause unfolding of the secondary structure of the peptide backbone. An important question is whether translocating proteins such as PE or TP40 may depend upon conformational flexibility to adopt a translocation-competent MG-like state at the acidic pH encountered in endosomes. Such conformational flexibility in TP40 which results in the formation of partially folded intermediates is evident in the fluorescence and CD data described above. Compactness of this intermediate, however, could not be examined because of self-association at acidic pH.

Tryptophan fluorescence measurements suggest that at pH 2 the tertiary structure of TP40 is not completely disrupted, as one would expect in a typical MG state, since the fluorescence λ_{max} is not consistent with a total solvent exposure. However, partially folded intermediates of β-lactamase at acidic pH values have also been found (in the presence of 0.5 M KCl) in which tryptophan residues are apparently buried (Goto and Fink, 1989).

2.4. Equilibrium Unfolding Induced by Guanidine Hydrochloride: Evidence for the Presence of a Molten Globule Intermediate

In order to determine if a MG-like intermediate can indeed be observed in the unfolding–refolding pathway of TP40, equilibrium unfolding induced by guanidine hydrochloride (Gdn·HCl) was studied (Gress et al., 1994). Disruption of secondary structure was monitored by far-UV CD, while that of tertiary structure was measured by tryptophan fluorescence and near-UV CD. The fluorescence spectra of both proteins are progressively red-shifted as the concentration of Gdn·HCl increases, indicating increasing solvent exposure of one or more tryptophan residues (Fig. 6). The midpoints of the transitions in λ_{max} occur at approximately 1.5 M and 1.4 M Gdn·HCl for TP40 and PE40Δcys, respectively. These transitions appear to be biphasic. For TP40, a relatively sharp change in λ_{max} (from 336 to 349 nm) is observed between 1 and 2 M chaotrope. This is followed by a broader transition, also manifested as a red-shift, to a λ_{max} of 354 nm at 4M Gdn·HCl. The midpoint of this transition occurs at approximately 2.1 M. This second transition accounts for approximately 10% of the total fluorescence quenching induced by Gdn·HCl. It thus appears that the intermediate state produced in the first, dominant, phase retains some residual tertiary structure which is disrupted at higher Gdn·HCl concentrations.

Far-UV CD spectra (202–260 nm) of TP40 and PE40Δcys were also measured as a function of Gdn·HCl concentration. The spectra of the fully folded forms of both proteins are characterized by a minimum at 206 nm and a negative shoulder around 220 nm (see Figs. 2 and 4). In the presence of increasing concentrations of Gdn·HCl, the 220 nm shoulder is progressively quenched in intensity while there is a gradual blue-shift of the 206-nm minimum accompanied by an increase in intensity in the 203–205 nm region (Fig. 7). These data are consistent with Gdn·HCl induced unfolding of the secondary structure of TP40. A plot of mean residue ellipticity as a function of Gdn·HCl concentration yields a value of 2.0 M for the midpoint of the transition which appears to be broader than the corresponding fluorescence transition. For PE40Δcys, a midpoint at 2.1 M Gdn·HCl is observed and the transition is also relatively broad. Although the presence of Gdn·HCl increases background noise in the far-UV, it was possible to obtain acceptable signal-to-noise ratios down to 202 nm using a 100-μm pathlength cell. The absence of absorption flattening in these measurements was confirmed by plotting mean residue ellipticity versus Gdn·HCl concentration at different wavelengths (214–222 nm), with all three plots yielding nearly identical midpoints for the unfolding transition. The fraction (f_{app}) of unfolded secondary and tertiary structures at a given Gdn·HCl concentration was calculated

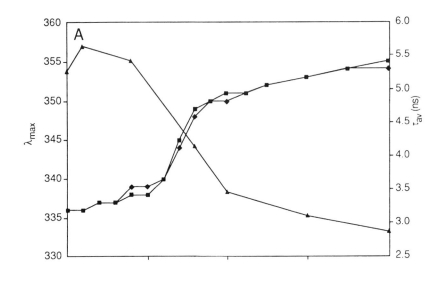

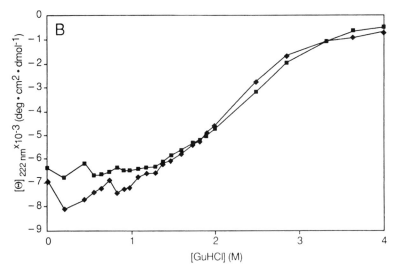

Figure 6. Unfolding of TP40 and PE40Δcys as a function of Gdn·HCl concentration as monitored by intrinsic tryptophan fluorescence and far-UV CD spectra. (A) ♦, λ_{max} in nm of the fluorescence emission spectrum of TP40; ■, λ_{max} in nm of the fluorescence emission spectrum of PE40Δcys; ▲, average tryptophan fluorescence lifetime (ns) of TP40. (B) CD mean residue ellipticity at 222 nm of TP40 (●) and PE40Δcys (♦).

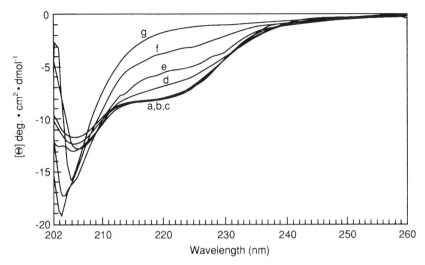

Figure 7. Far-UV spectra of TP40 in the (a) absence and presence of (b) 0.5 M, (c) 1.0 M, (d) 1.5 M, (e) 2.0 M, (f) 2.5 M, and (g) 4.0 M Gdn·HCl.

from the CD and fluorescence data, respectively, and plotted against the denaturant concentration. These plots (Fig. 8) are clearly noncoincident, with tertiary structure disruption appearing prior to secondary structure perturbation. The midpoints of these plots, i.e., Gdn·HCl concentrations at which $f_{app} = 0.5$, are summarized in Table VI. This observation suggests that the unfolding transition is not a two-state process and is consistent with the formation of one or more intermediates in the folding pathway. It is interesting to note that the second phase of the apparently two-phase fluorescence transition of TP40 manifests approximately the same midpoint as the far-UV CD transition, implying that they may reflect the same event.

The apparent hydrodynamic radii (r) of TP40 and PE40Δcys were measured by high-performance size-exclusion chromatography (HPSEC) as a function of Gdn·HCl concentration to probe their compactness. A number of proteins of known Stokes' radii (r) were eluted in the presence and absence of 6 M Gdn·HCl to serve as molecular size standards. Plots of r as a function of Gdn·HCl concentration are shown in Fig. 9 for TP40 and PE40Δcys. For TP40, values of r are estimated to be 3.8 and 5.7 nm at 0 and 4 M Gdn·HCl, respectively. Using these values as representative of fully folded and unfolded forms, the fraction of unfolded protein (f_{app}) was calculated at different Gdn·HCl concentrations. The resulting plot is shown in Fig. 8 (along with f_{app} calculated from CD and fluorescence measurements) and yields midpoints of 1.6 M and 1.7 M for TP40 and PE40Δcys, respectively (Table VI). At 1.3 M Gdn·HCl, a concentration at which the major fluorescence transition is nearly complete but the change in CD is relatively small, the values of r are 4.5 nm for TP40

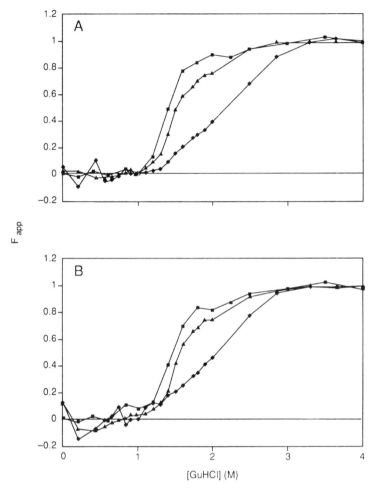

Figure 8. Fraction (f_{app}) of (A) unfolded TP40 and (B) PE40Δcys as a function of Gdn·HCl concentration. $f_{app} = (Y_{obs} - Y_{nat})/(Y_{unf} - Y_{nat})$, where Y_{obs} is the observed CD at 222 nm or fluorescence at λ_{max} or Stokes radius at a given Gdn·HCl concentration and Y_{nat} and Y_{unf} are the observed values for the native and completely unfolded forms, respectively. ■,f_{app} from fluorescence; ◆,f_{app} from CD; ▲,f_{app} from HPSEC.

and 4.3 nm for TP40Δcys. It thus appears that these proteins maintain at least a semicompact form at denaturant concentrations that cause major disruption of their tertiary configuration but are insufficient to substantially disrupt secondary structure. These results are entirely consistent with the formation of a MG-like intermediate. At intermediate Gdn·HCl concentrations (1.3–2.0 M), a relatively small population of a second species with an r-value of 8.3 nm eluted from the HPSEC column in addition to the smaller component. The amount of the presumably aggregated ($r = 8.3$ nm)

**Table VI. Gdn·HCl Denaturation
Midpoints of TP40 and PE40ΔCys
as Determined by Various Methods**

Protein	Gdn·HCl (M) for Half-Maximal Change		
	Fluorescence	CD	HP-SEC
TP40	1.4	2.1	1.6
PE40ΔCys	1.5	2.0	1.7

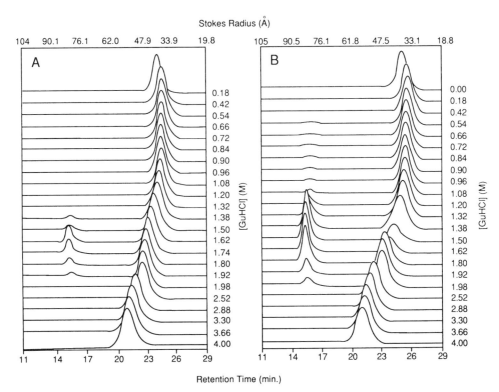

Figure 9. Determination of Stokes radii of (A) TP40 and (B) PE40Δcys as a function of Gdn·HCl concentration. The protein concentrations were 0.4 mg/ml. The *y*-axis is proportional to absorbance at 280 nm.

species reached a maximum at 1.7 M Gdn·HCl but then decreased with increasing Gdn·HCl concentration. TP40 and PE40Δcys again behaved in a parallel manner in this regard. This observation suggests that the partially unfolded intermediate(s) self-associate presumably via exposed hydrophobic surfaces. At higher Gdn·HCl concentrations, the more fully unfolded monomeric molecules are stabilized by interaction with the denaturant and self-association is no longer a thermodynamically favorable event.

Near-UV CD spectra of TP40 are shown in Fig. 10 as a function of Gdn·HCl concentration. The spectrum of fully folded TP40, i.e., in the absence of Gdn·HCl, is dominated by a broad, positive peak near 282 nm with a shoulder around 290 nm. A sharp decrease in the magnitude of this ellipticity is observed over this entire region (270–295 nm) when the Gdn·HCl concentration is increased from 1.0 to 1.3 M. This finding is consistent with the tryptophan fluorescence data and reinforces the conclusion that the unfolding of secondary and tertiary structures is noncooperative. An interesting observation derived from the aromatic CD spectra is that Gdn·HCl has a greater effect on the CD band near 280 nm than on the indole ^1L_b band in the 290–292 nm region. In the presence of 1.3 M Gdn·HCl, for example, the λ_{max} actually shifts from 282 to 290 nm. A more complete unfolding in 4 M Gdn·HCl leads to a featureless spectrum. It thus appears that the local structure around some fraction of the four tryptophan residues is probably maintained even in 1.3 M Gdn·HCl. This

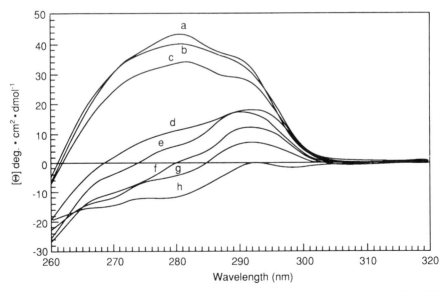

Figure 10.   Near-UV CD spectra of TP40 in the (a) absence of Gdn·HCl and in the presence of (b) 0.5 M, (c) 1.0 M, (d) 1.3 M, (e) 1.5 M, (f) 2.0 M, (g) 2.5 M, and (h) 4.0 M Gdn·HCl.

conclusion is consistent with the biphasic unfolding curve seen in the tryptophan fluorescence measurements.

2.5. Kinetics of Refolding

The kinetics of refolding of TP40 were measured by a combination of stopped-flow and conventional steady-state fluorescence. Refolding was achieved by diluting Gdn·HCl from 2.5 M (where approximately 90% of the fluorescence transition has occurred at equilibrium) to 0.7 M. Biphasic kinetics are observed with components manifesting half-lives of approximately 12 and 104 s. This suggests that the formation of tertiary structure may involve more than one intermediate and is again consistent with the previously observed two phases in equilibrium unfolding experiments.

The kinetics of changes in secondary structure content upon refolding TP40 by dilution from 4 M to 0.2 M GdnHCl were measured by monitoring the CD signal at 222 nm. The total change in CD resulting from refolding occurred within the dead time (10 s) of the measurement. Thus, the refolding of TP40 from Gdn·HCl manifests at least three distinguishable kinetic processes: a fast phase (half-life <10 s) in which the secondary structure forms, and at least two slower phases in which tertiary structure is restored, as detected by tryptophan fluorescence. The noncoincidence of the refolding of secondary and tertiary structures is consistent with the presence of partially folded or MG-like intermediates in the folding pathway.

The above unfolding–refolding data indicate, independently of the structural studies at low pH, that TP40 has sufficient structural flexibility to assume a MG-like intermediate and that the Gdn·HCl induced partially unfolded state(s) shows similarity to the low-pH-induced state(s), although their precise nature and relationship require further description.

2.6. Thermal Unfolding

The thermal stability of TP40 structure was studied at pH 7.2 by (1) measuring the temperature dependence of (1) the spectral shift (wavelength of spectral peak) of tryptophan fluorescence, (2) far-UV CD intensity at 206 nm, and (3) differential scanning calorimetry (DSC). The midpoints of the observed thermal transitions (T_m) were approximately 42°C and 55°C as determined by fluorescence and CD, respectively (Fig. 11). This difference in T_m values suggests that TP40's tertiary structure as determined by fluorescence is more sensitive to thermal perturbation than the protein's secondary structure as determined by CD. This is consistent with the presence of one or more intermediates in the thermal unfolding pathway of TP40. A T_m of 48°C was obtained from DSC which is intermediate between those detected by CD and fluorescence. The noncoincidence of T_m values obtained by CD and DSC is not

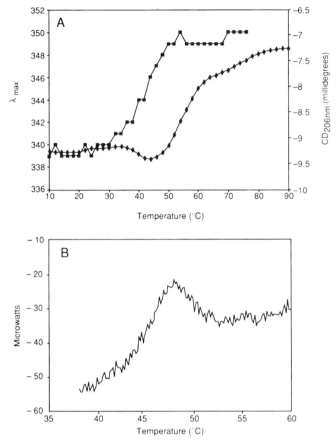

Figure 11.   Effect of temperature on TP40 conformation as measured at 0.1 mg/ml by (A) ■, tryptophan fluorescence at λ_{max} (nm), ♦, CD at 206 nm, and by (B) differential scanning calorimetry at 1.0 mg/ml.

clearly understood, but could arise from the kinetic nature of the DSC measurements and/or the (approximately 10-fold) higher protein concentration required for DSC measurements (~1 mg/ml). Note, however, that DSC detects the sum of all exo- and endothermic processes in the unfolding pathway and may, therefore, reflect the composite heats of multiple processes.

Thermal unfolding is also accompanied by aggregation of TP40, as measured by QLS and HPSEC. At 50°C, a D_h of approximately 11.5 nm was observed, compared to 3.8 nm at 23°C. The sample heated to 50°C (pH 7.2) also lost biological activity, as measured by cytotoxicity against A431 cells. This loss was irreversible since the activity was not regained after the sample was cooled to 4°C. On the other hand, a

TP40 sample incubated at 37°C for 18 hr was fully bioactive and manifested less than 1% aggregation, as monitored by HPSEC.

3. FORMULATION OF TP40 FOR CLINICAL ADMINISTRATION INTO THE HUMAN URINARY BLADDER

3.1. Considerations in Designing a Stable and Biologically Active Formulation

The solution stability upon storage of TP40 at pH near neutrality and at physiologic ionic strength was examined employing a simple buffer formulation containing 6.2 mM sodium phosphate and 150 mM NaCl (pH 7.2). QLS, velocity sedimentation, and equilibrium sedimentation studies had shown that TP40 did not aggregate under these conditions up to a concentration of at least 1 mg/ml. Storage at this concentration would subsequently allow us the flexibility to cover a wide concentration range in phase I clinical studies. This solution formulation, stored in sterile glass vials at either 4°C or (frozen) at −70°C, manifested little or no degradation or aggregation for up to 2 years as determined by SDS-PAGE and HPSEC. Furthermore, the *in vitro* cell-kill bioactivity was also fully retained (within the range of experimental error) over this period of time. A second consideration, as important as the stability issue, is maintenance of tumor-targeted cytotoxicity of TP40 in the urinary bladder during treatment. This critical event would require that the following conditions be met: (1) the pH of TP40 in the bladder be maintained such that EGFr binding of the TGF-α portion of TP40 is optimal, and (2) the structural integrity and flexibility of TP40 be retained to ensure maximal biological activity. A third consideration is the safety of the formulation to which the bladder wall would be exposed for significant periods of time in a clinical protocol involving a direct intravesical administration.

The interaction of TGF-α with EGFr is optimal between pH 6.5 and 8.0 and is drastically reduced at pH 5.5 (Haigler *et al.*, 1980). We found TP40 to retain *in vitro* A431 cell-killing activity in the pH range of 6.5–7.8 for at least 48 hr at 37°C. Furthermore, our structural studies described above have shown that structural integrity of the protein is maintained in this pH range. Therefore, a reasonable formulation goal for clinical studies was to maintain the pH of TP40 in the bladder, the initial site of therapeutic utilization, between 6.5 and 7.8.

Based on the above considerations, we reasoned that the formulation problem could be divided into two parts: (1) stability on storage and (2) maintenance of suitable buffering condition during the residence time of TP40 in urinary bladder so that its therapeutic potential can be maximized. The first condition was satisfactorily met by a 1-mg/ml TP40 solution buffered with 6.2 mM sodium phosphate containing 150 mM NaCl. The remarkable stability of this TP40 solution at storage temperatures of 4°C and −70°C has been described above. Approach to the second issue was guided by the clinical protocol and would require dilution of the above stock solution into another buffer prior to administration, as discussed below.

3.2. Selection of a Formulation for Intravesical Dosing in the Clinic

For phase I clinical study, a direct intravesical instillation was employed. Since the kinetics of TGF-α binding to EGFr is rapid, a 2-hr residence time for TP40 in the bladder was considered to be sufficient for interaction of this protein with the transformed EGFr bearing cells. The volume of urine accumulated in the bladder during this time would alter the pH of TP40, depending upon urine pH, to values outside of the desired range of 6.5–7.8, unless the drug is sufficiently buffered to resist large changes. It was estimated that, after a pretreatment voiding of the bladder, the maximum amount of urine accumulated (although highly variable from individual to individual) would not exceed 100 ml under the conditions of our clinical protocol. The clinical protocol called for administrtion of a 60-ml volume of TP40 solution into the bladder. The buffering capacity of this solution had to be sufficiently high to resist unacceptably large pH changes when diluted with up to ~100 ml of the patient's urine. Several buffer compositions were examined for their ability to maintain pH in the range of 6.5–7.8 when diluted with equal or twice the volume of test human urine samples. These samples were collected from 10 healthy volunteers under conditions (as described in the footnote to Table VII) closely resembling

Table VII. Buffering Capacity of Sodium Phosphate upon Mixing with Urine[a]

Urine pH	Buffer pH of 7.5	Buffer pH of 7.8	Buffer pH of 8.2
5.4	6.4	6.5	6.5
5.4	6.5	6.6	6.6
5.4	7.2	7.3	7.5
5.6	6.6	6.7	6.8
5.8	7.1	7.2	7.3
5.9	6.7	6.8	6.9
6.2	7.1	7.2	7.2
6.4	7.0	7.1	7.2
6.7	7.2	7.4	7.5
7.1	7.3	7.4	7.5

[a]The initial total concentration of sodium phosphate was 100 mM, made up by combining different concentrations of monobasic and dibasic phosphate required to achieve the desired pH values listed above. Urine was collected from healthy volunteers approximately 2 hr after their initial morning void. No food and minimal fluid were consumed during this 2-hr period. Two volumes of urine were diluted with one volume of buffer, resulting in a threefold dilution of the phosphate.

those to be followed in the clinical study. Most urine samples were acidic, their pH ranging from 5.4 to 7.1. Sodium phosphate, sodium bicarbonate and glycinamide, each at different concentrations and different pH values (between 7.5 and 8.2) were tested. Sodium phosphate at concentrations of 100 mM and above manifested the desired buffering ability. A solution containing 50 mM sodium phosphate and 150 mM glycinamide at pH 8.2 (but not 50 mM sodium phosphate alone) also provided adequate buffering in urine but did not show a significant advantage over a simpler formulation using 100 mM sodium phosphate alone. The final pH values obtained upon diluting 100 mM phosphate buffer solutions at three different initial pH values with twice their volume of test urine samples are shown in Table VII. Based on these results, a sodium phosphate buffer at pH 7.8 was identified as of sufficient capacity to meet our criterion of maintaining pH in the bladder in the desired range. TP40 incubated in this buffer maintained full A431 cell-killing bioactivity for at least 5 hr at room temperature, allowing adequate time for handling the material in the clinic. In subsequent phase I clinical study, patients' urine samples voided at the end of the 2-hr dwell time were found to retain *in vitro* cell-killing activity of TP40 (Goldberg *et al.*, 1995). Furthermore, TP40 buffered with 100 mM sodium phosphate (pH 7.8) was found to be well tolerated by patients at doses ranging from 0.15 to 9.6 mg/week for 6 weeks (Goldberg *et al.*, 1995).

At the lowest dose employed in the clinic (0.15 mg), the concentration of TP40 was 2.5 μg/ml. The possibility of loss of protein by adsorption at such low concentrations on the surface of the glass vial containing the dosing solution and during passage through the syringe/plastic bag/catheter assembly (used to deliver the drug to the patient's bladder) was measured. The amount of adsorptive loss of protein was no more than 10%, as detected by a micro-BCA assay.

3.3. Formulation Summary

The pharmaceutical formulation of TP40 developed for the clinic consisted of two parts: (1) the formulated drug at 1 mg/ml in phosphate (6.2 mM)-buffered saline (150 mM) and (2) the dosing diluent, 100 mM sodium phosphate at pH 7.8. Different doses ranging from 0.15 to 9.6 mg of total TP40 were obtained by diluting different volumes of (1) into 60 ml of (2). The dosing buffer maintains a pH in the bladder that is not only conducive to binding to EGFr's on the cell surface but also permits TP40 to remain in its folded and unaggregrated form. In this state, TP40 maintains its structural flexibility so that it may assume the partially unfolded structure that is required for translocation across endosomal membrane, where the pH is presumably close to 5. Upon entering the cytoplasm, neutral pH is regained and refolding to the native structure should occur, which then allows TP40 to carry out the final part of its pharmacological activity, i.e., ADP-ribosylation of EF-2 and consequent cell death.

4. CONCLUSION

A potentially chemotherapeutic protein has been designed to specifically target tumor cells that contain high concentrations of the EGFr. This conjugate protein, designated TP40, differs from TGF-α-PE40 in that the four cysteine residues of the PE40 segment in the latter have been replaced with alanines. This alteration eliminates the problem of disulfide scrambling between the TGF-α and PE40 portions and greatly facilitates large-scale manufacturing and purification. TP40 manifests a high degree of EGFr binding and substantial ADP ribosylation activity and, ultimately, cytotoxic activity against cells expressing EGFr, thereby fulfilling the principal requirements targeted in designing this protein. Although no direct method is available to measure translocation across membranes, the biophysical experiments described in this chapter suggest that the translocation efficiency of the PE40 domain of PE is not significantly compromised in this chimeric protein (TP40).

Finally, a formulation of TP40 safe for use in humans employing direct intravesical administration has been designed. This formulation has been used in a Phase I clinical trial of TP40 in 43 patients suffering from urinary bladder cancer that presented as solid tumors and/or superficial lesions or carcinoma *in situ* (CIS). The results of this trial have been recently published (Goldberg *et al.*, 1995). TP40 administered in this formulation containing 100 mM sodium phosphate at pH 7.8 was found to be safe at least under a clinical protocol which used a 2-hr bladder residence time. The critical requirement of maintaining a pH near neutrality in the bladder was met by this formulation, as judged by acceptable pH values of urine samples measured immediately following treatment. The idea of controlling pH of the drug solution administered in the bladder can potentially be extended to other chemotherapeutic agents, including nonpeptidyl molecules, which might have a pH-dependent activity or stability profile.

ACKNOWLEDGMENT. The authors wish to thank Ms. Laurie Rittle for her invaluable assistance in preparing this manuscript.

REFERENCES

Allured, V., Collier, R. J., Carroll, S. F., and McKay, D. B., 1986, Structure of exotoxin A of *Pseudomonas aeruginosa* at 3.0-Ångstom resolution, *Proc. Natl. Acad. Sci. U.S.A.* **83**:1320–1324.

Baldwin, R. L., 1991, Molten globules: specific or nonspecific folding intermediates?, *Chemtracts-Biochem. Mol. Biol.* **2**:379–389.

Christensen, H., and Pain, R. H., 1991, Molten globule intermediates and protein folding, *Eur. Biophys. J.* **19**: 221–229.

Dobson, C. M., 1992, Unfolded proteins, compact states and molten globules, *Curr. Opin. Struct. Biol.* **2**:6–12.

Draper, R. K., and Simon, M. I., 1980, The entry of diphtheria toxin into the mammalian cell cytoplasm: evidence for lysosomal involvement, *J. Cell Biol.* **87**:849–854.

Edwards, G. M., DeFeo-Jones, D., Tai, J. Y., Vuocolo, G. A., Patrick, D. R., Heimbrook, D. C., and Oliff, A., 1989, Epidermal growth factor receptor binding is affected by structural determinants in the toxin domain of transforming growth factor-alpha-*Pseudomonas* exotoxin fusion protein, *Mol. Cell Biol.* **9:**2860–2867.

Farahbakhsh, Z. T., and Wisnieski, B. J., 1989, The acid-triggered entry pathway of *Pseudomonas* exotoxin A, *Biochemistry* **28:**580–585.

George, H. A., Powell, A. L., Dahlgren, M. E., Herber, W. K., Maigetter, B., Burgess, W., Stirdivant, S. M., and Greasham, R. L., 1992, Physiological effects of TGF-α-PE40 expression in recombinant *Escherichia coli* JM 109, *Biotech. Bioeng.* **40:**437–445.

Goldberg, M. R., Heimbrook, D. C., Russo, P., Sarosdy, M. F., Greenberg, R. E., Giantonio, B. J., Linehan, W. M., Walther, M., Fisher, H. A. G., Messing, E., Crawford, E. D., Oliff, A. I., and Pastan, I. H., 1995, Phase I clinical study of the recombinant oncotoxin TP40 in superficial bladder cancer, *Clin. Cancer Res.* **1:**57–61.

Goto, Y., and Fink, A. L., 1989, Conformational states of β-lactamase: molten-globule states at acidic and alkaline pH with high salt, *Biochemistry* **28:**945–952.

Gress, J. O., Marquis-Omer, D., Middaugh, C. R., and Sanyal, G., 1994, Evidence for an equilibrium intermediate in the folding-unfolding pathway of a transforming growth factor-α-*Pseudomonas* exotoxin hybrid protein, *Biochemistry* **33:**2620–2627.

Haigler, H. T., Maxfield, F. R., Willingham, M. C., and Pastan, I., 1980, Dansylcadaverine inhibits internalization of ^{125}I-epidermal growth factor in BALB 3T3 cells, *J. Biol. Chem.* **255:**1239–1241.

Heimbrook, D. C., Stirdivant, S. M., Ahern, J. D., Balishin, N. L., Patrick, D. R., Edwards, G. M., DeFeo-Jones, D., FitzGerald, D. J., Pastan, I., and Oliff, A., 1990, Transforming growth factor-α-*Pseudomonas* exotoxin fusion protein prolongs survival of nude mice bearing tumor xenografts, *Proc. Natl. Acad. Sci. U.S.A.* **87:**4697–4701.

Jiang, J. X., and London, E., 1990, Involvement of denaturation-like changes in *Pseudomonas* exotoxin A hydrophobicity and membrane penetration determined by characterization of pH and thermal transitions, *J. Biol. Chem.* **265:**8636–8641.

Kline, T. P., Brown, F. K., Brown, S. C., Jeffs, P. W., Kopple, K. D., and Mueller, L., 1990, Solution structures of human transforming growth factor α derived from ^{1}H NMR data, *Biochemistry* **29:**7805–7813.

Kounnas, M. Z., Morris, R. E., Thompson, M. R., FitzGerald, D. J., Strickland, D. K., and Saelinger, C. B., 1992, The $α_2$-macroglobulin receptor/low density lipoprotein receptor-related protein binds and internalizes *Pseudomonas* exotoxin A, *J. Biol. Chem.* **267:**12420–12423.

Kuwajima, K., 1989, The molten globule state as a clue for understanding the folding and cooperativity of globular-protein structure, *Proteins: Struct. Funct. Genet.* **6:**87–103.

Linemeyer, D. L., Kelly, L. J., Menke, J. G., Gimenez-Gallego, G., DiSalvo, J., and Thomas, K. A., 1987, Expression in *Escherichia coli* of a chemically synthesized gene for biologically active bovine acidic fibroblast growth factor, *Bio/Technology* **5:**960–965.

Mach, H., Ryan, J. A., Burke, C. J., Volkin, D. B., and Middaugh, C. R., 1993, Partially structured self-associating states of acidic fibroblast growth factor, *Biochemistry* **32:**7703–7711.

Manavalan, P., and Johnson, W. C., Jr., 1987, Variable selection method improves the prediction of protein secondary structure from circular dichroism spectra, *Anal. Biochem.* **167:**76–85.

Massagué, J., 1990, Transforming growth factor-α, *J. Biol. Chem.* **265:**21393–21396.

Pastan, I., Chaudhary, V., and FitzGerald, D. J., 1992, Recombinant toxins as novel therapeutic agents, *Ann. Rev. Biochem.* **61:**331–354.

Pastan, I., and FitzGerald, D., 1989, *Pseudomonas* exotoxin: chimeric toxins, *J. Biol. Chem.* **264:**15157–15160.

Prestrelski, S. J., Arakawa, T., Wu, C.-S. C., O'Neal, K. D., Westcott, K. R., and Narhi, L. O., 1992, Solution structure and dynamics of epidermal growth factor and transforming growth factor α, *J. Biol. Chem.* **267:**319–322.

Sandvig, K., and Moskaug, J. Ø., 1987, *Pseudomonas* toxin binds Triton X-114 at low pH, *Biochem. J.* **245:**899–901.

Sanyal, G., Marquis-Omer, D., Gress, J. O., and Middaugh, C. R., 1993, A transforming growth factor-α-*Pseudomonas* exotoxin hybrid protein undergoes pH-dependent conformational changes conducive to membrane interaction, *Biochemistry* **32:**3488–3497.

Susi, H., and Byler, D. M., 1986, Resolution-enhanced Fourier transform infrared spectroscopy of enzymes, *Meth. Enzymol.* **130:**290–311.

Von Hoff, D. D., Marshall, M. H., Heimbrook, D. C., Stirdivant, S. M., Ahern, J. D., Herbert, W. K., Maigetter, R. Z., and Oliff, A., 1992, Activity of a recombinant transforming growth factor-α-*Pseudomonas* exotoxin hybrid protein against primary human tumor colony-forming units, *Invest. New Drugs* **10:**17–22.

Yamazaki, S., Sardana, M. K., and Lee, A. L., 1995, A rapid copper metal interaction high performance liquid chromatography assay for monitoring disulfide isomerization of TP40 (a recombinant fusion protein TGFα-PE40δcys), submitted.

Zalman, L. S., and Wisnieski, B. J., 1985, Characterization of the insertion of *Pseudomonas* exotoxin A into membranes, *Infect. Immun.* **50:**630–635.

11

Stability Characterization and Formulation Development of Recombinant Human Deoxyribonuclease I [Pulmozyme®, (Dornase Alpha)]

Steven J. Shire

1. BACKGROUND

Pulmozyme®, recombinant DNA derived human DNase I* (rhDNase), is the first new therapy in 30 years for the treatment of cystic fibrosis (CF). The rapid development time, 5 years from conception to market, was all the more remarkable because of the unique challenges faced with the development of a protein therapeutic for specific local delivery to the lung. In this chapter we discuss the rationale for development of this drug and the physical chemistry and biochemistry required to characterize the stability of the formulation on storage as well as during delivery by inhalation.

---

*The terminology DNase I and II mainly refers to mode of cleavage of DNA phosphodiester linkages. Hydrolysis of DNA by DNase I yields 5′-phosphate terminated polynucleotides, whereas DNase II yields 3′-phosphate terminated hydrolysis products.

Steven J. Shire • Department of Pharmaceutical Research and Development, Genentech, Inc., South San Francisco, California 94080.

Formulation, Characterization, and Stability of Protein Drugs, Rodney Pearlman and Y. John Wang, eds., Plenum Press, New York, 1996.

1.1. Cystic Fibrosis

Cystic fibrosis is the most common lethal inherited genetic disease in Caucasians occurring once in each 2500 births (Boat *et al.*, 1989). Clinical manifestations of the disease include obstruction of the airways and pancreatic ducts. In particular, the major cause of morbidity and mortality in CF is due to chronic obstruction of the airways by thick mucosal secretions. The recent discovery and cloning of the gene responsible for CF (Rommens *et al.*, 1989) has provided some insight into the basic molecular defect that causes CF. It had been noted previous to this discovery that cells from patients with CF did not have a normal efflux of chloride ions across respiratory epithelial cell membranes in response to elevated cyclic AMP levels (Sato and Sato, 1984). The amino acid sequence of the protein encoded by the CF gene, termed the cystic fibrosis transmembrane conductance regulator protein (CFTR), has been shown to be strikingly similar to that of other proteins involved in active transport across cell membranes (Riordan *et al.*, 1989). Recent experiments have shown that this protein can itself function as an ion channel, rather than just as a regulator of another endogenous channel (Anderson *et al.*, 1991). These observations were further supported by the finding that gene transfer experiments with full length, wild-type CFTR into CF cells resulted in normal chloride ion transfer across the membrane (Drumm *et al.*, 1990; Rich *et al.*, 1990). At present over 170 mutations of the CFTR gene have been described, although only about 20 of these mutations commonly occur in CF patients (Tsui and Buchwald, 1991; Abeliovich *et al.*, 1992). One deletion mutation in particular at F_{508} makes up 70% of all observed CF mutations (Tsui and Buchwald, 1991). The mutations manifest themselves as altered activity in response to effector agents such as cAMP, and also in terms of altered protein processing that affects proper presentation into the CF cell membrane. All these recent findings add support to an earlier hypothesis that an abnormal ion transport in CF patients leads to the dehydrated viscous mucus found in CF patients (Chernick and Barbero, 1959; Potter *et al.*, 1963).

1.2. Bovine DNase I as Treatment for Cystic Fibrosis

For reasons not completely understood, the dehydrated viscous mucus renders the patient susceptible to persistent bacterial infections which are difficult to treat with chronic antibiotic therapy. The viscous mucus may contribute to decreased mucocilliary clearance and persistent bacterial infection. It was recognized early on that the persistent bacterial infections result in a large concentration, (3 to 14 mg/g of sputum) of the patients own DNA from lysed neutrophils (Chernick and Barbero, 1959; Potter *et al.*, 1960). The increased concentration of DNA in the patients airways undoubtedly contributed further to the increased viscosity of mucosal secretions in CF patients. In fact, it was shown that incubation of purulent sputum with bovine pancreatic DNase I (bDNase) resulted in a large decrease in sputum viscosity (Armstrong and White, 1950; Chernick *et al.*, 1961). An early study using bDNase to treat chronic bronchitis patients demonstrated that the nuclease was capable of decreasing the viscosity of purulent sputum (Elmes and White, 1953). However, there was no clear clinical response in this study. Although no untoward effects were observed, it was concluded that the doses used were inadequate since the observed decrease of sputum viscosity lasted less than 12 hr. It is not clear from this study whether the dose was actually too low or whether the bDNase used was unstable since the enzyme was not characterized either before or after administration as an aerosol spray. Moreover, the aerosol for delivery was completely uncharacterized leaving open the question whether sufficient drug was deposited into the airways. Eventually, on the basis of the observed effects of purulent sputum from patients, bDNase was approved for human use in 1958 under the generic name dornase or the trade name Dornavac (Merck, Sharp and Dome Research Laboratories). A later study (Salomon et al., 1954) with dornase to treat various bronchopulmonary diseases had better characterization of bDNase activity before and after aerosolization, but again failed to physically characterize the aerosol (as discussed later in this chapter). The general conclusion from this study was that the treatment was well tolerated and that patients had beneficial effects within ½ to 1 hr after treatment. The reported beneficial effects included increased amounts of expectorated sputum compared to that before treatment and the change in the physical appearance of the sputum. However, the conclusions of this study were considerably weakened by the lack of an appropriate placebo control, or measurements of improvement in lung function. Additional studies were performed with dornase to treat patients with pneumonia (Spier et al., 1961) and also cystic fibrosis (Lieberman, 1968). These studies concluded that there was benefit to the patients in regard to noticeable thinning as well as an increased volume of expectorated sputum. The study on cystic fibrosis used cone-and-plate viscometry to quantify the decrease in sputum viscosity. Again, neither of these studies investigated stability of the bDNase nor provided data to demonstrate that an appropriate droplet-size distribution was generated to ensure sufficient deposition of drug within the airways. Altogether, the studies with bDNase did suggest that the drug had a reasonable safety profile and was effective in reducing the viscosity of purulent lung secretions. However, occasional adverse reactions were reported that could be attributed to an allergic reaction as a consequence of administration of a foreign protein or irritation due to contaminating proteases in the bDNase preparations (Lieberman, 1962; Raskin, 1968). In at least one clinical study, half of the patients given multiple doses of bDNase administered intravenously developed significant antibody titers (Johnson et al., 1954). As a consequence of these adverse reactions Dornavac was eventually withdrawn from the market.

1.3. Human DNase I as Treatment for Cystic Fibrosis

Although bDNase was effective in altering purulent sputum viscosity, the role of contaminating proteases in the observed reduction was uncertain. This was further exacerbated by the conflicting reports of the ability of various proteases to reduce viscosity of lung secretions (Chernick *et al.*, 1961; Lieberman, 1962). To specifically demonstrate that DNase was capable of altering the viscoelastic properties of sputum and to eventually test the product in human clinical trials without the potential adverse effects due to a foreign protein, human DNase I (rhDNase) was cloned from a human pancreatic cDNA library and expressed in human embryonic kidney 293 cells (Shak *et al.*, 1990). The expressed protein was purified and its enzymatic activity characterized. In particular, rhDNase was shown to decrease the viscosity of CF patient sputum by both a qualitative pourability assay as well as by quantitative viscometry using a Brookfield cone-and-plate viscometer. Correlation of a reduction in sputum DNA size (as determined by agarose gel electrophoresis) with a decrease in viscosity further supported the notion that the nuclease activity of rhDNase contributes significantly to the observed reduction in viscosity. Addition of trypsin and chymotrypsin did little to increase rhDNase ability to reduce CF sputum viscosity. Altogether, these results suggested that contaminating proteases were not required for the ability of DNase preparations to lower CF sputum viscosity.

The rhDNase used in clinical trials was expressed in Chinese hamster ovary cells (CHO), purified and formulated for delivery as an aerosol by jet nebulizers. Unlike previous clinical trials of bDNase, the stability of the rhDNase formulation before and after nebulization was characterized, as well as the physical properties of the aerosol (summarized in Section 4.1). Two Phase I dose-escalation studies were conducted at two different clinical centers (Aitken *et al.*, 1992; Hubbard *et al.*, 1992). In an open label study, without placebo controls, no acute adverse events in 12 healthy adults and 12 cystic fibrosis patients were detected (Aitken *et al.*, 1992). Patients were dosed three times a day, Monday through Friday, for 2 consecutive weeks. Serum concentrations of rhDNase after aerosol administration increased only slightly from 3 ± 2 to 5 ± 2 ng/ml after the last dose on day 12. Significantly, no antibody titers to rhDNase were detected after a single dose given on day 21. Similarly, Hubbard *et al.* (1992) in a phase I crossover study with placebo controls did not detect any acute adverse events. Preliminary indication of clinical efficacy in terms of improved lung function as assessed by forced expiratory volume in 1 s (FEV_1) was also obtained in both studies. Additional safety and efficacy data were obtained from randomized placebo-controlled Phase II clinical trials (Ramsey *et al.*, 1993; Ranasinha *et al.*, 1993) in which rhDNase was administered over a 10-day period. No life-threatening adverse effects were reported and in both studies there was an increase in forced vital capacity, FVC, as well as a 10–15% increase in FEV_1. One of the clinical trials was a dose-ranging study where either 0.6, 2.5, or 10 mg rhDNase was administered twice daily (Ramsey *et al.*, 1993). Overall, there was a dose-dependent response but it was relatively small, and in fact the magnitude of the changes in FEV_1 and FVC were not significantly different between the rhDNase dose groups on short-term administration. Expanded placebo controlled Phase III clinical trials involved a total of 968 patients over a 24-week treatment period (Aitken, 1993). Again, there were no life-threatening adverse responses, including no evidence of any asthmatic response. Although 5% of the patients receiving rhDNase did have low antibody titers, no clinical effect was observed. Patients receiving rhDNase had a significant increase of 6% in FEV_1 compared to placebo control. Moreover, patients given aerosolized rhDNase spent 1.2–1.4 fewer days in the hospital and had 2.4–2.7 fewer days of antibiotic treatment. These studies demonstrated conclusively that rhDNase was both an effective and safe drug for treatment of cystic fibrosis and resulted in FDA approval of rhDNase under the trade name Pulmozyme® on 12/30/93. Since then Pulmozyme® has been approved for use in over 35 countries. Recently, Pulmozyme® has been used in Phase II human clinical trials to treat patients with chronic pulmonary disease (Fick *et al.*, 1994). The results of that trial have been very promising and a more extensive placebo-controlled Phase III trial has been initiated.*

2. STRUCTURE AND PROPERTIES OF DNase I

Bovine DNase has been extensively characterized in numerous biochemical and biophysical studies (reviewed by Moore, 1981). A great deal less is known about the physical and chemical properties of rhDNase. Human DNase has been partially purified and characterized from plasma (Doctor, 1963), duodenal aspirates (Funakoshi *et al.*, 1977), and urine (Murai *et al.*, 1978). It has been claimed that human DNase from all these sources is immunologically equivalent and has essentially the same physical properties and enzymatic characteristics (Love and Hewitt, 1979; Ito *et al.*, 1984). This section reviews some of the key properties of bDNase and where appropriate relates them to what has been determined for the human protein.

2.1. Primary Structure of rhDNase and Homology with bDNase

rhDNase is a single polypeptide chain of 260 amino acid residues. The original sequence for bDNase was reported to contain 257 amino acid residues (Liao *et al.*, 1973). However, Oefner and Suck (1986) were unable to align the reported chemical sequence with the 2-Å resolution crystallographic electron density map of bDNase. In particular, it was found that better agreement was obtained if the tripeptide Ile-Val-Arg were inserted into the reported sequence at position 27. It was suggested that this tripeptide was deleted in the sequencing process because it was a repeat tripeptide in the sequence. Three further changes in the bDNase sequence were proposed (Thr_{14} to Ser_{14}, Gly_{224} to Pro_{224}, and Pro_{225} to Gly_{225}) in order to obtain better agreement between the electron density map and chemical sequence. An alignment of the two primary structures, after incorporation of these changes shows that there is only a

---

Note added in proof: The phase III trials for evaluation of Pulmozyme® in the treatment of chronic pulmonary disease were recently completed and did not support the use of Pulmozyme® in the treatment of this patient population.

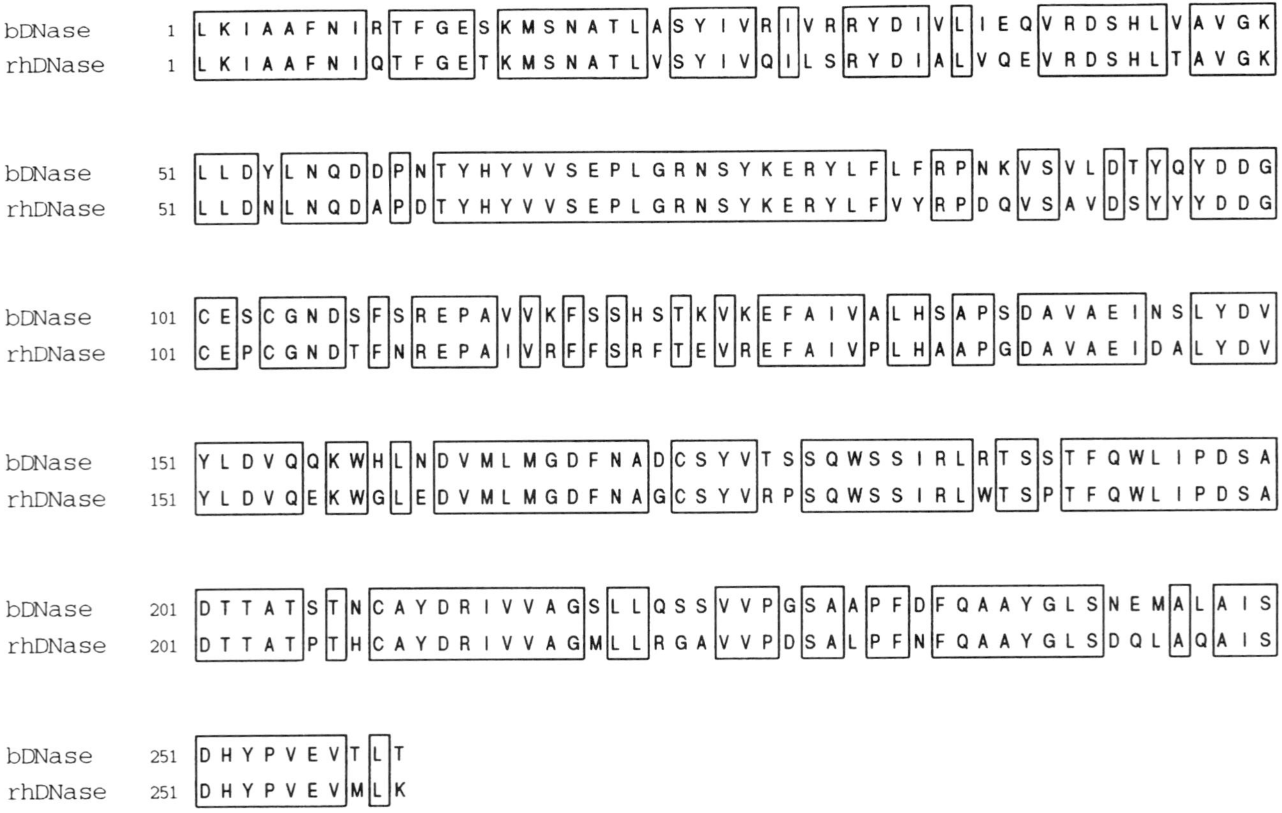

Steven J. Shire

Figure 1. Amino acid sequence homology of bovine (bDNase) and recombinant human (rhDNase) deoxyribonuclease I. Identical amino acids in both sequences are in boxed format.

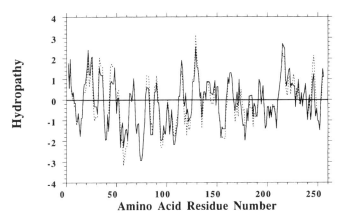

Figure 2. Hydropathy plot for bDNase and rhDNase. The hydropathy is an indication of relative hydrophilicity (positive values) and hydrophobicity (negative values) of the amino acid sequences. These plots were generated using a sliding window of 6 amino acid residues and the hydrophobicity scale of Hopp and Woods (1981).

77% sequence homology (Fig. 1). Most of the differences occur in hydrophilic regions on the surface of the protein. It has been suggested that some of the observed adverse reactions to administration of bDNase could be due to these differences in potentially immunogenic regions of the protein (Shak *et al.*, 1990). Although there is considerable diversity between the bDNase and rhDNase sequences, there does appear to be significant structural homology between these two proteins as shown by a number of observations. Despite the significant lack of amino acid sequence homology, the relative hydrophilicity and hydrophobicity of the two structures are very similar (Fig. 2). The four cysteine residues are in the same relative positions in the sequence alignment, suggesting that the same disulfide pairing occurs in both proteins (Cys_{173}-Cys_{209} and Cys_{101}-Cys_{104}). This was eventually verified using tryptic and mass spectral analysis under reducing and nonreducing conditions (unpublished observations, J. Frenz). Further support for the close structural homology between bDNase and rhDNase is the resistance to reduction in the presence of calcium of the Cys_{173}-Cys_{209} disulfide bond in rhDNase. The analogous bond in bDNase is also highly resistant to reduction (Price *et al.*, 1969c). In addition, a histidine residue at position 131 in bDNase has been shown to be essential for enzymatic activity (Price *et al.*, 1969b), and is conserved in rhDNase. Both proteins are also glycosylated with an N-linked carbohydrate at asparagine 18. However, rhDNase is also glycosylated at asparagine 106, whereas bDNase is not at the corresponding consensus Asn-X-Ser sequence (Frenz *et al.*, 1994). Moreover, the rhDNase oligosaccharides contain sialic acid as in bDNase but also consist of mannose 6-phosphate residues that have not been found in bDNase (Frenz *et al.*, 1994).

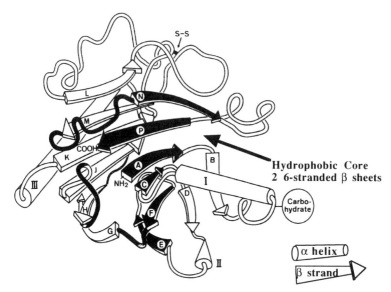

Figure 3. Ribbon diagram depicting the crystal structure of bDNase. The overall dimensions of the molecule are $45 \times 40 \times 35$ Å. The Cys_{170}-Cys_{206} disulfide bridge is shown, whereas the Cys_{98}-Cys_{101} disulfide is hidden from view. Two Ca^{2+} ions are bound under crystallization conditions. One of the sites is located near a flexible loop region that connects β strands G and H. The other site is is located in the loop formed by Asp_{198} to Cys_{206} close to the Cys_{170}-Cys_{206} disulfide bond. The calcium binding site associated with DNA binding and nuclease activity is near the active site His_{131}. This site is located between the two β-sheets of the molecule made up of strands E,F,C,A,P,N (sheet 1), and strands G,H,J,K,M,L (sheet 2). Adapted by permission from Suck *et al.* (1984).

2.2. Secondary and Tertiary Structure

As discussed previously, the tertiary structure of rhDNase is likely to be similar to that of bDNase.* The three-dimensional structure of bDNase (Fig. 3) determined by X-ray diffraction of single crystals shows that this protein is a compact molecule with overall dimensions of $45 \times 40 \times 35$ Å with a single carbohydrate chain extending ~15 Å from the surface at the start of helix I (Suck *et al.*, 1984; Oefner and Suck, 1986). The protein is classified as an αβ protein with two, 6-stranded β-pleated sheets packed against each other into a hydrophobic core. The α-helices and extensive loop regions flank the two antiparallel β-sheets. Assignment of residues in the crystal structure to a particular secondary structure was accomplished by analyzing the main-chain hydrogen bonding (Oefner and Suck, 1986) and resulted in an estimated structure of ~26% α-helix and ~34% β-sheet. The extensive loop regions of the bDNase molecule are stabilized by numerous intramolecular hydrogen bonds and salt

Note added in proof: The crystal structure of rhDNase has now been determined and is very similar to bDNase (Wolf, E., Frenz, J., and Suck, D., 1995, *Pro. Sci.* **4**:115).

bridges. The overall mean value for the isotropic temperature factor, B, is quite low at 11.9 Å^2, which reflects the structural stability and rigidity of the bDNase molecule. Of all the loop regions in the molecule, two regions at the exposed loop from Arg_{70} to Lys_{74} and Gly_{97} to Gly_{102} have distinctly higher B-values suggesting greater flexibility in those regions of the molecule. The first region is believed to be involved with binding to the DNA substrate while the second contains the Cys_{98}-Cys_{101} disulfide bond. One large, exposed loop from Ala_{168} to Ile_{193}, has a very low B-value. This was attributed to the stabilizing effects of the Cys_{170}-Cys_{206} disulfide bridge, and two salt bridges at Asp_{146}-Arg_{182} and Arg_{184}-Asp_{195}. Additional stabilization might also come from the intermolecular contacts across a twofold crystallographic axis as a result of crystal packing.

As discussed in the next section, divalent ions play an essential role in stabilizing the bDNase conformation as well as being essential for the activity of this enzyme. The crystallographic structure of bDNase shows at least two Ca^{2+} ions that are bound under the conditions for crystallization. One of the sites is located near the flexible loop region that contains the Cys_{98}-Cys_{101} disulfide bond, and the second site is located in the Asp_{198} to Cys_{206} loop very close to the Cys_{170}-Cys_{206} disulfide bond. Calcium is also found at the catalytic site in bDNase along with the conserved His_{131} residue required for activity. The nucleotide deoxythymidine-3′,5′-diphosphate (pdTp), in the presence of 5 mM Ca binds in the vicinity of His_{131} in a shallow groove between the two β-pleated sheets of the structure. The binding of calcium to this site appears to be weak in the absence of the nucleotide.

2.3. Physical and Chemical Properties

2.3.1. EFFECT OF BIVALENT METAL IONS ON STABILITY

It has been shown that bDNase conformation and stability are both highly dependent on the binding of calcium. The compact, rigid nature of bDNase confers significant stability on this protein, and calcium plays a significant role in maintaining this structure. Removal of calcium from bDNase at pH 7.5 induced changes in the far-UV circular dichroism spectrum, but not in the sedimentation coefficient determined by sedimentation velocity analysis (Poulos and Price, 1972). These results suggested that the molecule undergoes a conformational change that is detectable by CD but not a large enough change in shape or volume that would produce changes in sedimentation behavior. Large pH-induced changes in stokes radius of bDNase are reversed by addition of 20 mM Ca^{2+} (Lizarraga et al., 1978). In the presence of calcium the short disulfide bond between Cys_{98} and Cys_{101} can be reduced, whereas the disulfide bond between Cys_{170} and Cys_{206} is resistant to reduction (Price et al., 1969c; Liao et al., 1973). More significantly the reduction of the Cys_{170}-Cys_{206} bond results in inactivation of the enzyme, whereas the activity is retained after reduction of Cys_{98}-Cys_{101} (Price et al., 1969c). It has been reported that DNase isolated from human serum and pancreatic extracts retains activity after treatment with disulfide reducing agents in the presence of Ca^{2+} (Love and Hewitt, 1979). However, incubation with excess EGTA results in loss of activity upon reduction. Although, the identity of the essential disulfide bridge was not determined, these results are consistent with those observed for bDNase. In the presence of calcium, the bovine enzyme has been found to be highly resistant to proteolysis by contaminating pancreatic proteases (Price *et al.*, 1969a), and in particular, bDNase is highly resistant to inactivation by trypsin (Poulos and Price, 1972). Similarly, rhDNase digestion by trypsin is more difficult in the presence of calcium and requires removal of calcium to proceed to completion (J. Frenz, private communication).

2.3.2. EFFECT OF BIVALENT METAL IONS ON ACTIVITY

Bivalent metal ions are essential for the activity of bDNase. Hydrolysis of DNA proceeds by random, single-strand scission in the presence of Mg^{2+}. The replacement of Mg^{2+} with either Mn^{2+} or Ca^{2+} results in hydrolysis by simultaneous cleavage of both DNA strands. Significantly, the addition of both Mg^{2+} and Ca^{2+} ions results in a synergistic effect on bDNase activity (Wiberg, 1958). Price (1975) was able to demonstrate that in the presence of only Ca^{2+} at 0.1 mM or Mg^{2+} at 2.5 mM, bDNase has low specific activity, whereas when both metal ions are present bDNase has almost 700-fold greater specific activity. Similar synergistic effects of these bivalent metal ions have been reported for human DNase isolated from urine (Murai *et al.*, 1978), serum (Love and Hewitt, 1979), the pancreas (Funakoshi *et al.*, 1977), and rhDNase purified from the human 293 cell line (Shak *et al.*, 1990). It has been suggested that the bivalent metal ions serve two essential roles: one to bind to the enzyme and the other to bind to the DNA substrate (Lizarraga *et al.*, 1978; Moore, 1981). The Ca^{2+} ion may stabilize the DNase structure sufficiently to allow for effective recognition of the Mg^{2+}-DNA substrate (Lizarraga *et al.*, 1978). Further support for this hypothesis stems from the observation that the Mg^{2+} concentration required for bDNase activity is proportional to the DNA substrate concentration. Synergistic effects on bDNase activity were not found for other metal ions such as Zn^{2+}, Eu^{3+}, Sm^{3+}, Nd^{3+}, Cd^{2+}, Sn^{2+}, Fe^{2+}, Ni^{2+}, Cu^{2+}, Co^{2+}, and Mn^{2+} which were added at concentrations of 0.1 mM to bDNase preparations that contained 2.5 mM $MgCl_2$. The addition of 0.1 mM of the bivalent metal ions Sr^{2+} and Ba^{2+} to bDNase in 2.5 mM $MgCl_2$ resulted in preparations that were respectively ~63% and ~31% as active as bDNase with equivalent amounts of Ca^{2+} (Price, 1975). It has been shown that from 5 to 7 Ca^{2+} atoms bind to bDNase (Price, 1972). At a pH of 7.5, bDNase binds two Ca^{2+} ions strongly with an average K_d of 1.4×10^{-5} M and three more weakly with a K_d of 2×10^{-4} M. There are also two strong Mg^{2+} binding sites on bDNase with average K_d of 2.3×10^{-4} M. At pH 5.5, bDNase has only one strong Ca^{2+} binding site with a K_d of 2.2×10^{-5} M, and about five additional weak binding sites with K_d of 5×10^{-4}. The divalent cations Mg^{2+} and Mn^{2+} compete with Ca^{2+} for one of the two strong sites at pH 7.5 but are unable to bind to the one site at pH 5.5. This specific calcium binding site is likely the essential site required for bDNase activity. The fact that bDNase has activity in the presence of Sr^{2+} and Ba^{2+} ions suggests that these ions can also bind to the essential Ca^{2+} site. These metal ions are in the same column of the periodic table as Ca^{2+} and have similar properties.

3. ANALYTICAL CHARACTERIZATION

3.1. Analysis of Molecular Size

rhDNase migrates on SDS polyacrylamide gel electrophoresis as a broad band of apparent molecular weight between 31 and 38 kDa (data not shown). The spread in this band is typical of glycosylated proteins and reflects on the heterogeneity conferred on rhDNase by the N-linked glycosylation at Asn_{18} and Asn_{106}. This is confirmed by removal of carbohydrate by PNGase F, yielding a species that migrates as a narrow band with apparent molecular weight of 30 kDa (J. Frenz, unpublished results, data not shown). This apparent molecular weight is in good agreement with the molecular weight predicted from the amino acid sequence of rhDNase, 29.3 kDa. Little aggregated or fragmented rhDNase is found by size-exclusion chromatography; >99% of the protein migrates as one peak. Molecular weight of rhDNase determined by chromatography varies from 32 to 45 kDa, depending on the type and size cutoff of the chromatographic media (data not shown). Reported molecular weights for different human DNase preparations have also ranged from 30 to 40 kDa (Funakoshi *et al.*, 1977; Murai *et al.*, 1978; Love and Hewitt, 1979; Ito *et al.*, 1984). Determination of an accurate molecular weight for glycoproteins in solution by size-exclusion chromatography is difficult since the hydrodynamic volume of the glycoprotein is often being compared to unglycosylated standard proteins (Shire, 1994). In order to determine if our rhDNase preparations in solution were truly monomeric, we analyzed rhDNase by sedimentation equilibrium. The partial specific volume of 0.721 was computed from the amino acid and average carbohydrate composition using the additivity rule and values for the individual amino acid and carbohydrate residues (Cohn and Edsall, 1965; Gibbons, 1972; Perkins, 1986). The absorbance gradient in the centrifuge cell was analyzed with a single ideal species model (Shire, 1994). The excellent fit of the data to this model is shown by the random distribution of residuals (Fig. 4). The determined molecular weight of 33200 ± 1400 is in very good agreement with the molecular weight of 32653 based on the polypeptide sequence and average carbohydrate composition.

3.2. Analysis of Charge Heterogeneity

rhDNase exhibits considerable charge heterogeneity due to sialylation and phosphorylation of the N-linked oligosaccharides. Frenz *et al.* (1994) using anion-exchange chromatography with a polyethylenimine bonded phase, were able to effect separation of charge isoforms that result from the extents and positions of phospho-

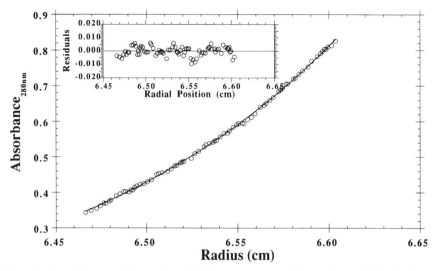

Figure 4.   Typical concentration gradient of rhDNase as a result of sedimentation equilibrium. Sedimentation was carried out at 15,000 rpm in an XLA analytical ultracentrifuge equipped with ultraviolet absorption optics. The absorbance monitored at 280 nm was fit to a single ideal species model (solid line). The residuals to the fit are shown in the inset.A magnitude and the random distribution of residuals suggests that a single ideal species model adequately accounts for the data.

rylation on the carbohydrate moieties of rhDNase. The proportion of these isoforms in the final product are dictated by cell fermentation conditions and do not change over time of storage. However, an additional charge heterogeneity results from a specific deamidation that occurs at Asn_{74}. The rate of deamidation of Asn residues in proteins is often pH-, ionic strength-, and temperature-dependent (Wright, 1991; Cleland *et al.*, 1993). The generation of deamidated product results in complex isoelectric focusing patterns (Fig. 5) as well as difficult separations by conventional ion exchange chromatography (Cacia *et al.*, 1993). However, effective separation of the deamidated and nondeamidated rhDNase was accomplished using "tentacle" ion-exchange chromatography (Cacia *et al.*, 1993). The "tentacle" ion-exchange resin contains from 5 to 50 repeating cation-exchange sulfate groups attached to a flexible polymeric backbone (Muller, 1990). The flexibility of the polymer chains allows the tethered charged species to conform to the complex topology of a protein surface, thereby maximizing the interaction between itself and charged groups of a protein. Interestingly, the tentacle ion-exchange chromatography was highly specific for the separation of the deamidated variant but was not able to separate the other charged species (Fig. 5). It was suggested that the polymeric nature of the tentacle ion-exchange resin may mimic certain characteristics of a DNA substrate (Cacia *et al.*, 1993). The crystal structure of a bDNase-synthetic oligonucleotide complex shows that the Asn_{74} residue is involved in the binding of the DNA substrate (Lahm

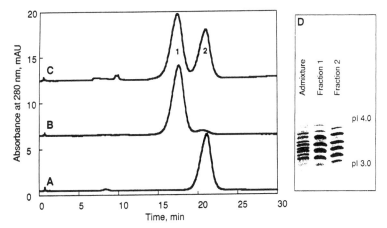

Figure 5.   Tentacle ion exchange chromatography of rhDNase (A), rhDNase deamidated at Asn$_{74}$ (B), and an admixture of both species (C). The deamidated (D) rhDNase (fraction 1) and rhDNase (fraction 2) were analyzed using isoelectric focusing from pH 3 to 5. The chromatography was performed on an HP1090M liquid chromatograph using a 5-μm, 1000-pore size, LiChrospher SO$_3^-$ column (EM Industries, Inc., Gibbstown, NJ). Details of the chromatography are given in Cacia *et al.* (1993). Reproduced by permission from Cacia *et al.* (1993).

and Suck, 1991). Therefore, the tentacle ion exchange resin may be functioning in an affinity rather than ion-exchange chromatography mode. This idea was further supported by successful separation of the deamidated variant by affinity chromatography using an anion-exchange resin with electrostatically immobilized DNA (Cacia *et al.*, 1993).

3.3. Analysis of Nuclease Activity

The classical assay for determining activity of bDNase preparations has been the hyperchromicity assay which is based on an increase in absorbance at 260 nm after hydrolysis of the DNA substrate (Kunitz, 1950). Kinetic data obtained by this spectrophotometric technique are often analyzed by Michaelis–Menten kinetics. The kinetics may actually be more complex since there are multiple hydrolysis sites on the DNA substrate, and a single individual clip may not result in a large hyperchromic shift. Nevertheless, it is possible to fit the initial rates as a function of DNA concentration with a Michaelis–Menten kinetic model (Cipolla *et al.*, 1994a). The K_m and V_{max} values for rhDNase were 36 ± 7 μg/ml and ~2 × 10^5 units/mg, respectively (1 unit is defined as the activity which causes an increase in absorbance at 260 nm of 0.001/min/ml at 25°C). The deamidation at Asn$_{74}$ did not appear to change the measured value for V_{max}, whereas the K_m value increased to 296 ± 52 μg/ml. This observation is consistent with the proposed role of Asn_{74} in binding of the DNA substrate in the crystal structure of the bDNase-synthetic oligonucleotide complex (Lahm and Suck, 1991). This also further supports the proposed structural homology between bDNase and rhDNase.

Hydrolysis of DNA by DNase has also been monitored by a variety of methods including radiometric, fluorometric, viscometric, potentiometric, and electrophoretic techniques (Kurnick, 1962). Most of the methods developed are imprecise and are not amenable for high throughput of samples. Sinicropi *et al.* (1994) have modified the assay developed by Kurnick which uses a DNA substrate complexed with the dye methyl green (Kurnick, 1950a). Methyl green intercalates between the stacked base pairs of double-stranded DNA resulting in a maximum of about one dye molecule per five base pairs (Kurnick and Mirsky, 1950; Korozumi *et al.*, 1963). Upon hydrolysis of the DNA by DNase, methyl green is released from the substrate complex and undergoes an isomerization at neutral pH (Kurnick, 1950b; Kurnick and Foster, 1950). This isomerization results in a fading of the dye's green color as assessed by a reduction in absorbance at 620 nm. Standard activity curves were constructed from dilutions of a reference standard, and the activity of the test sample was determined from these standard curves. The resulting concentration determinations were used to define 1 methyl green–DNA activity unit (1 MG unit) as the amount of activity equivalent to 1 μg of the rhDNase standard.

The modification of this assay resulted in a fast and precise throughput assay (less than 12% CV intra- and interassay variability) using microtiter plate methodology. A comparison with the hyperchromicity assay showed a strong correlation between the two assays (Sinicropi *et al.*, 1994). The activity of rhDNase and bDNase as a function of pH and divalent cation concentration was also explored using the modified assay. The pH and divalent cation optima were found to be similar for both of the nucleases. However, the specific activity of bDNase at 2400 ± 400 MG units/mg was greater than for rhDNase at 1000 MG units/mg. The activity of rhDNase was comparable to that determined for DNase isolated from human urine (Sinicropi *et al.*, 1994).

4. FORMULATION DEVELOPMENT

4.1. Aerosol Delivery of rhDNase: Characterization of DNase Aerosols

Most protein drugs that are currently marketed are delivered by injection. However, the site of action for rhDNase is in the airways, and in order to achieve a high local concentration of the drug, it is necessary to deliver rhDNase as an inhalation aerosol. Early clinical studies with bDNase used jet (Elmes and White, 1953; Salomon *et al.*, 1954; Spier *et al.*, 1961; Raskin, 1968) and ultrasonic nebulizers (Lieberman, 1968) to deliver bDNase aerosols. However, little was done to characterize the physical properties of the aerosols or the biochemical integrity of bDNase after nebulization. Aerosols generated using four different jet nebulizers driven by a Pulmo-Aide Model 5610D Compressor (De Vilbiss, Somerset, PA) were characterized in support of the human clinical trials conducted in the United States (Cipolla *et al.*, 1994a,b).

The distribution of the size of droplets in an aerosol is critical in determining deposition of an inhalation aerosol drug. Droplets larger than 6 μm will deposit mainly in the oropharynx, whereas droplets less than 1 μm are likely to be exhaled during normal tidal breathing. Accordingly, the mass percent respirable fraction is defined as the percent of the total droplet mass from 1 to 6 μm. The particle size distribution of nebulized rhDNase at 1 mg/ml was similar for the four jet nebulizers initially tested (Fig. 6) and was between 46% and 51%. The nebulizer efficiency is defined as the percent of the total amount of drug loaded into the nebulizer that is actually delivered as an aerosol to the mouthpiece of the nebulizer. The observed nebulizer efficiency for the four jet nebulizers, ranging from 44% to 55% was typical

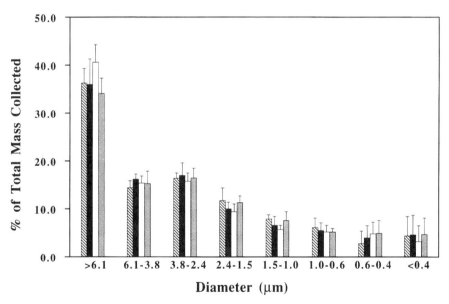

Figure 6.   Droplet size distribution of rhDNase aerosols. Aerosols were generated over 10 min using four different jet nebulizers loaded with 2.5 ml of rhDNase at 1 mg/ml. The droplet size distribution was determined with a seven-stage cascade impactor (In-Tox Products, Albuquerque, NM). Nebulizers used were: (▨) Respirgard II model 124030 (Marquest, Englewood, CA) modified by removal of the expiratory one-way valve, (■) Acorn II model 124014 (Marquest, Englewood, CA), (□) Airlife Misty with Tee Adapter model 0020308 (Baxter-American Pharmaseal Co., Valencia, CA), and (▩) Up-Draft II model 1734 (Hudson RCI, Temecula, CA.). The error bars are the standard deviations that result from seven to eight independent determinations. Used by permission from Cipolla *et al.* (1994b).

for other drugs delivered by jet nebulization (Byron, 1990). The delivery efficiency, defined as the percent of the initial rhDNase dose delivered to the mouthpiece in the respirable range of 1 to 6 μm was between 20% and 28%. Characterization of rhDNase before and after nebulization showed that there was no reduction in activity and no generation of aggregates as assessed by the DNA–methyl green activity assay and HPLC sizing chromatography, respectively. The rhDNase tertiary and secondary structures also were unaltered after nebulization as determined by near- and far-UV circular dichroism spectrophotometry (data not shown). Altogether, these studies showed that all four jet nebulizers that were tested were essentially equivalent in their ability to deliver respirable doses of intact, fully active, nonaggregated rhDNase (Cipolla *et al.*, 1994a,b). Additional studies designed to characterize rhDNase aerosols generated by seven additional jet nebulizers coupled with different air compressor systems showed that large differences exist in the droplet size distribution and delivery efficiency of aerosols produced by the different delivery systems (Cipolla *et al.*, 1994c). The structural integrity and activity of rhDNase in aerosols produced by jet nebulizers remained unaltered. However, some ultrasonic nebulizers caused denaturation of the rhDNase, probably due to the elevated temperature during ultrasonic nebulization.

4.2. Choice of Formulation Components

4.2.1. REQUIREMENT FOR AN ISOTONIC FORMULATION WITHOUT BUFFER SALTS

Since rhDNase is administered as an aerosol for local pulmonary delivery, a formulation is required that is compatible with its delivery to the upper airways of the lung. The osmolality and pH of nebulizer solutions are critical variables that affect bronchoconstriction and subsequent adverse reactions during pulmonary delivery of drugs (Fine *et al.*, 1987; Balmes *et al.*, 1988; Beasley *et al.*, 1988; Desager *et al.*, 1990; Snell, 1990; Sant'Ambrogio *et al.*, 1991). It has also been recommended that, whenever possible, nebulizer solutions should be formulated as isotonic solutions at pH >5 (Beasley *et al.*, 1988). Recent studies have shown that if the formulation is not isotonic then the droplet-size distribution of an aerosol may be altered during delivery as the result of a loss or uptake of water vapor from the airways (Gonda *et al.*, 1982; Gonda and Phipps, 1991). It is also not uncommon to find that buffer components can cause adverse reactions such as cough (Godden *et al.*, 1986; Auffarth *et al.*, 1991) and, therefore, we have attempted to formulate rhDNase as an unbuffered isotonic solution. The control of the pH in an unbuffered formulation is a major concern, especially since many protein degradation pathways are highly pH dependent (Cleland *et al.*, 1993). However, it has been shown that rhDNase formulated at 1 mg/ml provides sufficient buffering capacity so that the pH of the formulated drug product is quite stable over the recommended storage life of the drug (Cipolla *et al.*, 1994a).

4.2.2. REQUIREMENT FOR CALCIUM

The requirement of calcium and other bivalent cations for bDNase and rhDNase activity, substrate specificity, and stability was previously discussed. In particular, bDNase has one specific calcium binding site at pH 5 that appears to be essential for activity. The binding of calcium to rhDNase at pH 5–6 was studied to determine if the calcium binding properties of the bovine and human protein were similar. rhDNase preparations at concentrations ranging from 1.25 to 1.58 mM were exhaustively dialyzed against 150 mM NaCl at pH 5–6. The total concentration of calcium in the dialyzed rhDNase solutions, $[Ca^{2+}]_{AA}$, was determined by atomic absorption spectroscopy and the data analyzed with the following binding equation:

$$n = A + \frac{NK_a[Ca^{2+}]_{free}}{1 + K_a[Ca^{2+}]_{free}}$$

where n = total number of calcium binding sites/rhDNase, i.e., $[Ca^{2+}]_{bound}/[rhDNase]$ with association constant K_a, A = number of tightly bound sites/rhDNase, and N = number of weakly bound sites/rhDNase.

The calculated charge based on amino acid composition for rhDNase at pH 5 is approximately -5 and at 150 mM NaCl the Donnan effect will be small (Cantor and Schimmel, 1980). In this situation, with exhaustive dialysis, the concentration of unbound calcium at equilibrium is the concentration of calcium in the solution used for dialysis. The amount of bound calcium $[Ca^{2+}]_{bound}$, can then be estimated as the difference between the concentration determined by atomic absorption spectrophotometry, $[Ca^{2+}]_{AA}$, and the concentration of Ca^{2+} in the solution used for dialysis. The analysis suggests the binding equation is a good representation of the binding data with one strong binding site ($A = 1.3 \pm 0.03$) and four weak binding sites ($N = 4.2 \pm 0.3$) with an association constant of 0.4 ± 0.05 mM^{-1} (Fig. 7). These results are comparable to what has been observed for bDNase at pH 5, and by analogy with bDNase suggest that there is one tightly bound calcium ion in rhDNase that is essential for activity. After treatment with EDTA, there are 1–1.5 calcium ions that remain bound to rhDNase, and subsequent formulation into a phosphate buffer results in a loss of activity compared to an untreated sample (Fig. 8). Deamidation is a major degradation route as discussed in more detail in the next section. It has been established that phosphate catalyzes deamidation in many peptides (Capasso *et al.*, 1991); however, the rate of deamidation was similar with and without the phosphate buffer (data not shown). Presumably the phosphate buffer effectively competes with any remaining calcium bound to the protein, and removal of this essential and tightly bound calcium results in loss of activity. It has also been shown, again in analogy with bDNase, that trypsin is unable to fully digest rhDNase unless sufficient calcium is

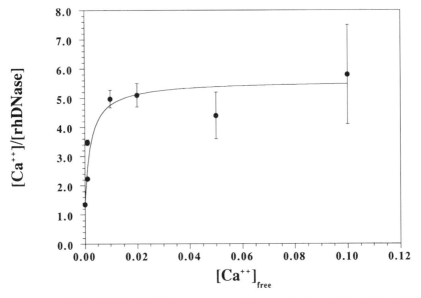

Figure 7. Equilibrium dialysis of rhDNase at concentrations ranging from 1.25 to 1.58 mM. The rhDNase solutions were exhaustively dialyzed against 150 mM NaCl at pH 5–6. The total concentration of calcium in the dialyzed rhDNase solutions, $[Ca^{2+}]_{AA}$, was determined by atomic absorption spectroscopy. The data were analyzed as described in the text.

removed by treatment with EDTA (Frenz, J., Genentech, Inc., personal communication, 1992). These observations strongly suggest that the binding of calcium stabilizes the conformation and is essential for the activity of rhDNase. The optimum amount of calcium for bDNase activity was determined to be ~0.5 mM and it was claimed that bDNase activity is inhibited at about 1 mM calcium (Price, 1975). Sinicropi *et al.* (1994) showed using the DNA–methyl green activity assay that rhDNase had a near maximum reaction velocity with the inclusion of 2.4 mM $CaCl_2$ and 2.4 mM $MgCl_2$ in the final reaction mixture. The addition of 1 mM calcium (~33-fold molar excess compared to rhDNase) was shown to be sufficient to maintain stability at the recommended storage temperature of 2–8°C (Cipolla *et al.*, 1994a).

4.3. Solution Stability

4.3.1. MAJOR ROUTE OF DEGRADATION

A variety of assays including size-exclusion chromatography, SDS polyacrylamide gel electrophoresis (SDS-PAGE), tentacle ion-exchange chromatography,

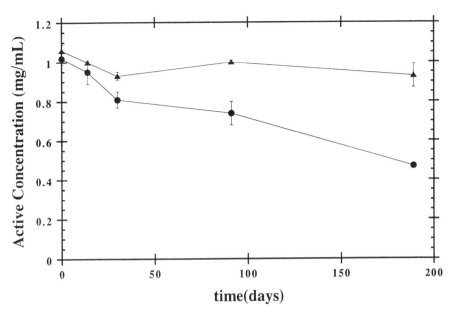

Figure 8. Effect of calcium on activity of rhDNase stored at 25°C at ~pH 6. rhDNase was either formulated in 150 mM NaCl and 1 mM CaCl$_2$ (solid triangles) or treated with EDTA and formulated in isotonic 10 mM PO$_4$ (solid circles). The active concentration was determined by the DNA–methyl green activity assay. Reproduced by permission from Cipolla *et al.* (1994a).

and the DNA–methyl green activity assay were used to monitor product stability. As previously discussed, the tentacle ion-exchange chromatography detects a specific deamidation at Asn$_{74}$ (Cacia *et al.*, 1993). Aggregation of rhDNase, as detected by native size-exclusion chromatography and SDS-PAGE, is minimal (<1%). The deamidation at Asn$_{74}$ is a major route of degradation of rhDNase as detected by the methyl green activity assay. This degradation route, however, does not lead to a completely inactive molecule but rather a protein with 40–50% of the activity of the nondeamidated protein. The correlation between deamidation and activity as assessed by the methyl green activity assay is shown in Fig. 9 for rhDNase formulated in 5 mM Tris, 150 mM NaCl at pH 8 and stored at 37°C. This decrease in activity appears to be related to a decrease in binding of the substrate as shown by determination of K_m using the hyperchromicity assay. The deamidation of Asn in proteins often proceeds through a cyclic imide intermediate that hydrolyzes to either an aspartate or isoaspartate amino acid residue (Wright, 1991; Cleland *et al.*, 1993). The formation of isoaspartate appears to be thermodynamically favored as shown by analysis of various proteins and peptides. The conversion of an asparagine to isoaspartate not only results in the formation of a negatively charged species, but also results in the placement of an extra methylene group in the peptide backbone. This potentially

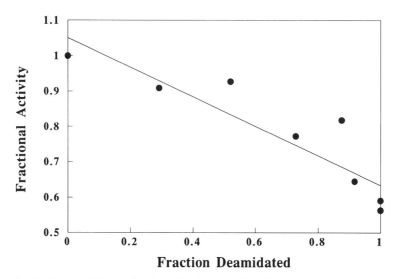

Figure 9. Fractional activity as a function of fraction deamidated for rhDNase at pH 8 and 37°C. The fractional activity is computed as the active concentration as determined by the DNA-methyl green activity assay divided by the concentration determined using the UV absorbance at 280 nm (absorptivity for a 1-cm pathlength = 1.7 mg/ml cm^{-1}). Fraction deamidated is computed as $C_{deam,t}/C_{deam,t=0}$, where $C_{deam,t}$ and $C_{deam,t=0}$ are concentrations of deamidated rhDNase at time t and 0, respectively. The solid line is the result of a linear regression analysis (intercept = 1.0, slope = −0.42, and linear correlation coefficient, $R = 0.907$).

could alter the conformation of the protein, affecting activity and stability. However, the global secondary structure of fully deamidated and nondeamidated rhDNase as assessed by far-UV circular dichroism is similar (Fig. 10).

4.3.2. KINETIC ANALYSIS AND pH RATE PROFILE

The rate of deamidation of rhDNase was measured using tentacle ion-exchange chromatography (Cipolla *et al.*, 1994a). The chromatography data resulted in linear, pseudo-first-order kinetics, and the rate constants were determined at pH 5,6,7 and 8 at 2–8, 15, 25, and 37°C. The pseudo-first-order rate constants for deamidation were obtained using real-time data after 88 days of storage and are presented along with the standard errors from a linear regression analysis (Table I). The errors in the determined rate constants of deamidation at 2–8°C and 15°C at pH values below 7 were large (± 100%) because of the small degree of deamidation. In some cases the experimental error was larger than the observed change in deamidation resulting in apparent positive slopes. As expected, the pseudo-first-order rate constants for deamidation (Table I) are highly pH dependent and decrease with a reduction in pH (Fig. 11) as has been previously observed for deamidation of peptides (Robinson and

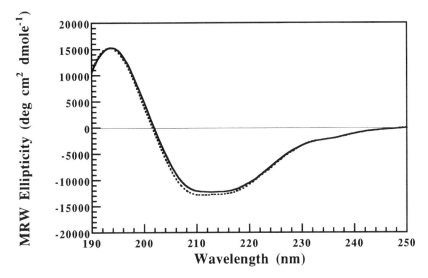

Figure 10. Far-UV circular dichroism spectra of rhDNase (solid line) and rhDNase deamidated at Asn$_{74}$ (dashed line).

Table I. First-Order Rate Constants (days^{-1}) for Deamidation of rhDNase as Assessed by Tentacle Ion-Exchange Chromatography[a]

Formulation[b]	2–8°C	15°C	25°C	37°C
Acetate, pH 5	+	~0	7 ± 1 $\times 10^{-4}$	3.7 ± 0.15 $\times 10^{-3}$
Succinate, pH 5	3.6 ± 10 $\times 10^{-4}$	7 ± 7 $\times 10^{-5}$	5.6 ± 1.5 $\times 10^{-4}$	3.8 ± 1.5 $\times 10^{-3}$
Citrate, pH 5	+	+	7.3 ± 1.4 $\times 10^{-4}$	4.0 ± 1.3 $\times 10^{-3}$
Histidine, pH 6	3 ± 3 $\times 10^{-4}$	1.3 ± 0.2 $\times 10^{-3}$	3.6 ± 0.15 $\times 10^{-3}$	1.4 ± 0.03 $\times 10^{-2}$
Succinate, pH 6	+	7 ± 7 $\times 10^{-5}$	1.6 ± 0.1 $\times 10^{-3}$	9.96 ± 0.16 $\times 10^{-3}$
Maleate, pH 6	+	2.4 ± 1 $\times 10^{-4}$	1.3 ± 0.08 $\times 10^{-3}$	9.66 ± 0.65 $\times 10^{-3}$
Tris, pH 7	1.9 ± 0.5 $\times 10^{-3}$	5.7 ± 0.8 $\times 10^{-3}$	1.3 ± 0.08 $\times 10^{-2}$	3 ± 0.15 $\times 10^{-2}$
Tris, pH 8	1.1 ± 0.1 $\times 10^{-2}$	2.3 ± 0.13 $\times 10^{-2}$	4.8 ± 0.3 $\times 10^{-2}$	1.3 ± 0.03 $\times 10^{-1}$

[a]+ Indicates that slope was positive. The origin and significance of such a result is discussed in the text.
[b]Buffers consist of 5 mM buffer salt, 150 mM NaCl, and 1 mM CaCl$_2$.

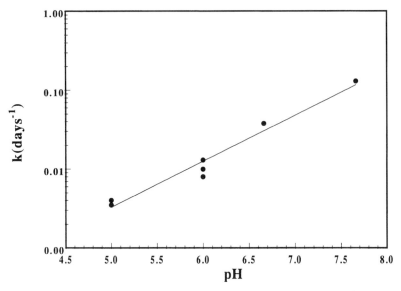

Figure 11. The dependence of pH on the rate of deamidation where the solid circles are for the deamidation rate constants at 37°C of rhDNase at 3.9 mg/ml in 5 mM buffer, 1 mM $CaCl_2$, and 150 mM NaCl, at pH 5.0 (acetate, succinate, and citrate), pH 6.0 (histidine, succinate, and maleate), pH 7.0 and pH 8.0 (Tris). The Tris buffer pH values, measured at room temperature, have been corrected for the temperature dependence of the Tris ionization constant.

Rudd, 1974; Wright, 1991; Cleland *et al.*, 1993). Although the rate constant for deamidation at pH 5 is smaller than at pH 8 (~0.004 versus 0.1 day^{-1} at 37°C storage), precipitation occurs at 37°C at pH 5. These data suggested that the formulation pH should be kept low enough to effectively control the rate of deamidation but not too low since precipitation could occur upon storage.

The kinetics of deamidation can also be used to provide further support for deamidation as the major degradation route in rhDNase. When the differences in methyl green activity between deamidated and nondeamidated rhDNase at pH ~7.7 and 37°C are taken into account, the first-order plots (Fig. 12) yield similar pseudo-first-order rate constants, 0.078 ± .005 day^{-1} and 0.069 ± 006 day^{-1} for deamidation and loss in methyl green activity, respectively (Cipolla *et al.*, 1994a).

4.3.3. ACCELERATED STABILITY AND ARRHENIUS KINETICS

The pseudo-first-order rate constants for deamidation can be determined with good precision at high pH values above 15°C. However, storage at 2–8°C results in very low rates of deamidation, especially for the more acidic formulations. These

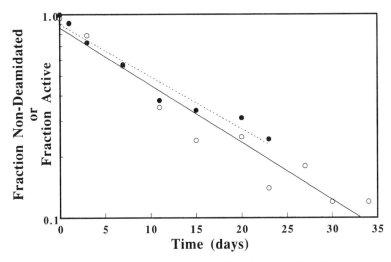

Figure 12. Kinetics at pH ~7.7 and 37°C of activity loss (filled circles) and deamidation (open circles) of rhDNase as determined by methyl green activity assay and tentacle ion-exchange chromatography respectively. The dashed line is the result of a fit of the activity data to first-order kinetics ($k = 0.069 \pm 0.006$ day^{-1} and $R^2 = 0.986$).The fraction of active rhDNase was computed by taking into account the fact that deamidated rhDNase has ~50% of the methyl green activity of nondeamidated rhDNase. Fraction nondeamidated is computed as $C_{nondeam,t}/C_{nondeam,t=0}$, where $C_{nondeam,t}$ and $C_{nondeam,t=0}$ are concentrations of nondeamidated rhDNase at time t and 0, respectively. The solid line is the result of a fit of the deamidation data to first-order kinetics ($k = 0.078 \pm 0.005$ day^{-1} and $R_2 = 0.992$).

determined values tend to have large errors because of the small changes that are being monitored with the ion-exchange assay. In some instances the errors were larger than the change in the measured percent deamidation resulting in a physically impossible positive slope for the first-order plot (Table I). This problem can be circumvented if the deamidation reaction follows Arrhenius kinetics. A comparison of rate constants determined from real-time data after 88 days at 2–8°C with rate constants determined from Arrhenius kinetics is summarized in Table II. Overall the agreement appears to be quite good, especially at pH 7 and 8 where the real-time rate constants have small standard errors. These results suggest that accelerated stability studies and evaluation by Arrhenius kinetics is possible for assessment of deamidation rates of this one particular Asn in rhDNase as monitored by the tentacle ion-exchange assay. The activation energy in kcal/mole obtained from the slopes of the Arrhenius plots are also given in Table II. The values for all formulations tend to range from ~20–30 kcal/mole with the exception of the Tris formulations with values of 13–14 kcal/mole. Some of this difference is probably the result of the well-known temperature-dependent pH shifts of Tris buffers which were not taken into account in these studies. Since the dpH/dT for Tris is -0.028/°C the pH at 37°C will be 0.34 pH

Table II. Comparison of Rate Constants at 5°C
Obtained from Arrhenius Kinetics and Stability Data
after 88 Days at 2–8°C Storage

Formulation[a]	$k_{88\ days}$ (days^{-1})	$k_{arrhenius}$ (days^{-1})	ΔE^b (kcal/mole)
Tris, pH 8	$1.1 \pm 0.1 \times 10^{-2}$	9.3×10^{-3}	14
Tris, pH 7	$1.9 \pm 0.5 \times 10^{-3}$	2.5×10^{-3}	13.4
Succinate, pH 6	$+^c$	7.3×10^{-6}	28
Maleate, pH 6	$+$	3.6×10^{-5}	29.9
Histidine, pH 6	$3 \pm 3 \times 10^{-4}$	3.8×10^{-4}	19.0
Succinate, pH 5	$3.7 \pm 10 \times 10^{-5}$	3.6×10^{-5}	29.3
Citrate, pH 5	$+$	3.1×10^{-5}	26.0
Acetate, pH 5	$+$	3.2×10^{-5}	25.5

[a]Buffers consist of 5 mM buffer salt, 150 mM NaCl, and 1 mM $CaCl_2$.
[b]Energy of activation. Succinate at pH 6 and 5 were evaluated without the 15°C data because of the large error in the values at 15°C.
[c]+ indicates that slope was positive. The origin and significance of such a result is discussed in the text.

unit lower and at 15°C it will be 0.28 pH unit greater than at 25°C. The difference in the rates of deamidation as a function of pH is accentuated at the higher temperatures and therefore the larger shift down in pH at 37°C storage will result in an Arrhenius plot with a decreased slope. The observed values of 20–30 kcal/mole for all formulations except Tris are consistent with those previously reported for deamidation of an Asn in a model hexapeptide at pH 5 and 7.5 (Patel and Borchardt, 1990).

4.4. Choice of Container Closure

4.4.1. BLOW-FILL-SEAL TECHNOLOGY

All the above considerations led us to formulate rhDNase at 1 mg/ml in an unbuffered isotonic liquid formulation containing 150 mM NaCl and 1 mM $CaCl_2$. The container-closure system for this formulation was originally a 5-cc glass vial with siliconized, Teflon-coated, gray, butyl rubber stoppers. The average pH of the formulation in the glass vials was 7.0, and the formulation showed good stability over 1.5 years at 2–8°C (Cipolla *et al.*, 1994a). An alternative to glass vials is the plastic packaging technology of Automatic Liquid Packaging Incorporated (ALP, Inc.) This process takes granular pellets of blowable thermoplastic material and in one self-contained machine extrudes, blow-molds, fills, and seals plastic vials or ampules in one continuous operation. This blow-fill-seal technology has already been used for the packaging of aerosol products such as normal saline and the bronchodilator, metaproterenol sulfate (Alupent). The advantages of such a system include more convenient patient usage, contact of one material with drug since stopper enclosures are not required, reduction of breakage of vials, elimination of vial preparation procedures and rapid throughput of the filling operations.

4.4.2. STABILITY IN PLASTIC AMPOULES

The blow-fill-seal technology can result in the exposure of product to temperatures as high as 37°C for several minutes. Before undertaking an actual fill at ALP Inc. a preliminary experiment was set up to test the quality of rhDNase in plastic ampoules after a 15-min exposure to 37°C (Meserve *et al.*, 1994). Plastic pellets used to make the plastic ampoules are available from more than one manufacturer. Therefore, two low-density polyethylene plastics, Escorene and Dupont 20, were used to make plastic ampoules at ALP, Inc. The plastic ampoules previously filled and sealed with water were drained, washed with deionized water and air-dried. The empty ampoules were filled with rhDNase at 4 mg/ml and resealed with a gas torch. The ampoules were placed in an incubator at 37°C for 15 min and the rhDNase then analyzed by assessment of color and clarity, UV absorption spectroscopy, ELISA, DNA–methyl green activity assay, and gel-sizing chromatography. The stability of rhDNase in plastic ampoules before and after incubation at 37°C for 15 min is shown in Table III and shows that the protein is fully active without any aggregate formation after the 15-min exposure at 37°C. The secondary and tertiary structure of rhDNase after 15 min at 37°C was investigated by circular dichroism spectrophotometry (data not shown). The near-UV CD of rhDNase at 37°C shows decreased intensity of the CD bands compared with the spectrum of rhDNase at 20°C (Fig. 13). This decrease in intensity is likely due to increased mobility of the aromatic amino acid residues. There were no wavelength shifts, suggesting that the polarity of the environments of the aromatic amino acid residues were not greatly altered. After decreasing the sample temperature to 20°C, the near-UV CD spectrum is indistinguishable from that of a sample which had never been heated to 37°C. This result suggests that any

Table III. Stability of rhDNase (4mg/ml) before and after Incubation in Plastic Ampoules at 37°C for 15 min

Sample	Color & clarity[a]	UV (mg/ml)	ELISA (mg/ml)	MG[b] (mg/ml)	% Monomer
rhDNase, 2–8°C in glass vial	co/PO	3.88	4.01 ± 0.34	3.64 ± 0.20	100%
rhDNase, 37°C, 15 min in Dupont 20 plastic ampoule	co/PO	3.93	3.88 ± 0.22	3.95 ± 0.15	100%
rhDNase, 37°C, 15 min in Escorene plastic ampoule	co/PO	3.92	3.78 ± 0.16	3.88 ± 0.12	100%

[a]co = colorless; PO = clear with occasional particulates observed.
[b]Methyl green-DNA activity.

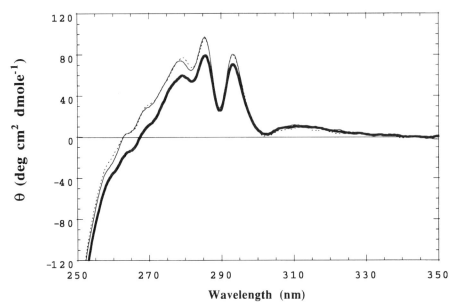

Figure 13. Near-UV circular dichroism spectra of rhDNase at 20°C (solid line), 37°C (bold solid line), and at 20°C after 15 min at 37°C (dotted line). All spectra were taken at a concentration of ~0.5 mg/ml in a thermostated 1-cm cylindrical cell using an Aviv 60DS spectropolarimeter. The data are the result of averaging three scans with a 5-s averaging time for each data point taken at 0.25-nm intervals. Ellipticity values were converted to mean residue weight ellipticity using a mean residue weight of 112.8 for rhDNase.

structural alterations or increased flexibility of the protein structure as monitored by the aromatic amino acid residues is completely reversible with short-term exposure to temperatures up to 37°C. The near- and far-UV CD of rhDNase at 4 mg/ml before and after incubation of the protein in the plastic ampoules at 37°C for 15 min as compared to the rhDNase in glass vials within experimental error, are unaltered (data not shown). This result shows that rhDNase conformation is not affected by a 15-min incubation at 37°C in plastic ampoules.

The preliminary experiments showed that rhDNase can be exposed to the surface of a plastic ampoule at the elevated temperatures that might be encountered during the filling operation. rhDNase was vialed originally in glass vials for the clinical studies, and therefore a direct stability comparison was made between rhDNase in glass vials and rhDNase filled into plastic ampoules using the blow-fill-seal technology at ALP, Inc. The ALP, Inc. manufacturing process uses low-density polyethylene resins which are gas permeable. This property of the resin may result in water vapor transfer with concomitant alteration in drug concentration. It is also possible that permeation of oxygen could result in oxidation of the protein if this were

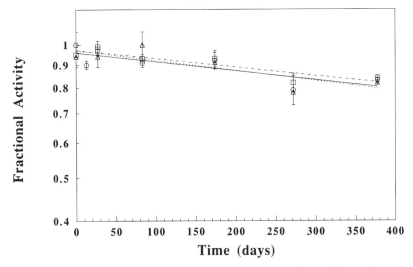

Figure 14.   Stability of rhDNase at 25°C in plastic ampoules made with Dupont 20 resin. The fractional activity is computed as the active concentration as determined by the DNA–methyl green activity assay divided by the concentration determined using the UV absorbance at 280 nm (absorptivity = 1.7 cm^{-1} ml/ mg). The data were analyzed by pseudo-first-order kinetics for unfoiled ampoules (open circles, solid line, $k = 4.7 \times 10^{-5}$ day^{-1}), foiled ampoules (open squares, dashed line, $k = 4.5 \times 10^{-5}$ day^{-1}), and ampoules foiled in the presence of a nitrogen atmosphere (open triangles, dotted line, $k = 5.2 \times 10^{-5}$ day^{-1}).

a major degradation route. This problem can be addressed by packaging the plastic ampoules in a gas-impermeable foil pouch which can be filled with nitrogen. The stability study was therefore also designed to determine if the stability in plastic ampoules is different when the ampules are foiled with or without a nitrogen atmosphere (Meserve *et al.*, 1994). The stability assays included tentacle ion-exchange and gel-sizing chromatography, color and clarity determination, SDS-PAGE, and the methyl green–DNA activity assay. The presence of a foil barrier with a nitrogen atmosphere did not have any appreciable protective effect on the activity of rhDNase (Fig. 14) or aggregate formation as assessed by SDS-PAGE and gel-sizing chromatography or color and clarity of product (data not shown). These data suggest that a foil barrier is not required to maintain stability and quality of rhDNase. However, the low-density polyethylene resins do allow for water vapor transfer with potential alteration of drug concentration (Fig. 15). Moreover, exposure to intense fluorescent light (~1600 foot-candles) can result in aggregate formation as detected by SDS-PAGE (data not shown). Thus, an additional attribute of the foil barrier is its ability to decrease exposure to light.

The rate of deamidation was similar for rhDNase stored at 2–8°C in foiled and unfoiled plastic ampoules but substantially different from protein stored in glass vials

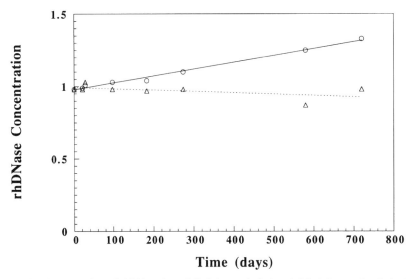

Figure 15. Concentration of rhDNase in unfoiled (open circles) and foiled (open triangles) plastic ampoules stored at 37°C. The concentration was determined using UV absorption spectroscopy at 280 nm.

(Fig. 16). The pseudo-first-order rate constants at 2–8, 25, and 37°C were at least threefold greater for rhDNase stored in glass vials than in plastic ampoules (Table IV). This difference in deamidation rate can be accounted for by the ~0.5-unit difference in pH of rhDNase in glass versus plastic ampoules (Fig. 17). The pH of rhDNase in a plastic ampoule quickly increases by 0.3–0.4 pH unit in less than 2 hr when transferred directly into a glass vial and remains constant after the initial increase (data not shown). Thus the difference in pH between rhDNase stored in glass vials and plastic ampoules is likely due to the leaching of ions, possibly sodium, from the glass surface. The subsequent replacement of these ions by protons from the water will lead to a significant increase in pH, especially considering the low buffer capacity of the formulation.

5. SUMMARY AND CONCLUSIONS

Most proteins have been formulated and delivered by injection. rhDNase is one of the first protein drugs to be formulated for local delivery to the lung. We have successfully formulated rhDNase as a liquid that is stable for 2 years in plastic ampoules at 2–8°C. Many aspects of the successful development of this drug have been summarized in this chapter, including characterization of the major degradation route, rationale for choice of formulation and container-closure components, and

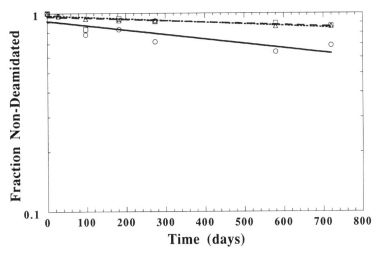

Figure 16. Kinetics at 2–8°C of deamidation of rhDNase formulated in 150 mM NaCl, 1 mM CaCl$_2$ stored in glass vials (open circles), foiled Dupont 20 plastic ampoules (open squares), and unfoiled Dupont 20 plastic ampoules (open triangles). The fraction of nondeamidated rhDNase is computed as C$_{nondeam,t}$/C$_{nondeam,t=0}$, where C$_{nondeam,t}$ and C$_{nondeam,t=0}$ are concentrations of nondeamidated rhDNase at time t and 0, respectively.

characterization of rhDNase aerosols. In particular, it has been shown that the formulated protein can be delivered as an aerosol by using current jet nebulizer technology. Although the recirculation of protein solutions under high shear rates in the nebulizer bowl could potentially denature the protein (Byron, 1990; Niven *et al.*, 1992) we have demonstrated that rhDNase is unaltered during the nebulization process. The choice of plastic ampoules manufactured by a blow-fill-seal technology was predicated on the large throughput for fills afforded by this technology and improved patient convenience. An additional, unforeseen benefit was the improved stability of the product in plastic versus glass containers mainly due to the lower pH of the unbuffered rhDNase formulation after filling into plastic ampoules.

Table IV. First-Order Rate Constants (days^{-1}) for Deamidation of rhDNase as Assessed by Tentacle Ion-Exchange Chromatography

Container	2–8°C	25°C	37°C
Glass	$5.7 \pm 1.6 \times 10^{-4}$	$7.2 \pm 0.8 \times 10^{-3}$	$2.6 \pm 1.2 \times 10^{-2}$
Unfoiled plastic	$2.0 \pm 0.3 \times 10^{-4}$	$2.2 \pm 0.1 \times 10^{-3}$	$8.2 \pm 0.9 \times 10^{-3}$
Foiled plastic	$1.7 \pm 1.1 \times 10^{-4}$	$1.7 \pm 0.3 \times 10^{-3}$	$7.4 \pm 0.8 \times 10^{-3}$

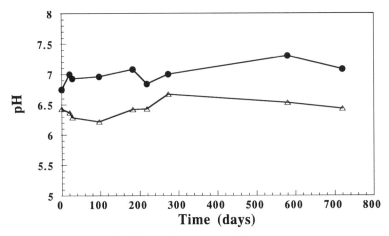

Figure 17. pH of rhDNase at 2–8°C stored in glass vials (filled circles) and plastic ampoules (open triangles).

ACKNOWLEDGMENTS. It would be impossible to acknowledge all the people at Genentech that have contributed to the successful and rapid development of Pulmozyme. Please excuse any inadvertent omissions of names and contributors. The author would like to personally thank his co-workers, including David Cipolla, Igor Gonda, Kim Chan, and Andy Clark, for much of their input and discussions over the past few years. Suzanne Weck made many important contributions, and her calcium binding (Fig. 7) and circular dichroism experiments (Fig. 10) have been presented in this chapter. Special thanks are extended to Kathy Meserve for her technical help in the stability assessment of rhDNase vialed in plastic ampoules. Many thanks go to John Frenz for valuable discussions and sharing with me unpublished results. I wish to also thank Tom Bewley for critical reading of the manuscript. I would like to thank both Steve Shak and Rodney Pearlman for their encouragement and support throughout all phases of this project.

REFERENCES

Abeliovich, D., Lavon, I. P., Lerer, I., Cohen, T., Springer, C., Avital, A., and Cutting, G., 1992, Screening for five mutations detects 97% of cystic fibrosis (cf) chromosomes and predicts a carrier frequency of 1:29 in the Jewish Ashkenazi population, *Am. J. Hum. Genet.* **51:**951–956.

Aitken, M. L., 1993, Clinical trials of recombinant human in cystic fibrosis patients, *Monaldi Arch. Chest. Dis.* **48:**653–656.

Aitken, M. L., Burke, W., McDonald, G., Shak, S., Montgomery, A. B., and Smith, A., 1992, Recombinant human DNase inhalation in normal subjects and patients with cystic fibrosis. A phase 1 study, *JAMA* **267:**1947–1951.

Anderson, M. P., Rich, D. P., Gregory, R. J., Smith, A. E., and Welsh, M. J., 1991, Generation of c-AMP-activated chloride currents by expression of CFTR, *Science* **251**:679–682.

Armstrong, J. B., and White, J. C., 1950, Liquefaction of viscous purulent exudates by deoxyribonuclease, *Lancet* **2**:739–740.

Auffarth, B., de Monchy, J. G. R., van der Mark, T. W., Postma, D. S., and Koeter, G. H., 1991, Citric acid cough threshold and airway responsiveness in asthmatic patients and smokers with chronic airflow obstruction, *Thorax* **46**:638–642.

Balmes, J. R., Fine, J. M., Christian, D., Gordon, T., and Sheppard, D., 1988, Acidity potentiates bronchoconstriction induced by hypoosmolar aerosols, *Am. Rev. Respir. Dis.* **138**:35–39.

Beasley, R., Rafferty, P., and Holgate, S. T., 1988, Adverse reactions to the non-drug constituents of nebulizer solutions, *Br. J. Clin. Pharmacol.* **25**:283–287.

Boat, T., Welsh, M. J., and Beaudet, A., 1989, Cystic fibrosis, *The Metabolic Basis of Inherited Disease* (C. Scriver, A. Beudet, W. Sly, and D. Valle, eds.), McGraw-Hill, New York, pp. 2649–2860.

Byron, P. R., 1990, Aerosol formulation, generation, and delivery using nonmetered systems, in: *Respiratory Drug Delivery* (P. R. Byron, ed.), CRC Press, pp. 143–165.

Cacia, J., Quan, C. P., Vasser, M., Sliwkowski, M. B., and Frenz, J., 1993, Protein sorting by high-performance liquid chromatography. I. Biomimetic interaction chromatography of recombinant human deoxyribonuclease I on polyionic stationary phases, *J. Chromatogr.* **634**:229–239.

Cantor, C. R., and Schimmel, P. R., 1980, *Biophysical Chemistry. Part III: The Behavior of Biological Macromolecules*, W. H. Freeman, San Francisco.

Capasso, S., Mazzarella, L., and Zagari, A., 1991, Deamidation via cyclic imide of asparaginyl peptides: Dependence on salts, buffers and organic solvents, *Peptide Res.* **4**:234–238.

Chernick, W. S., and Barbero, G. J., 1959, Composition of tracheobronchial secretions in cystic fibrosis of the pancreas and bronchiectasis, *Pediatrics* **24**:739–745.

Chernick, W. S., Barbero, G. J., and Eichel, H. J., 1961, In-Vitro evaluation of effect of enzymes on tracheobronchial secretions from patients with cystic fibrosis, *Pediatrics* **27**:589–596.

Cipolla, D., Gonda, I., Meserve, K., Weck, S., and Shire, S. J., 1994a, Formulation and aerosol delivery of recombinant deoxyribonucleic acid derived human deoxyribonuclease I. in: *ACS Symposium Series 567, Formulation and Delivery of Proteins and Peptides* (J. L. Cleland and R. Langer, eds.), American Chemical Society, Washington, DC, pp. 322–342.

Cipolla, D., Gonda, I., and Shire, S. J., 1994b, Characterization of aerosols of human recombinant deoxyribonuclease I (rhDNase) generated by jet nebulizers, *Pharm. Res.* **11**:491–498.

Cipolla, D. C., Clark, A. R., Chan, H.-K., Gonda, I., and Shire, S. J., 1994c, Assessment of aerosol delivery systems for recombinant human deoxyribonuclease, *STP Pharma Sci.* **4**:50–62.

Cleland, J. L., Powell, M. F., and Shire, S. J., 1993, The development of stable protein formulations: a close look at protein aggregation, deamidation and oxidation, *Crit. Rev. Ther. Drug Carr. Syst.* **10**:307–377.

Cohn, E. J., and Edsall, J. T., 1965, *Proteins, Amino Acids and Peptides as Ions and Dipolar Ions*, Hafner, New York.

Desager, K. N., Van Bever, H. P., and Stevens, W. J., 1990, Osmolality and pH of antiasthmatic drug solutions, *Agents Actions* **31**:225–228.

Doctor, V. M., 1963, Studies on the purification and properties of human plasma deoxyribonuclease, *Arch. Biochem. Biophys.* **103**:286–290.

Drumm, M. L., Pope, H. A., Cliff, W. H., Rommens, J. M., Marvin, S. A., Tsui, L.-C., Collins, F. C., Frizzell, R. A., and Wilson, J. M., 1990, Correction of the cystic fibrosis defect *in vitro* by retrovirus mediated gene transfer, *Cell* **62**:1227–1233.

Elmes, P. C., and White, J. C., 1953, Deoxyribonuclease in the treatment of purulent bronchitis, *Thorax* **8**:295–300.

Fick, R. B., Anzueto, A., Mahutte, K., and Members of the rhDNase-COPD Study Group, 1994, Recombinant DNase mortality reduction in acute exacerbations of chronic bronchitis, *Clinical Research* **42**:294A.

Fine, J. M., Gordon, T., Thompson, J. E., and Sheppard, D., 1987, The role of titratable acidity in acid aerosol-induced bronchoconstriction, *A. Rev. Respir. Dis.* **135**:826–830.

Frenz, J., Quan, C. P., Cacia, J., Democko, C., Bridenbaugh, R., and McNerney, T., 1994, Protein sorting by high performance liquid chromatography. 2. Separation of isophosphorylates of recombinant human DNase I on a polyethylenimine column, *Anal. Chem.* **66:**335–340.

Funakoshi, A., Tsubota, Y., Wakasugi, H., Ibayashi, H., and Takagi, Y., 1977, Purification and properties of human pancreatic deoxyribonuclease I, *J. Bioch.* **82:**1771–1777.

Gibbons, R. A., 1972, Physico-chemical methods for the determination of the purity, molecular size and shape of glycoproteins, *Glycoproteins, Part A* (A. Gottschalk, eds.), Elsevier, Amsterdam, pp. 31–140.

Godden, D. J., Borland, C., Lowry, R., and Higenbottam, T. W., 1986, Chemical specificity of coughing in man, *Clin. Sci.* **70:**301–306.

Gonda, I., Kayes, J. B., Groom, C. V., and Fildes, F. J. T., 1982, Characterization of hygroscopic inhalation aerosols, in: *Particle Size Analysis* (N. G. Stanley-Wood, ed.), Wiley, New York, pp. 31–43.

Gonda, I., and Phipps, P. R., 1991, Some consequences of instability of aqueous aerosols produced by jet and ultrasonic nebulizers, in: *Aerosols*, 1 (S. Masuda and K. Takahashi, eds.), Pergamon Press, New York, pp. 227–230.

Hopp, T. P., and Woods, K. R., 1981, Prediction of protein antigenic determinants from amino acid sequences, *Proc. Natl. Acad. Sci. USA* **78:**3824–3828.

Hubbard, R. C., McElvaney, N. G., Birrer, P., Shak, S., Robinson, W. W., Jolley, C., Wu, M., Chernick, M. S., and Crystal, R. G., 1992, A preliminary study of aerosolized recombinant human deoxyribonuclease I in the treatment of cystic fibrosis, *N. Engl. J. Med.* **326:**812–815.

Ito, K., Minamiura, N., and Yamamoto, T., 1984, Human urine Dnase. I: Immunological identity with human pancreatic DNase I and enzymic and proteochemical properties of this enzyme, *J. Biochem.* **95:**1399–1406.

Johnson, A. J., Goger, P. R., and Tillet, W. S., 1954, The intravenous injection of bovine crystalline pancreatic desoxyribonuclease into patients, *J. Clin. Invest.* **33:**1670–1686.

Korozumi, T., Kurihara, K., Hachimori, Y., and Shibata, K., 1963, Interaction of methyl green with deoxyribonucleic acid as observed by a new method of using hydrogen peroxide, *J. Biochem.* **53:** 135–142.

Kunitz, M., 1950, Crystalline desoxyribonuclease. I. Isolation and general properties. Spectrophotometric method for the measurement of desoxyribonuclease activity, *J. Gen. Physiol.* **33:**349–362.

Kurnick, N. B., 1950a, The determination of desoxyribonuclease activity by methyl green; application to serum, *Arch. Biochem.* **29:**41–53.

Kurnick, N. B., 1950b, Methyl green-pyronin. I. Basis of selective staining of nucleic acids, *J. Gen. Physiol.* **33:**243–264.

Kurnick, N. B., 1962, Assay of deoxyribonuclease activity, *Methods Biochem. Anal.* **9:**1–38.

Kurnick, N. B., and Foster, M., 1950, Methyl green III. Reaction with desoxyribonucleic acid, stoichiometry, and behavior of the reaction product, *J. Gen. Physiol.* **34:**147–159.

Kurnick, N. B., and Mirsky, A. E., 1950, Methyl green-pyronin. II. Stoichiometry of reaction with nucleic acids, *J. Gen. Physiol.* **33:**265–274.

Lahm, A., and Suck, D., 1991, DNase I–induced DNA conformation. 2 Å structure of a DNase I–octamer complex, *J. Mol. Biol.* **221:**645–667.

Liao, T. H., Salnikow, J., Moore, S., and Stein, W. H., 1973, Bovine pancreatic deoxyribonuclease A. Isolation of cyanogen bromide peptides; complete covalent structure of the polypeptide chain, *J. Biol. Chem.* **248:**1489–1495.

Lieberman, J., 1962, Enzymatic dissolution of pulmonary secretions, *Am. J. Dis. Child.* **104:**342–348.

Lieberman, J., 1968, Dornase aerosol effect on sputum viscosity in cases of cystic fibrosis, *J. Am. Med. Assoc.* **205:**114–115.

Lizarraga, B., Sanchez-Romero, D., Gil, A., and Melgar, E., 1978, The role of Ca^{2+} on pH-induced hydrodynamic changes of bovine pancreatic deoxyribonuclease A, *J. Biol. Chem.* **253:**3191–3195.

Love, J. D., and Hewitt, R. R., 1979, The relationship between human serum and human pancreatic DNase I, *J. Biol. Chem.* **254:**12588–12594.

Meserve, K., Weck, S., and Shire, S. J., 1994, Stability of recombinant deoxyribonuclease I (rhDNase) in plastic vials manufactured by the automatic liquid packaging (ALP) system, *Pharm. Res.* **11:**S-74.

Moore, S., 1981, Pancreatic DNase, in: *The Enzymes* (P. D. Boyer, ed.), Academic Press, New York, Chapter 15.

Muller, W., 1990, New ion exchangers for the chromatography of biopolymers, *J. Chromatogr.* **510**: 133–140.

Murai, K., Yamanaka, M., Akagi, K., Anai, M., Mukai, T., and Omae, T., 1978, Purification and properties of deoxyribonuclease from human urine, *Biochim. Biophys. Acta* **517**:186–194.

Niven, R. W., Butler, J. P., and Brain, J. D., 1992, How air jet nebulizers may damage "sensitive" drug formulations. Abstracts 11th Annual Meeting of the American Association for Aerosol Research, San Francisco, CA.

Oefner, C., and Suck, D., 1986, Crystallographic refinement and structure of DNase I at 2 Å resolution, *J. Mol. Biol.* **192**:605–632.

Patel, K., and Borchardt, R. T., 1990, Chemical pathways of peptide degradation. II Kinetics of deamidation of an asparaginyl residue in a model hexapeptide, *Pharm. Res.* **7**:703–711.

Perkins, S. J., 1986, Protein volume and hydration effects, *Eur. J. Biochem.* **157**:169–180.

Potter, J., Matthews, L. W., Lemm, J., and Spector, S., 1960, The composition of pulmonary secretions from patients with and without cystic fibrosis, *Am. J. Dis. Child.* **100**:493–495.

Potter, J. L., Matthews, L. W., Lemm, J., and Spector, S., 1963, Human pulmonary secretions in health and disease, *Ann. N.Y. Acad. Sci.* **106**:692–697.

Poulos, T. L., and Price, P. A., 1972, Some effects of calcium ions on the structure of bovine pancreatic deoxyribonuclease A, *J. Biol. Chem.* **247**:2900–2904.

Price, P. A., 1972, Characterization of Ca^{++} and Mg^{++} binding to bovine pancreatic deoxyribonuclease A, *J. Biol. Chem.* **247**:2895–2899.

Price, P. A., 1975, The essential role of Ca^{2+} in the activity of bovine pancreatic deoxyribonuclease, *J. Biol. Chem.* **250**:1981–1986.

Price, P. A., Liu, T.-Y., Stein, W. H., and Moore, S., 1969a, Properties of chromatographically purified bovine pancreatic deoxyribonuclease, *J. Biol. Chem.* **244**:917–933.

Price, P. A., Moore., S., and Stein, W. H., 1969b, Alkylation of a histidine residue at the active site of bovine pancreatic deoxyribonuclease, *J. Biol. Chem.* **244**:924–928.

Price, P. A., Stein, W. H., and Moore, S., 1969c, Effect of divalent cations on the reduction and re-formation of the disulfide bonds of deoxyribonuclease, *J. Biol. Chem.* **244**:929–932.

Ramsey, B. W., Astley, S. J., Aitken, M. L., Burke, W., Colin, A. A., Dorkin, H. L., Eisenberg, J. D., Gibson, R. L., Harwood, I. R., Schidlow, D. V., *et al.*, 1993, Efficacy and safety of short-term administration of aerosolized recombinant human deoxyribonuclease in patients with cystic fibrosis, *Am. Rev. Respir. Dis.* **148**:145–151.

Ranasinha, C., Assoufi, B., Shak, S., Christiansen, D., Fuchs, H., Empey, D., Geddes, D., and Hodson, M., 1993, Efficacy and safety of short-term administration of aerosolised recombinant human DNase I in adults with stable stage cystic fibrosis, *Lancet* **342**:199–202.

Raskin, P., 1968, Bronchospasm after inhalation of pancreatic dornase, *Am. Rev. Respir. Dis.* **98**:597–598.

Rich, D. P., Anderson, M. P., Gregory, R. J., Cheng, S. H., Paul, S., Jefferson, D. M., McCann, J. D., Klinger, K. W., Smith, A. E., and Welsh, M. J., 1990, Expression of cystic fibrosis transmembrane conductance regulator corrects defective chloride channel regulation in cystic fibrosis airway epithelial cells, *Nature* **347**:358–363.

Riordan, J. R., Rommens, J. M., Kerem, B., Alon, N., Rozmahel, R., Grzelczak, Z., Zielenski, J., Lok, S., Plavsic, N., Chou, J., Drumm, M. L., Iannuzzi, M. C., Collins, F. S., and Tsui, L., C., 1989, Identification of the cystic fibrosis gene: genetic analysis, *Science* **245**:1073–1080.

Robinson, A. B., and Rudd, C. J., 1974, Deamidation of glutaminyl and asparaginyl residues in proteins and peptides, *Curr. Top. Cell. Recog.* **8**:247–295.

Rommens, J. M., Iannuzzi, M. C., Kerem, B. S., Drumm, M. L., Melmer, G., Dean, M., Rozmahael, R., Cole, J. K., D., Hidaki, N., Zsiga, M., Buchwald, M., Riordan, J. R., Tsui, L., and Collins, F. S., 1989, Identification of the cystic fibrosis gene: chromosome walking and jumping, *Science* **245**:1059–1065.

Salomon, A., Herchfus, J. A., and Segal, M. S., 1954, Aerosols of pancreatic Dornase in bronchopulmonary disease, *Ann. Allergy* **12**:71–79.

Sant'Ambrogio, G., Anderson, J. W., Sant'Ambrogio, F. B., and Mathew, O. P., 1991, Response to laryngeal receptors to water solutions of different osmolality and ionic composition, *Resp. Med.* **85** (Suppl. A):57–60.

Sato, K., and Sato, F., 1984, Defective beta adrenergic response of cystic fibrosis sweat glands in vivo and in vitro, *J. Clin. Invest.* **73**:1763–1771.

Shak, S., Capon, D. J., Hellmiss, R., Marsters, S. A., and Baker, C. L., 1990, Recombinant human DNase I reduces the viscosity of cystic fibrosis sputum, *Proc. Natl. Acad. Sci. USA* **87**:9188–9192.

Shire, S. J., 1994, Analytical ultracentrifugation and its use in biotechnology, in: *Modern Analytical Ultracentrifugation* (T. M. Schuster and T. M. Laue, eds.), Birkhauser, Boston, pp. 261–297.

Sinicropi, D., Baker, D. L., Prince, W. S., Shiffer, K., and Shak, S., 1994, Colorimetric determination of DNase I activity with a DNA-methyl green substrate, *Anal. Biochem.* **222**:351–358.

Snell, N. J. C., 1990, Adverse reactions to inhaled drugs, *Resp. Med.* **84**:345–348.

Spier, R., Witebsky, E., and Paine, J. R., 1961, Aerosolized pancreatic dornase and antibiotics in pulmonary infections, *J. Am. Med. Assoc.* **178**:878–886.

Suck, D., Oefner, C., and Kabsch, W., 1984, Three-dimensional structure of bovine pancreatic DNase I at 2.5 Å resolution, *EMBO* **3**:2423–2430.

Tsui, L. C., and Buchwald, M., 1991, Biochemical and molecular genetics of cystic fibrosis, *Adv. Hum. Genet.* **20**:153–266.

Wiberg, J. S., 1958, On the mechanism of metal activation of deoxyribonuclease I, *Arch. Biochem. Biophys.* **73**:337–358.

Wright, H. T., 1991, Deamidation of asparaginyl and glutaminyl residues in proteins, *CRC Crit. Rev. Biochem. Mol. Biol.* **26**:1–52.

Index

Acidic fibroblast growth factor (aFGF), 59, 141,
    181
Adrenocorticotropin (ACTH), 12
Adsorption, 197, 198, 200, 210, 233, 236, 238,
    389
Aerosol: *see* Formulation, aerosol
Agglutinin, 13
Aggregate. 167, 192, 210, 311, 355
    covalent, 213, 225, 232, 323
    insoluble, 169, 207
    noncovalent, 225, 232, 264, 290, 408, 411
    soluble, 167, 207, 375
Aggregation, 3, 22, 90, 108, 147, 164, 184, 192,
    225, 323, 335, 408, 411
    characterization of, 167, 168, 290
    influence of excipients on, 165, 167, 184
    influence of pH on, 164, 203, 228, 375
    influence of temperature on, 164, 192, 202,
        322, 386
Aldolase, 14
Alpha helix, 149, 185, 254, 285, 291, 306, 309,
    332, 400
Amino acid composition, 259, 262, 280, 311,
    314, 377, 409
Amino acid sequence: *see* Sequence, primary
Amylin antagonist, 15
Amyloid-related serum protein (ARSP), 16
Analytical characterization: *see* Characterization,
    analytical
Analytical ultracentrifuge, 191, 255, 256, 291,
    294, 404
    equilibrium sedimentation, 255, 375, 387, 403,
        404
    velocity sedimentation, 376, 387, 401
Angiogenin, 17
Antibody 4D5, heavy chain, 21
Antibody 4D5, light chain, 23
Antibody 17-1A, heavy chain, 24

Antibody 17-1A, light chain, 26
Antibody E25 (heavy chain), 28
Antibody E25 (light chain), 27
Antibody Light Chain-κ (mouse), 30
Antibody OKT3, heavy chain, 31
Antibody OKT3, light chain, 32
Antibody OKT4a, heavy chain (humanized), 34
Antibody OKT4a, light chain (humanized), 35
Antifibrin monoclonal antibody, 343
Anti-HER2, heavy chain, 18
Anti-HER-2, light chain, 20
Antioxidant, 156, 173, 273
Arrhenius kinetics, 164, 262, 296, 414, 416
Atrial natriuretic peptide (ANP) (human), 36
Autooxidation, 8, 194, 208

Backbone cleavage, 2
Basic fibroblast growth factor (bFGF), 61, 141
Beta elimination, 170, 200
Beta sheet, 182, 149, 185, 255, 285, 316, 369, 400
Bioassay, 81, 158, 207, 247, 260, 262, 266, 279,
    289, 298, 305, 333
Biological activity, 19, 155, 157, 164, 177, 181,
    182, 184, 196, 200, 205–207, 211, 221,
    225, 261, 275–277, 289, 298, 305, 309,
    310, 329, 386, 387
Blow-fill seal technology, 416, 417
Brain-derived neurotrophic factor (BDNF) (hu-
    man), 37
Bulking agent, 293, 296, 315, 357, 359, 361

Calbindin (bovine), 38
Calmodulin, 39
Carbohydrate composition, 310
Carbonic anhydrase C, 40
Carrier proteins: *see* Stabilizer, carrier proteins
CD4 (human), 42
CD4-IgG, 43

CD4-PE40, 45

Cell binding activity, 365, 367

Cell growth inhibition assay (GIA), 228–232

Cell proliferation assay, 62, 141, 143, 228, 238, 333

Chaotropic agent, 169, 172, 176, 290, 379

Characterization, 201, 213, 222, 304
  analytical, 225, 311, 347, 395, 403, 408, 420
  biochemical, 201
  biological, 7, 304
  biophysical, 182, 191, 201, 259, 315, 365, 368, 397
  chemical, 252, 270, 306
  physicochemical, 144, 151, 183, 200, 202, 205, 208, 280, 289, 344

Chelating agent, 143, 156, 208, 345, 346, 352

Chloroperoxidase (*Caldariomyces fumago*), 48

Cholera-B subunit protein (*Vibrio cholerae*), 49

Chromatography, high performance liquid chromatography (HPLC), 65, 164, 259
  affinity HPLC, 150, 157, 159
  chelating HPLC, 149, 176
  hydrophobic interaction chromatography (HIC), 8, 369
  ion exchange (IEX), 143, 149, 159, 198, 200, 235, 249, 307, 319, 321, 331, 347, 403–406, 411, 415
  reversed phase (RP), 79, 81, 89, 104, 149, 157, 164, 168, 169, 171, 204, 225, 230, 259, 262, 266–269, 283, 288, 289, 294, 296, 317, 334, 335, 407
  size exclusion chromatography (SEC), 150, 161, 168, 170, 206, 207, 211, 319, 336–338

Chymotrypsin hydrolysis, 396

Ciliary neurotrophic factor (CNTF) (human), 50

Circular dichroism spectroscopy (CD), 155, 185, 203, 255, 283, 315

Conformation, 2, 46, 67, 100, 110, 112, 119, 144, 149–156, 159, 171–177, 183–186, 191, 194–197, 200, 202–208, 213, 276, 283, 284, 289, 306, 310, 315, 332, 333, 370, 378, 386, 401, 410, 412, 418

Controlled release: *see* Formulations, controlled release

Covalent aggregates: *see* Aggregate, covalent

Crystallin-A (chicken), 51

Cyclic imide: *see* Deamidation

Cyclodextrin, 173, 174, 194, 195, 208, 212, 360

Cytochrome *c*, 53

Deamidation, 2, 13, 16, 112, 150, 183, 202, 204, 207, 315, 319, 410
  asparagine, 3, 5, 202–205, 404, 411

Deamidation (*cont.*)
  cyclic imide formation, 2, 13, 15, 118, 150, 411
  examples of, 12–133
  glutamine, 5, 325
  mechanism (pathway), 3,5, 6,13, 414
  pH effect , 202, 416
  rate of, 5, 205, 325, 404, 414, 419
  temperature effect, 208, 414

Degradation, 2,4, 11, 119–113, 142, 150, 158, 196, 232, 240, 260, 267, 269, 270, 296, 318
  chemical , 2, 4, 5, 202, 261
  examples of, 12–113
  kinetics (rate), 3, 8, 113–119, 262, 263
  pathway (mechanism), 3, 4, 12, 112, 150, 162, 261, 265, 318, 323, 408–411, 419–421
  product, 8 150, 159, 161, 240, 260, 265, 267, 270
  examples of, 12–112

Delivery System: *see* formulation

Demineralized bone matrix (DBM), 175, 239

Denaturation, 3, 167, 200, 336, 343, 382
  chemical, 147, 148, 187
  pH-induced, 145, 147, 153
  surface-induced , 235
  temperature effect on, 147, 153, 154, 186, 285, 343

Deoxyribonuclease I [rhDNase (human)Dornase Alpha] (Pulmozyme®), 55, 393

Differential scanning calorimetry (DSC), 153, 186, 198, 201, 385

Dimer, 149, 168, 182 , 203, 223, 254, 256, 287, 320, 326, 349, 352, 353
  cysteine, 160
  covalent, 158–160, 208, 276, 287
  disulfide linked, 149, 169
  dissociable, 169
  noncovalent, 226
  nondissociable, 169

Disulfide
  bond, 203, 247, 276, 306
  exchange, 170, 231, 233, 314
  formation, 156, 309
  scrambling, 170

Dosage form: *see* formulation

Edman degradation, 49, 50, 70, 281, 283

Electrophoresis
  isoelectric focusing gel electrophoresis (IEF), 204, 207, 287, 317
  native PAGE, 226, 229
  sodium dodecyl sulfate-polyacrylamide gel electrophoresis (SDS-PAGE), 207, 225, 286, 294, 316, 334

Enzyme linked immunosorbent assay (ELISA): see Immunoassay
Epidermal growth factor (EGF 1-48) (human), 56
Epidermal growth factor (murine), 57
Epitope, 295, 309, 344, 349
Erythrocyte protein 4.1 (human), 58
Excipient, 9, 28, 151, 164, 165, 173, 196, 200, 206, 213, 340, 347, 348, 355, 356, 361, 362

Fibroblast growth factor, acidic (human) (a-FGF), 59, 181
Fibroblast growth factor, basic (human) (b-FGF), 61, 141
Filgrastim: see Granulocyte-colony stimulating factor
Flexibility, 2, 3, 9–11, 118–120, 160, 205, 378, 386–389, 404, 418
Flexibility plot, 10
    examples, 12–112
Fluorescence spectroscopy, 144, 146, 148, 153, 167, 169, 172, 185, 186, 188–189, 193, 194, 196–198, 202, 204, 206, 315
Formulation, 173, 200, 209, 238, 240, 290, 322, 331
    aerosol, 406–409, 416, 421
    aqueous solution, 173, 331
    bone, 239
    controlled release, 239
    freeze-dried, 173, 175, 210, 211, 234, 236, 331
    gastrointestinal formulation, 240
    gel, 175, 265
    long acting, 239, 294
    parenteral, 8, 16, 81, 95, 96, 294
    powder, 174
    topical, 202, 205
Fourier transform infrared (FTIR) spectroscopy, 148, 149, 173, 369
Free radical, 8
Freeze drying (lyophilization), 109, 173, 175, 200, 232, 347–349, 354, 355, 358–362
Freeze-thaw stress, 232, 322, 238
Front face fluorescence, 197, 198

Globular protein, 144, 285, 315
Glucagon, 62
Glycosaminoglycans (GAG), 141, 143, 170, 171, 173, 174, 176, 177, 220
Glycosylation, 3, 105, 141, 275, 283–285, 290, 304, 310, 311, 319, 322, 323, 325, 331–335, 339, 403
Granulocyte-colony stimulating factor (human) (G-CSF, Filgrastim) (Neupogen®), 63, 303

Granulocyte-macrophage colony-stimulating factor (human) (GM-CSF, Sargramostim) (Leukine®), 329
Growth hormone (bovine), 64
Growth hormone (human), 66
Growth hormone (porcine), 68
Growth hormone releasing factor (GHRF) variant (human), 69

Half-life, 5, 6, 204, 278, 294, 330, 334, 385
Hemoglobin (human), 70
Heparin, 154, 171, 175, 181, 183, 186-190
Heterodimer, 329
Heterogeneity, 3, 17, 30, 42, 50, 52, 54, 71, 73, 75, 94, 97, 110, 113, 119, 156, 184, 188, 287, 403, 404
High performance liquid chromatography: see Chromatography
Hirudin, 71
Histone, 73
Homodimer, 224, 226
Hot spots, 2, 3, 112, 113, 117–126
Human serum albumin (HSA), 237
Hyaluronic acid, 175
Hydrolysis, 3, 5–7, 9, 11, 12, 15, 37, 40, 49, 50, 56, 67, 69, 77, 78, 82, 84, 92, 95, 96, 100, 101, 106, 109, 117–119, 200, 207, 280, 281, 312, 314, 340, 357, 402, 405, 406
Hydropathy (plot), 119, 120, 399
    examples, 9–112
Hydrophobic interaction chromatography (HIC): see Chromatography
Hypoxanthine-guanine phosphoribosyltransferase (HXGT), 74

Immunoassay
    enzyme-linked immunosorbent assay (ELISA), 227, 237, 294
    radioimmunoassay, 261
Immunoscintigraphy, 343, 344, 362
Impurities, 176, 262, 348
Infrared spectroscopy (IR), 173, 310
Insulin (human), 75
Insulin-like growth factor-I (IGF-I), 76
Insulinotropin, 78
Interferon alpha-2b (human) (IFN-α-2b), 79
Interferon-β-1b (IFN-β-1b) (Betaseron®), 80, 275
Interferon gamma (human) (γ-IFN), 81
Interleukin-1 receptor antagonist (IL-1RA), 82
Interleukin-1 α (IL-1α), 84
Interleukin-1 β (human) (IL-1β), 85

Interleukin-1 β (murine), 86
Interleukin-2 (IL-2), 88
Interleukin-11 (human), 90
Isoelectric focusing gel electrophoresis: *see* Electrophoresis
Isotonic, 20, 24, 105, 158, 203, 210, 294, 408, 411, 416

Kinetics, 3, 7, 54, 59, 71, 78, 102, 11, 175, 184, 188, 201, 204, 261, 263, 264, 309, 310, 385, 388, 405, 412, 414–416, 419
Kjeldahl, 146
Kyte-Doolittle scale, 5, 10, 11, 119

Light degradation, 8, 265, 267, 419
Light scattering, 184, 190, 195–197, 207, 320
Liposome, 295, 374, 375
Liquid chromatography/mass spectroscopy LC/MS, 160, 162
Lung surfactant (human) SP-C, 91
Lyophilized formulation: *see* Formulation, freeze-dried
Lysozyme (hen egg white), 92

Mass spectroscopy, 162, 207, 252, 260, 265, 267, 283, 313, 314, 318, 332
Mechanism of
    action, 151, 196, 219–221, 224, 280, 308
    inactivation, 183, 200, 206, 213, 229
    interaction, 194, 375
    stabilization, 233
Metal ions, 8, 156, 175, 208, 264, 267, 352, 401, 402
Methionine, 8, 9, 40, 117, 142, 159, 161, 262–264, 270, 281, 282, 306, 317, 318, 402
    oxidation, 39, 40, 117, 262–267, 288, 289, 294, 295, 324
    sulfone, 8, 313
    sulfoxide, 8, 260, 265, 313
Methyl cellulose, 240, 269
Mitogenic activity, 181, 196, 207
Molten globule state , 186
Monomer, 62, 107, 143, 149, 150, 156, 159, 160, 167, 171, 172, 175, 196, 207, 210, 211, 223–236, 254–256, 276, 291, 306, 320, 332, 335, 337, 352–356, 360–364, 375–377, 384, 403, 427
Multimer formation, 156, 159
Mutant, 152, 160, 203, 204, 218, 311, 367
Mutein, 148, 151, 159, 172, 174, 277
Myelin basic protein (MBP), 93

Native confomation (structure), 100, 144, 147-150, 157, 159, 168, 172–176, 183–188, 191, 196, 197, 200, 201, 204, 206, 252, 253, 259, 261, 264, 275–278, 284–289, 304, 309, 321, 370, 378, 383, 389
Nebulizer, 396, 406–408, 420
Neocarzinostatin, 94
Nerve growth factor (human) (NGF), 95
Nonglycosylated, 275, 310
Nuclear magnetic resonance (NMR) spectroscopy, 182, 199, 283, 284, 310, 369

Oligomer, 208, 213, 276, 277, 286–289, 295, 296, 332, 224, 375
Oligosaccharide, 189, 310, 330, 399, 403
Osmolality, 231, 408; *see also* Isotonic
Oxidation, 2–4, 8, 9, 11, 12–113, 117–120, 132, 149, 158, 159, 183, 194, 195, 200, 204, 208, 261, 262, 265, 269, 281, 289, 306, 312, 322, 324, 345–348, 351–355, 418
    cysteine, 149, 156, 158, 159, 172, 191, 193, 195, 200, 202- 208, 213, 309
    light-induced, 265, 290, 345
    metal-catalyzed, 8, 264, 265
    methionine, 133, 263–265, 288, 289, 295, 318, 324
    peroxide-induced, 8, 9, 20, 108, 133, 163, 227, 264, 269, 324, 325
    prevention of, 156, 158, 172, 196, 265, 268, 270, 354

Parathyroid hormone, 97
Parenteral: *see* Formulation, parenteral
Particulate matter, 322, 340, 350, 359, 361, 417
Peptide
    digest, 253, 311
    map, 253, 282, 312
Peroxide: *see* Oxidation
Pharmacokinetics, 250, 251, 278, 330
Photo-oxidation: *see* Oxidation, light induced
pH rate profile, 53, 55, 57, 142, 262, 412
Plastic ampules, 210, 416–422
Polyanion binding site, 183, 192, 198
Polylactide-co-glycolide (PLG), 239, 240, 295
Polymer, 174–176, 184, 192–194, 205, 206, 211, 294, 344, 404
Polysorbate (Tween®), 20, 24, 67, 165, 174, 234–239, 292, 322, 324, 325, 359, 360
Potency: *see* Biological activity
Precipitate, 146–148, 167–172, 198, 290, 348
Preformulation, 183, 212, 213, 228, 344, 346, 350, 355

Preservative, 67, 151, 166, 174, 331, 340
Proteolysis, 14, 112, 201, 220, 253, 284, 322, 325, 347, 378, 402
Purity, 143, 248, 259, 276, 268, 295, 317, 345, 348, 349, 356, 368
Pyroglutamic acid formation, 3, 7, 8, 49, 268

Quasielastic light-scattering (QLS), 7, 375
Quenching, 144, 146, 147, 185, 286, 315, 316, 375, 379

Racemization, 2, 3, 6, 200
Radioimmunoassay, 261, 305
Radio-immunoscintigraphic agent, 243, 344, 345, 362, 365
Radiolabel, 175, 295, 343–351, 358, 360, 361, 364
Radionuclide, 343, 345, 346
Rate, 5, 6, 40, 52, 76, 91, 95, 164, 185, 191, 202, 233, 236, 263, 309, 325, 405
    constant, 6, 9, 54, 104, 188, 265, 412–415, 420, 421
    of aggregation, 165, 167, 176, 184, 185, 192
    of deamidation, 5, 57, 58, 70, 76, 100, 112, 188, 404, 409, 412–416, 419
    of degradation, 262, 263, 296, 323
    of oxidation, 80, 262, 263, 265, 352
    pH rate profile, 54, 57, 261, 412
    of reaction, 3, 5, 8, 16, 59, 65, 69, 72, 82, 156, 261
    of unfolding, 188, 201
Reactivity, 264, 310, 345, 349
Real time
    stability, 208
    storage, 164, 208, 232, 296, 347, 362, 387, 393, 410, 416
Rearrangement, 229–231, 325
Receptor interaction 309, 332
Reconstituted solution, 104, 136, 206, 227–239, 294, 331, 348, 359
Reduction, 3, 157, 211, 224, 226, 237, 248, 300, 345, 348, 353, 399, 401
Relaxin, 98, 247
Residual moisture, 340, 347, 350, 354, 355, 358
Reversed phase-high performance liquid chromatography (RP-HPLC): see Chromatography
Ribonuclease A, 99
Ribonuclease U2 (RNase U2) (Ustilago sphaerogena), 100

Safe-T-Therm®, 322, 323
Sargramostim: see Granulocyte-macrophage colony-stimulating factor
Secretin, 101

Sequence, 5, 8, 9, 11, 117, 142, 145, 164, 184, 192, 205, 222, 223, 252, 285, 306, 330, 399
    amino acid (primary), 2, 3, 9, 11, 12, 118–120, 142, 184, 198, 224, 248, 253, 275, 277–284, 304, 307, 311–313, 330, 394, 397, 399, 403
    analysis, 3, 10, 204, 283, 311, 312, 314
    examples of, 12–112
    homology, 142, 172, 182, 222, 248, 249, 309, 397–399
Serine hydroxymethyltransferase (SHMT) (rabbit), 102
Shelf-life, 3, 6, 7, 9, 54–56, 60, 67, 73, 77, 78, 84–88, 91, 95, 96, 102, 108, 109, 164, 170, 239, 286, 289, 323, 330, 332, 344, 357, 361
Size exclusion chromatography (SEC): see Chromatography
Sodium dodecyl sulfate-polyacrylamide gel electrophoresis (SDS-PAGE): see Electrophoresis
Solubility, 186, 258, 259, 284, 292–294
Specific activity, 203, 228, 276, 278, 333, 402, 407
Stability, 7, 61, 62, 76, 85, 104, 105, 108, 160, 165, 175, 193, 196, 200, 210, 212, 228, 231, 258, 265, 279, 296, 306, 310, 316, 342, 344, 355, 361, 396, 400, 409, 411
    accelerated, 102, 153, 202, 208, 325, 414
    aqueous solution, 4, 16, 120, 228, 232, 261, 284, 332, 352, 387, 410
    chemical, 108, 202, 207, 317, 355
    conformational, 183, 184, 186, 200
    container effect on, 417
    effect of temperature, 102, 154, 164, 170, 187, 198, 204, 279, 285, 385
    freeze-thaw, 227
    indicating, 150, 164, 206, 259, 295, 323
    prediction, 2, 7
    solid phase, 174, 210, 234, 322
Stabilizer, 175, 183, 188, 201, 213, 224, 292
    antioxidant, 156, 270
    buffer, 25, 153, 173
    carrier proteins, 235, 237, 238, 293–298
    chelator, 143, 156
    cosolvent, 166, 197, 270
    polyanions, 145, 154, 167, 171, 173, 175, 189, 192, 198, 201, 204, 213
    lyophilization, 231, 238, 362
    polymers, 189, 192, 233
    salts, 400, 402, 410
    surfactants, 165, 166, 235–238, 291, 296–298

Structure, 2, 11, 144–150, 166, 181, 182, 184,
       213, 223, 252, 315, 369, 397, 401, 418;
       see also Sequence
   crystal (X-ray), 11, 144, 145, 189, 200, 205,
       223, 254, 258, 264, 306, 331, 369, 400,
       401, 404
   native, 172, 183, 197, 201, 389
   primary, 12–112, 142, 223, 249, 252, 253, 278,
       280, 285, 289, 306, 311, 312, 330, 397
   secondary, 8, 149, 185, 186, 194, 254, 255,
       258, 283, 285, 306, 331, 369, 371, 372,
       379, 382, 385, 389, 400, 408, 412, 417
   tertiary, 150, 159, 182, 254, 283, 284, 308,
       325, 331, 372, 378, 379, 382–385, 399,
       408, 417
Substituent effect, 3, 5, 7
Succinimide formation, 4, 20, 57, 145, 159, 161,
       163, 176
Sulfated polysaccharides, 154, 181, 183, 192,
       194
Surfactant, 9, 57, 91, 92, 165, 166, 226,
       290–293, 296
Superoxide radical, 8

Technetium-99, 344
Tetramer, 75, 168, 189, 291
Thermal unfolding: *see* Unfolding
Thrombopoietin (TPO), 107
Tissue factor-243, 104
Tissue plasminogen activator (human) (t-PA),
       108
TP40, 365
Transamination, 3

Transforming growth factor beta (TGF-β), 106,
       219
Trimer, 156, 168, 286, 287
Trypsin (bovine), 109
Tryptic digest , 268, 284
Turbidity, 164, 165, 184, 185, 192, 202, 208,
       350, 359
Tween®: *see* Polysorbate

Ultraviolet spectroscopy (UV), 154, 164, 185,
       315
Unfolding, 56, 144, 146, 150, 154, 168, 183,
       186–189, 197, 202, 207, 370–373, 378,
       380, 384–386, 390
   denaturant-induced, 166, 167, 184, 186, 188,
       191, 197, 397
   kinetics, 360
   thermal-induced, 184, 186, 189, 194–197, 200,
       202, 203, 206, 386
USP Particulate Test, 340
USP Preservative Effectiveness Test, 340

V8 digest, 312, 318, 325
Vascular endothelial growth factor (VEGF), 111
Viscosity, 175, 206
Volume of distribution, 251, 278

Water content, 211, 238
Western blot, 226, 227, 232, 238, 287, 295

X-ray diffraction crystallography, 11, 144, 145,
       164, 182, 189, 199, 200, 205, 223, 254,
       258, 264, 306, 331, 369, 400, 401, 404